Atlas of
HEART DISEASES

CARDIOPULMONARY DISEASES AND CARDIAC TUMORS

Volume III

Atlas of
HEART DISEASES

CARDIOPULMONARY DISEASES AND CARDIAC TUMORS

Volume III

VOLUME EDITOR

Samuel Z. Goldhaber, MD

Associate Professor of Medicine
Harvard Medical School
Physician, Cardiovascular Division
Brigham and Women's Hospital
Boston, Massachusetts

SERIES EDITOR

Eugene Braunwald, MD, MD (Hon), ScD (Hon)

Hersey Professor of the Theory and Practice of Medicine
Harvard Medical School
Chairman, Department of Medicine
Brigham and Women's Hospital
Boston, Massachusetts

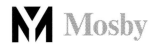

St. Louis Baltimore Boston Carlsbad Chicago Naples New York Philadelphia Portland
London Madrid Mexico City Singapore Sydney Tokyo Toronto Wiesbaden

Developed by Current Medicine Inc., Philadelphia

CURRENT MEDICINE

20 NORTH THIRD STREET • PHILADELPHIA, PA 19106

Development Editors........ *Maureen McNally*
and Rachel Delp

Art Director .... *Paul Fennessy*

Designer .... *Lisa Caro*

Illustration Director .... *Larry Ward*

Illustrators .... *Laura Pardi Duprey,*
Liz Kazanecki, Lisa Antonucci Messina,
and Larry Ward

Production Manager .... *David Myers*

North American and worldwide
sales and distribution:
MOSBY-YEAR BOOK, INC.
11830 Westline Industrial Drive
St. Louis, MO 63146

In Canada: TIMES MIRROR
PROFESSIONAL PUBLISHING LTD.
130 Flaska Drive
Markham, Ontario
Canada L6G 1B8

Cardiopulmonary diseases and cardiac tumors / volume editor, Samuel Z. Goldhaber.
        p. cm. – (Atlas of heart diseases; v. 3)
        Includes bibliographical references and index.
    ISBN 1-878132-23-7 (hard-cover)
    1. Cardiopulmonary system–Diseases–Atlases. 2. Heart–Cancer–Atlases.
    I. Goldhaber, Samuel Z. II. Series.
    [DNLM: 1. Pulmonary Heart Disease–therapy–atlases.
    2. Thrombophlebitis–atlases. 3. Heart Neoplasms–atlases.
    WG 200 A881 1995 v. 3]
RC682.A818 1995 vol. 3
[RC702]
616. 1'2 s–dc20
[616. 1'2]
DNLM/DLC   94-30333
for Library of Congress   CIP

Library of Congress Cataloging-in-Publication Data
ISBN 1-878132-23-7

Printed in Singapore by Imago Productions (FE) Ltd.

10   9   8   7   6   5   4   3   2   1

SERIES PREFACE

Disorders of the cardiovascular system are the most common causes of death and serious morbidity in the industrialized world. In 1991, more than 40% of all deaths in the United States were attributed to cardiac and vascular diseases. These conditions accounted for almost 5 million years of potential life lost.

Despite these sobering statistics, progress in cardiovascular medicine has been immense, and is, in fact, accelerating. Our understanding of the pathobiology of most forms of heart disease has advanced steadily, and there have been enormous advances in the diagnosis, treatment, and prevention of cardiovascular disorders. For example, during just one decade, from 1981 to 1991, the overall death rates from cardiovascular disease declined by 26% and death rates from acute myocardial infarction and stroke declined by 32%. Similar progress has been made in other major cardiovascular disorders, including hypertension, valvular and congenital heart disease, congestive heart failure, and the arrhythmias.

The physician responsible for the care of patients with cardiovascular disease now has a number of vehicles available for obtaining up-to-date information, including excellent journals and textbooks of every conceivable size, scope, and depth. In developing new strategies for transmitting information about these conditions, it is important to consider that cardiovascular medicine is the most "visual" of medical specialties. Cardiovascular diagnosis is based on the recognition and understanding of a variety of graphic waveforms, images, decision trees, and gross and microscopic anatomy. Treatment increasingly involves the intelligent use of algorithms, which are also most effectively portrayed visually. Likewise, mechanical correction of cardiovascular disorders, whether catheter-based or surgical, can best be described pictorially. This *Atlas of Heart Diseases* has been designed to provide a detailed and comprehensive visual exposition of all aspects of cardiovascular medicine. Several thousand images, accompanied by detailed captions, have been carefully selected by expert authors and reviewed by the 12 distinguished Volume Editors. These images are now available separately in print and slide form and also will soon be formatted for CD-ROM use.

Many people deserve credit for the successful completion of this ambitious effort. The expertise and hard work of the authors and the devoted efforts of the Volume Editors naturally form the foundation of the *Atlas of Heart Diseases*. Great credit is also due to Abe Krieger, President of Current Medicine, who conceived the *Atlas* series; to Maureen McNally, the extremely effective Development Editor; and to Kathryn Saxon, who coordinated the efforts in my office.

All of us who have been engaged in this project hope that each individual volume, and the entire *Atlas*, will be useful to physicians of all specialties who are responsible for the care of patients with cardiovascular disorders, to investigators and teachers of cardiovascular medicine, and ultimately to the millions of patients worldwide with disorders of the heart and circulation.

Eugene Braunwald, MD

PREFACE

Many common cardiovascular disorders afflict the heart as a result of pathologic processes that initially injure the pulmonary vessels or lung parenchyma. By definition, patients with cor pulmonale have enlargement of the right heart due to underlying pulmonary vascular or alveolar abnormalities. Pulmonary embolism and primary pulmonary hypertension, like cor pulmonale, frequently cause hemodynamic compromise of right ventricular function. Less often, high altitude pulmonary edema or clinical manifestations of cardiac tumors will bring patients to the attention of cardiovascular disease specialists.

In this Volume, expert physicians from the United States, Canada, United Kingdom, and France present pictorial updates of the most recent advances in the diagnosis and treatment of cardiopulmonary diseases and cardiac tumors. Pathophysiology, diagnostic imaging modalities, and treatment algorithms all receive heavy emphasis. The Series Editor and the Publisher have encouraged the use of original unpublished drawings, diagrams, and clinical case illustrations from personal collections. Therefore, throughout this Volume, a multitude of original echocardiograms, ultrasounds with color Doppler imaging, angiograms, and computed tomography and magnetic resonance scans, as well as photographs of gross and microscopic pathology, can be found. The authors have presented their topics with a combination of images and detailed figure legends as though they were talking to the reader with slide illustrations and explaining their significance during Grand Rounds lectures.

This Volume is divided into four sections: cardiopulmonary diseases, surgical interventions, venous thrombosis and insufficiency, and cardiac tumors. In the first section, cor pulmonale, pulmonary embolism, primary pulmonary hypertension, and high altitude pulmonary edema are covered thoroughly. The second section updates the reader with an interest in cardiopulmonary illnesses and cardiac tumors on the latest "high-tech" surgical interventions. This awareness will permit members of specialized cardiac care centers to function more effectively as multidisciplinary teams that offer complementary services in advanced diagnostic imaging as well as in an array of contemporary medical and surgical therapies. The third section provides a detailed examination of venous thrombosis and insufficiency, a major and often overlooked cause of medical and social disability. The final section focuses on cardiac tumors. As the detection and treatment of cancer improves, the duration of survival is increasing among patients with both primary tumors and tumors metastatic to the heart.

Regarding the work on this particular Volume, special mention is warranted for individuals whose help was essential on both a professional and personal level. The chapter authors took time from their vast array of commitments to assign high priority and place on the fast track their time-consuming and meticulously crafted contributions to the *Atlas*. Dr. Braunwald, who has been a mentor to me for more than two decades, served as the inspiration and catalyst for this ambitious project. Maureen McNally, the Development

Editor, and my secretary Joan Macauley, have worked with extraordinary diligence and equanimity to ensure the successful completion of this undertaking. Finally, Dr. Thomas W. Smith, Chief of our Cardiovascular Division, has set a standard of excellence that encourages the pursuit of this type of academic endeavor.

As this venture progressed from inception to publication, my family has been extraordinarily understanding of my commitment and enthusiastic about the final results. I wish to extend special apprecia-tion and affection to my wife, Reeve, and to my children, Alissa and Benjamin. My hope is that the images and figure legends in this Volume will help enhance the care of patients with cardiopulmonary diseases and cardiac tumors. Hopefully those involved in treating patients with these intriguing illnesses will be inspired to continue investigating the many unsolved issues that confront us.

Samuel Z. Goldhaber, MD

CONTRIBUTORS

DAVID H. ADAMS, MD
Assistant Professor of Surgery
Harvard Medical School
Division of Cardiac Surgery
Brigham and Women's Hospital
Boston, Massachusetts

MICHAEL F. ALLARD, BSc, MD, FRCP(C)
Assistant Professor
University of British Columbia
Department of Pathology and
  Laboratory Medicine
St. Paul's Hospital
Vancouver, British Columbia

JOHN M. ARMITAGE, MD
Associate Professor of Surgery
University of Pittsburgh Medical Center
Division of Cardiothoracic Surgery
Presbyterian University Hospital
Pittsburgh, Pennsylvania

WILLIAM R. AUGER, MD
Assistant Professor of Medicine
University of California, San Diego
Pulmonary/Critical Care Division
UCSD Medical Center
San Diego, California

SHELINA BABUL, BSc
University of British Columbia
Department of Pathology and
  Laboratory Medicine
St. Paul's Hospital
Vancouver, British Columbia

RICHARD N. CHANNICK, MD
Assistant Professor of Medicine
University of California, San Diego
Pulmonary/Critical Care Division
UCSD Medical Center
San Diego, California

PAT O. DAILY, MD
Director of Cardiac Surgery
Sharp Memorial Hospital
San Diego, California

JOHN C. ENGLISH, BSc(Hon), MD, FRCP(C)
Clinical Instructor
University of British Columbia
Department of Pathology and
  Laboratory Medicine
Vancouver Hospital and Health
  Sciences Center
Vancouver, British Columbia

PETER F. FEDULLO, MD
Associate Professor of Medicine
University of California, San Diego
Pulmonary/Critical Care Division
UCSD Medical Center
San Diego, California

SAMUEL Z. GOLDHABER, MD
Associate Professor of Medicine
Harvard Medical School
Physician, Cardiovascular Division
Brigham and Women's Hospital
Boston, Massachusetts

STUART W. JAMIESON, MB, FRCS
Professor
University of California, San Diego
Head, Division of Cardiothoracic Surgery
UCSD Medical Center
San Diego, California

ROBERT KORMOS, MD
Director of Mechanical Circulatory Support
Division of Cardiothoracic Surgery
Presbyterian University Hospital
Pittsburgh, Pennsylvania

EVAN LOH, MD
University of Pennsylvania Medical Center
Hospital of the University of
  Pennsylvania
Cardiovascular Division
Philadelphia, Pennsylvania

BRUCE M. McMANUS, MD
Professor and Head
Department of Pathology
University of British Columbia
Vancouver, British Columbia

GUY MEYER, MD
Department of Pulmonary Medicine
  and Cardiovascular Surgery
Laennec Hospital
Paris, France

KENNETH M. MOSER, MD
Professor of Medicine
University of California, San Diego
Director, Pulmonary/Critical Care Division
UCSD Medical Center
San Diego, California

JOSEPH F. POLAK, MD
Associate Professor of Radiology
Harvard Medical School
Department of Radiology
Brigham and Women's Hospital
Boston, Massachusetts

PHILIPPE REYNAUD, MD
Department of Pulmonary Medicine
  and Cardiovascular Surgery
Laennec Hospital
Paris, France

**C. VAUGHAN RUCKLEY, MB,
ChM, FRCSE, FRCPE**
Professor of Vascular Surgery
The University of Edinburgh
Department of Surgery
Royal Infirmary of Edinburgh
Edinburgh, Scotland

ROBERT B. SCHOENE, MD
Associate Professor of Medicine
University of Washington School
  of Medicine
Director, Pulmonary Function
  and Exercise Laboratory
Harborview Medical Center
Seattle, Washington

LORRAINE SKIBO, MD
Assistant Professor
Department of Radiology
Stanford University
Chief, Section of Interventional
  Radiology
Department of Veterans Affairs
  Medical Center
Palo Alto, California

HERVÉ SORS, MD, MSc
Professor of Pneumology
Department of Pulmonary Medicine
  and Cardiovascular Surgery
Laennec Hospital
Paris, France

DANIEL TAMISIER, MD
Department of Pulmonary Medicine
  and Cardiovascular Surgery
Laennec Hospital
Paris, France

GLENN P. TAYLOR, MD, FRCP(C)
Associate Professor
Department of Pathology and
  Laboratory Medicine
University of British Columbia
Department of Pathology
British Columbia Children's Hospital
Vancouver, British Columbia

JANET E. WILSON, BSc, MT(ASCP)
University of British Columbia
Department of Pathology and
  Laboratory Medicine
St. Paul's Hospital
Vancouver, British Columbia

CONTENTS

CHAPTER 4

PRIMARY PULMONARY HYPERTENSION

Richard N. Channick

CHAPTER 5

HIGH ALTITUDE PULMONARY EDEMA

Robert B. Schoene

SECTION II: SURGICAL INTERVENTIONS

CHAPTER 6

ACUTE PULMONARY EMBOLECTOMY

Guy Meyer, Daniel Tamisier, Philippe Reynaud, and Hervé Sors

SECTION III: VENOUS THROMBOSIS AND INSUFFICIENCY

CHAPTER 11

DIAGNOSIS OF VENOUS THROMBOSIS
Joseph F. Polak

CHAPTER 12

TREATMENT OF VENOUS THROMBOSIS
Samuel Z. Goldhaber

CHAPTER 13

PREVENTION OF VENOUS THROMBOSIS
Samuel Z. Goldhaber

Cardiopulmonary Diseases

COR PULMONALE

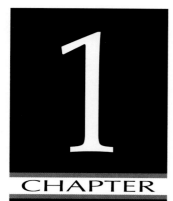

1

CHAPTER

Evan Loh

The term *cor pulmonale* describes a spectrum of cardio-pulmonary syndromes that are characterized by pulmonary hypertension, right ventricular hypertrophy, and right ventricular dilatation. Cor pulmonale includes a diverse range of etiologies, pathophysiologic mechanisms, and clinical characteristics. The common denominator of all syndromes is pulmonary hypertension. Right ventricular hypertrophy and dilatation are most often caused by parenchymal lung disease; however, derangements of ventilatory drive, respiratory pumping mechanisms, or the pulmonary vascular bed can also cause these disorders. Arterial hypoxemia, hypercapnia, and respiratory acidosis can further contribute to increased afterload of the right ventricle. Systemic manifestations of cor pulmonale are related to alterations in cardiac output, gas exchange in the lung, and venostasis.

The earliest discussions of the relationship between the right side of the heart and the lungs were described in *Exercito de Motu Cordis et Sanguinis in Animalibus Cordis* by William Harvey [1]. Harvey was the first to describe the limitations of the right ventricle and its passive role in providing blood to the lungs as follows:

> *"So it appears that whereas one ventricle, the left, suffices for distribution of the blood for the body, and withdrawing it with the vena cava, as is the case in all animals lacking lungs, nature was compelled, when she wished to filter blood throughout the lungs to add the right ventricle. . . Thus the right ventricle may be said to be made for the sake of transmitting blood through the lungs, not for nourishing them."*

McGinn and White [2] were the first to use the clinical term *acute cor pulmonale* in the discussion of a case of massive thromboembolism in 1935. Because pulmonary vascular disease, pulmonary hypertension, and cor pulmonale have few specific manifestations, especially early in their course, the diagnosis of cor pulmonale is often difficult. Treatment is directed primarily at the underlying pulmonary or ventilatory disorder rather than at the right ventricular failure. Supplemental oxygen is often necessary to avoid hypoxemia. Corticosteroids, anticoagulants, vasodilators, and other specific therapeutic agents can be used as indicated to treat the specific underlying pulmonary and pulmonary vascular disorders. When medical therapies fail, lung or heart-lung transplantation is a consideration for selected individuals.

This chapter provides a pictorial discussion of the conditions that produce secondary pulmonary hypertension by acting primarily on gas exchange as well as the causes of secondary pulmonary hypertension that are associated with complex congenital heart disease and primary pulmonary hypertension, all of which lead to cor pulmonale. Further, the pathophysiology, assessment and work-up, clinical presentation, and therapeutic interventions for patients with cor pulmonale are presented.

DEFINITION AND NATURAL HISTORY

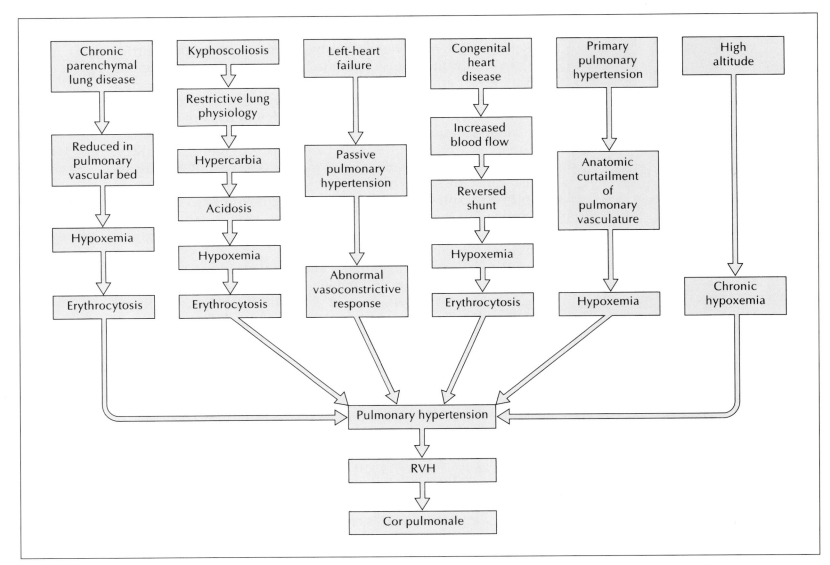

FIGURE 1-1. Flow diagram demonstrating the etiology and pathophysiology of cor pulmonale. General categories of disease states and the various pathophysiologic mechanisms that lead to development of the disorder are shown. Note that the final common pathway for the group of diseases that comprise cor pulmonale is advanced, long-standing pulmonary hypertension. RVH— right ventricular hypertrophy.

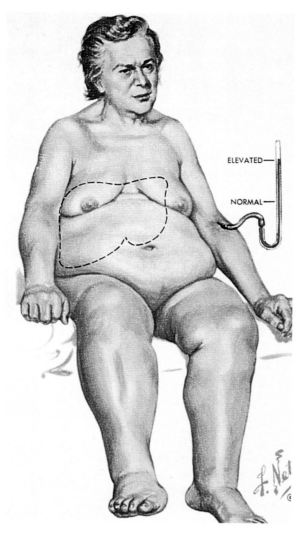

FIGURE 1-2. A patient with advanced cor pulmonale demonstrating marked peripheral cyanosis, increased venous filling pressure with hepatomegaly, abdominal distention secondary to ascites, severe peripheral edema, and engorgement of the jugular veins. Causes of diseases that would be consistent with this presentation include primary and secondary pulmonary hypertension with associated right ventricular failure. This collective clinical presentation is referred to as *cor pulmonale*. (*From* Netter [3]; with permission.)

ELEVATED—

NORMAL—

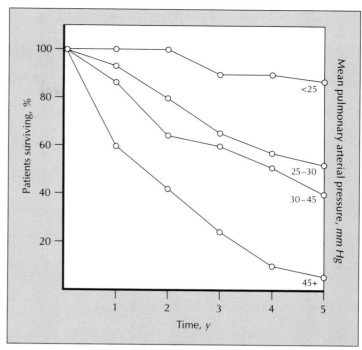

FIGURE 1-3. Correlation between survival (in years) and baseline mean pulmonary arterial pressure in patients with pulmonary hypertension secondary to parenchymal lung disease. A higher initial presenting mean pulmonary artery pressure was associated with significantly higher mortality. These findings suggest that regardless of the etiology of pulmonary hypertension, mean pulmonary artery pressure remains the single best determinant of long-term survival. For more survival statistics of patients with primary pulmonary by hypertension based on initial presenting left and right ventricular hemodynamics, *see* Chapter 4. (*Adapted from* Bishop [4]; with permission.)

PULMONARY BLOOD FLOW, PRESSURE, AND RESISTANCE

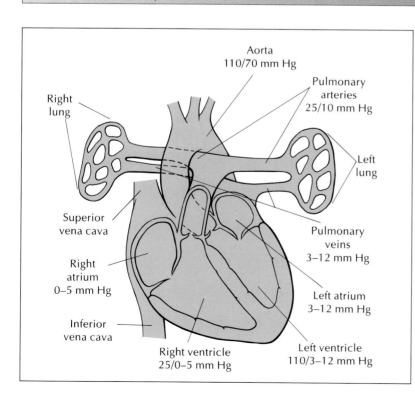

Aorta
110/70 mm Hg

Pulmonary
arteries
25/10 mm Hg

Right
lung

Left
lung

Superior
vena cava

Pulmonary
veins
3–12 mm Hg

Right
atrium
0–5 mm Hg

Left atrium
3–12 mm Hg

Inferior
vena cava

Right ventricle
25/0–5 mm Hg

Left ventricle
110/3–12 mm Hg

FIGURE 1-4. Normal pressure relationships between the pulmonary and systemic circulations. Note the normal range of pressures in the chambers of the right side of the heart and pulmonary arteries. (*Adapted from* Fowler [5]; with permission.)

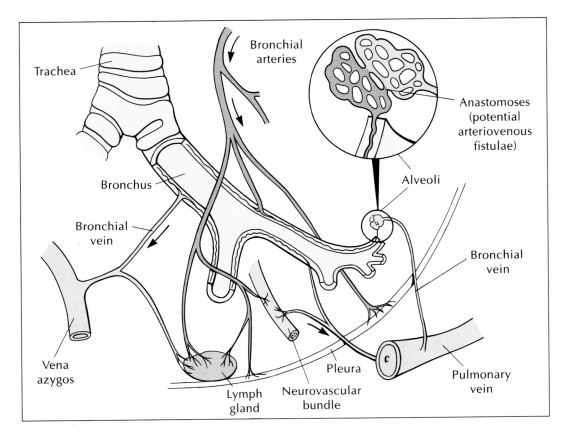

FIGURE 1-5. Bronchial (systemic) circulation in the lungs. When occlusion of a pulmonary artery occurs, anastomoses (**inset**) between bronchial and pulmonary vessels and through the walls of pulmonary vessels (vasa vasorum and neurovascular bundles) allow systemic perfusion of alveolar tissues normally served by that artery. Bronchial veins from airways, draining via the azygos into systemic veins, are affected by high systemic venous pressure. Dilatation of the anastomoses between the bronchial and pulmonary circulation in the presence of pulmonary hypertension results in collateral vessels, which cause intrapulmonary right-to-left shunting and contribute to systemic hypoxemia. Hypoxemia then causes impairment of endothelium-dependent vasorelaxation, further aggravating pulmonary hypertension. (*Adapted from* Butler [6]; with permission.)

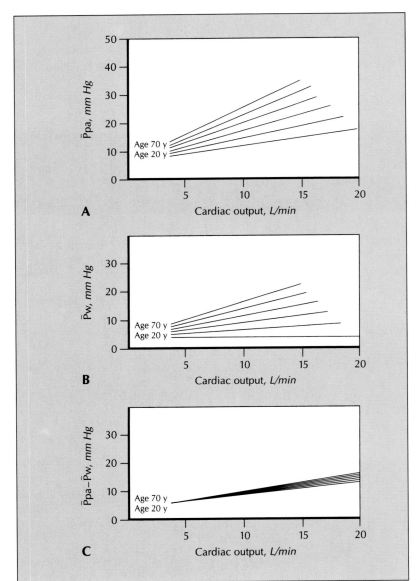

FIGURE 1-6. Relationship between pulmonary vascular pressures and cardiac output in normal subjects aged 20 to 70 years.
　A, Mean pulmonary artery pressure ($\bar{P}pa$) as a function of age and cardiac output (rest and exercise).
　B, Mean pulmonary wedge pressure ($\bar{P}w$) as a function of age and cardiac output (rest and exercise).
　C, Driving pressure (pulmonary artery minus wedge pressure) as a function of age and cardiac output (rest and exercise). Although mean pulmonary artery pressure and wedge pressure both rise with age, the transpulmonary pressure gradient remains unchanged with age and responds normally to increases in cardiac output with vasodilation. Thus, age does not seem to affect flow-mediated vasodilatory control of pulmonary artery pressure. (*Adapted from* Tartulier and coworkers [7]; with permission.)

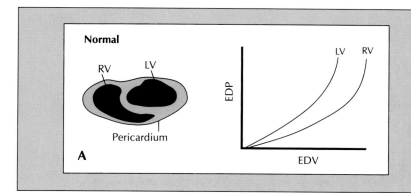

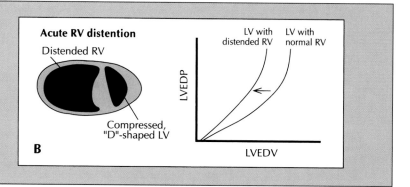

FIGURE 1-7. Interdependence of the right (RV) and left (LV) ventricles. **A,** Under normal conditions, the RV is much more distensible than the LV. **B,** In patients who develop acute cor pulmonale, there is a sudden and large increase in RV volume. Because of space limitations imposed by the pericardium, the distended RV impinges upon and compresses the LV cavity. The increase in RV volume causes the interventricular septum to shift toward the LV, thus causing a decrease in the dimension of the septum to free wall of the LV.

The distention of the RV decreases the overall LV end-diastolic volume (LVEDV), even though the LV end-diastolic pressure (LVEDP) remains the same (*arrow*). As the LV becomes progressively less compliant, increases in LVEDP do not normally augment LVEDV. Therefore, the LV is unable to compensate for its loss of volume. Eventually, the LV cavity is obliterated, resulting in low forward cardiac output and hemodynamic collapse. (*Adapted from* Weber and coworkers [8]; with permission.)

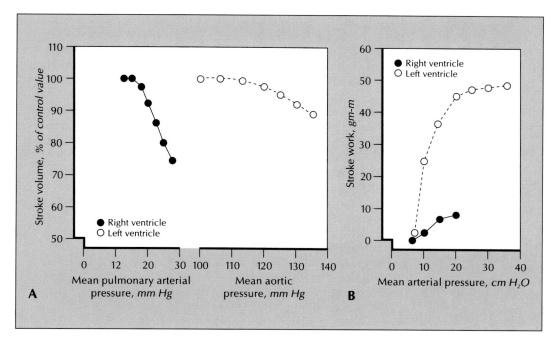

FIGURE 1-8. Effects of increasing preload and afterload on right and left ventricular function. The responses to alterations in afterload (**A**) and preload (**B**) of the right and left ventricles differ greatly. The hemodynamic data in *panel A* were obtained by constricting the main pulmonary artery and aorta of mongrel dogs. Note the much steeper decline in right compared with left ventricular stroke volume as a function of increasing afterload. In contrast, increasing preload (*panel B*) results in a much greater increase in left ventricular stroke work than in right. Therefore, these data demonstrate that the right ventricle is much more sensitive to acute changes in afterload than is the left ventricle. Conversely, the left ventricle is much more sensitive than the right to changes in preload. (*Adapted from* McFadden and Braunwald [9]; with permission.

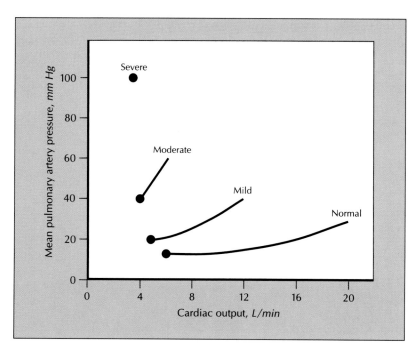

FIGURE 1-9. The relationship between mean pulmonary artery pressure and cardiac output in normal subjects as well as in those with mild, moderate, or severe elevation of pulmonary vascular resistance. *Solid circles* indicate values at rest. Note that as pulmonary vascular resistance increases, resting pulmonary artery pressure increases and resting forward cardiac output decreases. Further, an increase in cardiac output causes progressively steeper and greater increases in pulmonary artery pressure, suggesting an abnormality in flow-mediated vasodilation and autoregulation of pulmonary artery tone. With increases in cardiac output secondary to mild exercise in patients with moderate to severe pulmonary hypertension, pulmonary artery pressure rises precipitously, resulting in acute right ventricular failure. Right ventricular distention causes a shift of the septum toward the left ventricle, causing leftward displacement of the left ventricular volume-pressure curve, as shown in Fig. 1-7B. (*Adapted from* Butler [6]; with permission.)

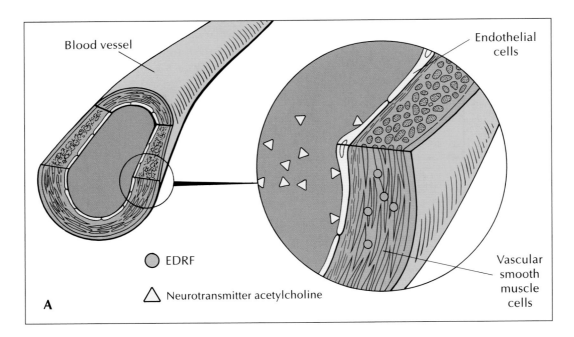

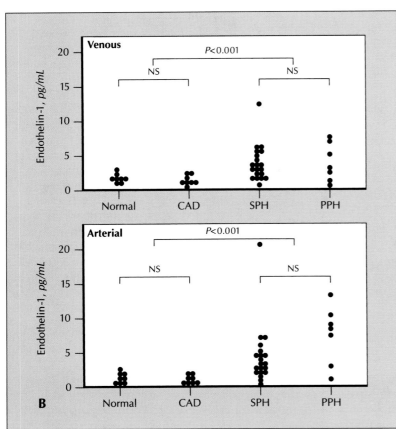

FIGURE 1-10. Endothelial control of pulmonary artery tone.

A, The normal pulmonary artery dilates when a neurotransmitter, such as acetylcholine, binds to endothelial cells on the vessel's inner walls. These cells release endothelium-derived relaxing factor (EDRF), whose active moiety has been identified as nitric oxide, which then diffuses to adjacent vascular smooth muscle cells, causing them to relax. Because acetylcholine stimulates the endothelium to release EDRF and cause vasodilation, the loss of response to acetylcholine can be used as a bioassay of EDRF release and overall endothelial function [10]. Constriction of pulmonary arteries and focal vascular injury are prominent features of pulmonary hypertension. Inhibition of EDRF augments pulmonary hypertension in newborn lambs [11]. In pulmonary arterial rings of patients undergoing heart-lung transplantation for end-stage chronic obstructive lung disease, the endothelium-dependent pulmonary relaxation that is normally achieved in response to acetylcholine is impaired [12].

B, Endothelin, a 21–amino-acid peptide also produced by the endothelium, causes potent vasoconstriction and smooth muscle proliferation. Plasma endothelin-1 levels are normal in patients with coronary artery disease (CAD) but elevated in patients with primary (PPH) and secondary (SPH) pulmonary hypertension [13]. Immunocytochemical analysis has shown that endothelin-1 is localized primarily to endothelial cells of pulmonary arteries with medial thickening and intimal fibrosis [14]. Endothelin-1 mRNA is increased at these same sites in patients with pulmonary hypertension. These findings suggest that local production of endothelin-1 contributes to the vascular abnormalities associated with secondary and primary pulmonary hypertension. (*continued*)

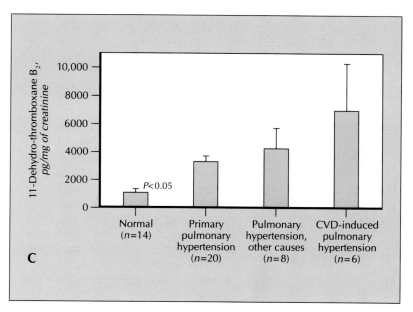

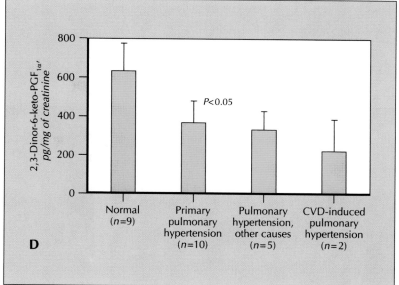

C

D

FIGURE 1-10. (*continued*) C, Thromboxane A_2 is a potent vasoconstrictor and stimulus for platelet aggregation, whereas prostacyclin, released by vascular endothelial cells, antagonizes the effects of thromboxane A_2. In patients with pulmonary hypertension, the stable urinary metabolite of thromboxane A_2 (11-dehydrothromboxane B_2) is increased [15].

D, In contrast, these same patients had depressed levels of the stable urinary metabolite of prostacyclin (2,3-dinor-6-keto-prostaglandin $F_{1\alpha}$). Whether these metabolic abnormalities are the causes or result of primary pulmonary hypertension is uncertain. It is possible that patients with primary pulmonary hypertension sustain an inflammatory and immunologic injury in which the pulmonary endothelium is merely an innocent bystander [16]. An excess production of thromboxane A_2, compared with prostacyclin, may be the result of this endothelial injury. CVD—collagen vascular disease. (Part A *adapted from* Snyder and Bredt [10]; part B *adapted from* Stewart and coworkers [13]; parts C and D *adapted from* Christman and coworkers [15]; with permission.)

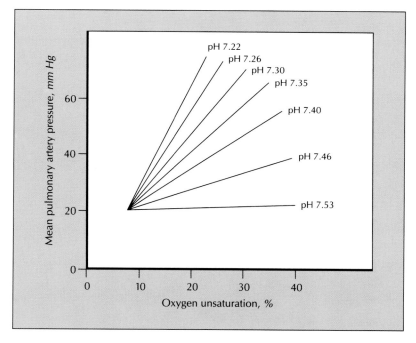

FIGURE 1-11. The interrelationships among pulmonary artery pressure, arterial blood oxyhemoglobin saturation, and hydrogen ion concentration. These data suggest that both hypoxemia and acidosis are important modulators of basal pulmonary artery tone. (*Adapted from* Enson and coworkers [17]; with permission.)

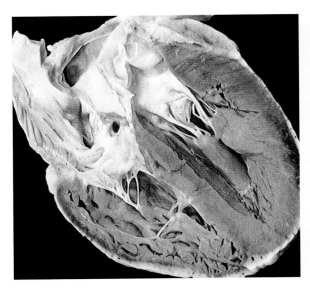

FIGURE 1-12. Normal appearance of a human heart sectioned in an apical four-chamber view. Normal thickness of the left ventricular wall is less than 1 cm; the right ventricular wall is less than 0.5 cm. (Courtesy of G. Winters, MD, Brigham and Women's Hospital, Boston, MA.)

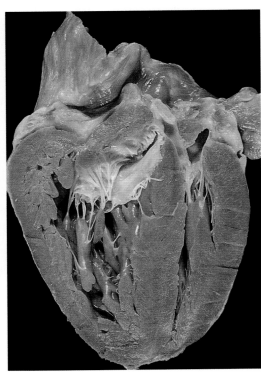

FIGURE 1-13. Atrial septal defect with cor pulmonale. Pulmonary hypertension is common in adults with atrial septal defect. Occasionally, severe Eisenmenger's physiology will develop. This image illustrates the findings at postmortem examination in a patient with a secundum atrial septal defect. Note the marked ventricular hypertrophy with prominent trabeculations throughout the right ventricle. Typically in such patients, concentric right ventricular hypertrophy is superimposed on the previously volume-loaded right ventricle, producing a large, thick-walled, hypokinetic chamber. The preterminal clinical course is characterized by right ventricular failure, pulmonary and tricuspid regurgitation, and right-to-left shunting. (Courtesy of R. Mitchell, MD, Brigham and Women's Hospital, Boston, MA.)

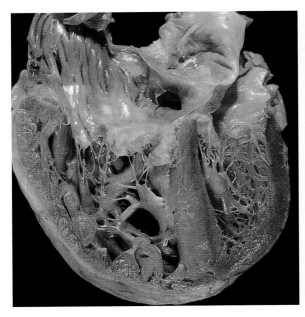

FIGURE 1-14. Gross appearance of the heart of a patient with primary pulmonary hypertension. The gradual development of significant pulmonary hypertension causes compensatory development of right ventricular hypertrophy, which minimizes right ventricular wall stress. Note the increased thickness and trabeculation of the right ventricular wall. (Courtesy of R. Mitchell, MD, Brigham and Women's Hospital, Boston, MA.)

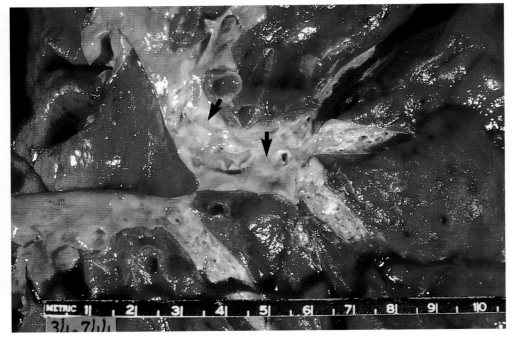

FIGURE 1-15. Cross-section demonstrating atherosclerosis of the pulmonary artery in a patient with longstanding pulmonary hypertension. The pathologic development of this process is identical to that observed in the aorta of a patient with longstanding, essential hypertension. Given the normally low pressure of the pulmonary vascular system, calcification of the pulmonary artery is very unusual and only observed in cases of advanced, longstanding pulmonary hypertension. Calcium deposits and atheromas are indicated (*arrows*). (Courtesy of J. Godleski, MD, Brigham and Women's Hospital, Boston, MA.)

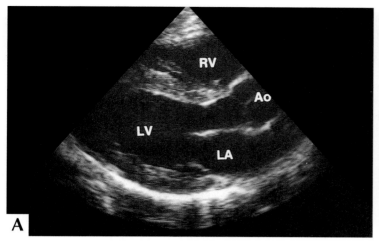

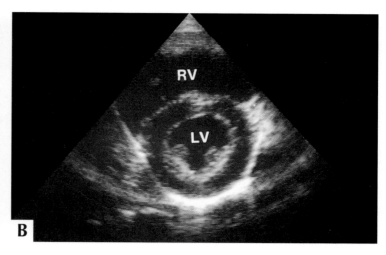

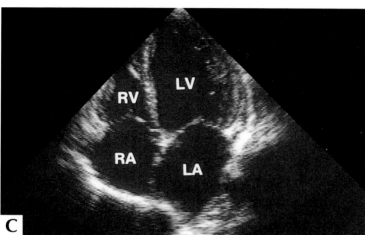

FIGURE 1-16. Echocardiographic features of a normal heart.
A, Standard parasternal long-axis view demonstrating the right ventricle (RV), left ventricle (LV), aortic outflow tract (Ao), and left atrium (LA).
B, Standard short-axis view of the right and left ventricles.
C, Standard apical four-chamber view. RA—right atrium. (*Adapted from* Kislo [18]; with permission.)

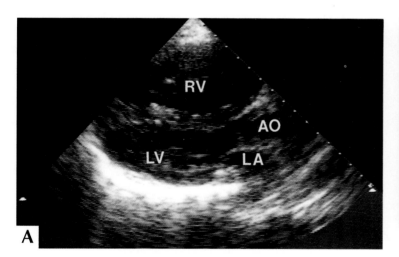

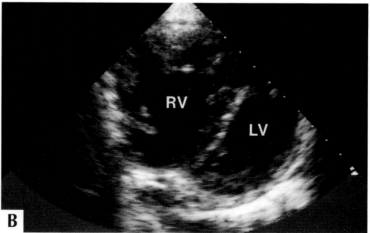

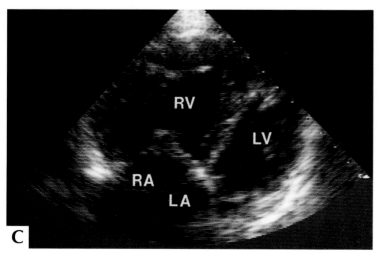

FIGURE 1-17. Echocardiographic features of the heart in a patient with cor pulmonale. **A,** Parasternal long-axis view from a patient with advanced primary pulmonary hypertension complicated by cor pulmonale. Note the abnormal flattening of the interventricular septum and its abnormal bulging into the left ventricle (LV), consistent with volume and pressure overload of the right ventricle (RV). **B,** Short-axis view demonstrating a markedly enlarged RV with RV hypertrophy. Abnormal bowing of the interventricular septum into the LV gives a characteristic *D* configuration of the LV, consistent with volume and pressure overload of the RV. **C,** Apical four-chamber view also demonstrating RV hypertrophy and abnormal septal bowing as described in panels *A* and *B*. AO—aorta; LA—left atrium; RA—right atrium.

PATHOGENESIS

PATHOPHYSIOLOGY OF PULMONARY HYPERTENSION

A   INCREASED RESISTANCE TO PULMONARY VENOUS DRAINAGE

Elevated left ventricular diastolic pressure
  Left ventricular systolic failure
  Left ventricular diastolic dysfunction
  Constrictive pericarditis
Left atrial hypertension
  Mitral valve disease
  Cor triatriatum
  Left atrial myxoma or thrombus
Pulmonary venous obstruction
  Congenital stenosis of pulmonary veins
  Anomalous pulmonary venous connection with obstruction
  Pulmonary veno-occlusive disease
  Mediastinal fibrosis

B   INCREASED RESISTANCE TO FLOW THROUGH PULMONARY VASCULAR BED

Decreased cross-sectional area of pulmonary vascular bed secondary to parenchymal diseases
  Chronic obstructive pulmonary disease
  Restrictive lung disease
  Collagen-vascular diseases (scleroderma, systemic lupus erythematosus, rheumatoid arthritis)
  Fibrotic reactions (Hamman-Rich syndrome, desquamative interstitial pneumonitis, pulmonary hemosiderosis)
  Sarcoidosis
  Neoplasm
  Pneumonia
  Status after pulmonary resection
  Congenital pulmonary hypoplasia
Decreased cross-sectional area of pulmonary vascular bed secondary to Eisenmenger's syndrome
Other conditions associated with decreased cross-sectional area of the pulmonary vascular bed
  Primary pulmonary hypertension
  Hepatic cirrhosis and/or portal thrombosis
  Chemically induced aminorex fumarate, *Crotalaria* alkaloids
  Persistent fetal circulation in the newborn

C   INCREASED RESISTANCE TO FLOW THROUGH LARGE PULMONARY ARTERIES

Pulmonary thromboembolism
Peripheral pulmonic stenosis
Unilateral absence or stenosis of the pulmonary artery

D   HYPOVENTILATION

Obesity-hypoventilation syndromes
Pharyngeal-tracheal obstruction
Neuromuscular disorders
  Myasthenia gravis
  Poliomyelitis
  Damage to central respiratory center
Disorders of the chest wall
Pulmonary parenchymal disorders associated with hypoventilation

E   MISCELLANEOUS CAUSES OF PULMONARY HYPERTENSION

Residence at high altitude
Isolated partial anomalous pulmonary venous drainage
Tetralogy of Fallot
Hemoglobinopathies
Intravenous drug abuse
Alveolar proteinosis
Takayasu's disease

FIGURE 1-18. Clinical causes of pulmonary hypertension that either result in or are associated with cor pulmonale, including (**A**) increased resistance to pulmonary venous drainage; (**B**) increased resistance to flow through pulmonary vascular bed; (**C**) increased resistance to flow through large pulmonary arteries; (**D**) hypoventilation; and (**E**) miscellaneous causes. (*Adapted from* McFadden and Braunwald [9]; with permission.)

EXACERBATION OF PULMONARY HYPERTENSION BY ENDOTHELIAL DYSFUNCTION

PHYSIOLOGIC EFFECT	MECHANISMS
Promote vasoconstriction	Decreased EDRF (nitric oxide)
	Increased endothelin
	Increased thromboxane A_2
	Decreased prostacyclin
Increase platelet activation	Decreased EDRF
	Decreased prostacyclin
Amplify vascular thrombosis	Decreased thrombomodulin (the endothelial surface site for activation of protein C by thrombin)
	Decreased synthesis of heparan sulfate (a glycosaminoglycan similar to heparin)
	Increased release of plasminogen activator inhibitor type I
	Decreased release of tissue-type plasminogen activator
Migration and replication of vascular smooth-muscle cells	Growth factors
	Cytokines

FIGURE 1-19. Endothelial dysfunction exacerbates and accelerates the processes that cause pulmonary hypertension [19]. Factors that appear to promote pulmonary vasoconstriction, increase platelet activation, and amplify vascular thrombosis are part of the process. EDRF—endothelium-derived relaxing factor.

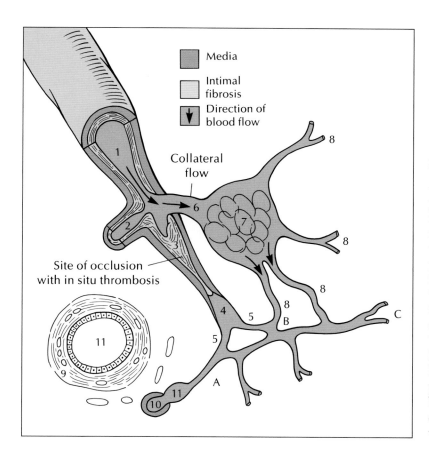

FIGURE 1-20. Diagram demonstrating the origin and probable connections of small, thin-walled collateral blood vessels in the lung in advanced cases of pulmonary hypertension. Such connections create functional arteriovenous fistulae and right-to-left shunting that contribute to the hypoxemia observed in patients with advanced cor pulmonale. 1—Dilated muscular pulmonary artery with thin wall media and intimal fibrosis considered part of the generalized dilatation proximal to the site of vascular occlusion; 2—Hypertrophied muscular pulmonary artery arising as a side branch of the muscular pulmonary artery with an accumulation of intimal fibrous tissue at the site of origin; 3—Terminal muscular pulmonary artery occluded by fibrous tissue and/or thrombosis in situ; 4—Terminal dilated pulmonary arteriole; 5—Capillaries in alveolar walls arising from the pulmonary arteriole; 6—Dilated, thin-walled, veinlike branch of hypertrophied parent muscular pulmonary artery; 7—Localized angiomatoid lesion; 8—Capillaries in alveolar walls arising from dilatation lesions; 9—Dilated thin-walled vessels in submucosa of small bronchus with vascular smooth muscle proliferation; 10—Small bronchial artery in fibrotic coat of a small bronchus giving rise to thin-walled branches (*see* Fig. 1-5); 11—cross-sectional view of the small bronchial artery with medial hyperlasia; A—Bronchopulmonary anastomosis at capillary level; B—Anastomosis between capillaries arising from parent muscular pulmonary artery and dilatation lesions; C—Possible anastomosis between thin-walled vessels of the pulmonary artery and those of the pulmonary vein. (*Adapted from* Harris and Heath [20], with permission.)

CLASSIFICATION OF PULMONARY HYPERTENSION

TYPE	MECHANISM	EXAMPLES
Passive	Impedance to pulmonary venous drainage	Mitral stenosis
Hyperkinetic	Increased pulmonary blood flow	Atrial septal defect Ventricular septal defect
Obstructive	Impedance to flow through large pulmonary arteries	Pulmonary thromboembolism Unilateral absence or stenosis of a pulmonary artery
Obliterative	Impedance to flow through small pulmonary blood vessels	Primary pulmonary hypertension Pulmonary veno-occlusive disease Collagen vascular diseases
Vasoconstrictive	Impedance to flow from hypoxia-induced vasoconstriction	Chronic mountain sickness Sleep apnea syndrome
Polygenic	Two or more of the causes listed above	Chronic obstructive pulmonary diseases (obliterative and vasoconstrictive) Interstitial pulmonary fibrosis (obliterative and vasoconstrictive)

FIGURE 1-21. Classification of pulmonary hypertension based on type, pathophysiologic mechanisms, and clinical examples. (*Adapted from* Butler [6]; with permission.)

HISTOPATHOLOGIC DIFFERENTIATION

	MUSCULAR PULMONARY ARTERIES				
DISEASE	TYPE OF INTIMAL PROLIFERATION	MEDIAL HYPERTROPHY	PLEXIFORM LESIONS	FIBRINOID NECROSIS	ARTERITIS
Primary pulmonary hypertension	Concentric onion-skin type	Severe in early stages	Common	Frequent	Frequent
	Occasional thrombi near fibrinoid necrosis	Less severe in late stages			
Recurrent pulmonary thromboembolism	Fresh, organizing and recanalized thrombi; eccentric pads of intimal fibroelastosis	Slight	Absent	Absent	Rare
Pulmonary veno-occlusive disease	Usually absent or slight	Slight	Absent	Rare	Rare

FIGURE 1-22. Histopathologic differentiation of pulmonary hypertension, recurrent pulmonary thromboembolism, and pulmonary veno-occlusive disease, all of which may present clinically as unexplained pulmonary hypertension. Respective histopathologic features as they relate to the development of advanced pulmonary hypertension are presented. The histopathologic changes that occur both in pulmonary arteries as well as in pulmonary veins and venules are described. (*Adapted from* Harris and Heath [20]; with permission.)

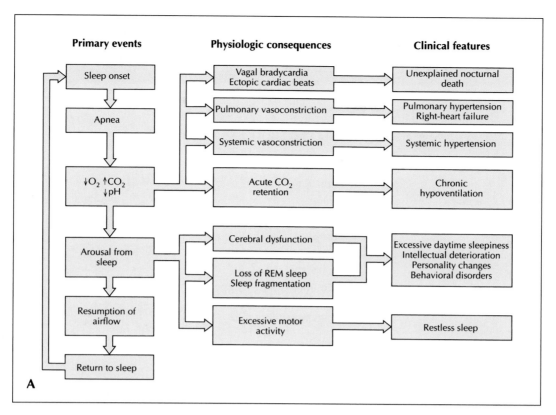

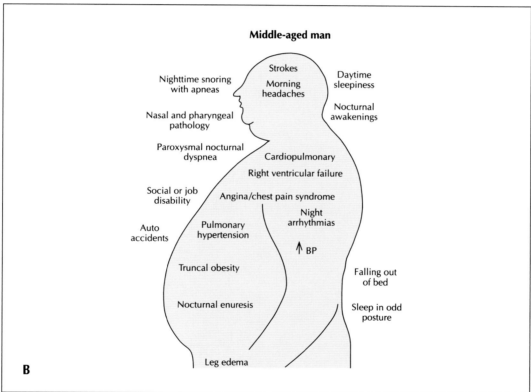

FIGURE 1-23. The pathophysiology and clinical features of the obstructive sleep apnea syndrome complicated by cor pulmonale. Hypoxemia is a powerful stimulus for the development of pulmonary hypertension. The chronic hypoxemia of advanced sleep apnea results in pulmonary hypertension leading to the clinical syndrome of cor pulmonale.

A, Progression of primary events associated with obstructive sleep apnea. These events cause abnormalities in cardiopulmonary physiology that subsequently result in the clinical presentation of pulmonary hypertension with cor pulmonale, chronic hypoventilation, and unexplained nocturnal death.

B, Pathophysiologic profile of a patient with obstructive sleep apnea and advanced cor pulmonale. The typical patient is an obese middle-aged man who snores severely and has episodes of protracted apnea, paroxysmal nocturnal dyspnea, abdominal distention, and nocturnal enuresis. Continuous monitoring of nocturnal arterial saturation confirms severe abnormalities in the arterial saturation and conduction system of the heart associated with these episodes of apnea. (*Adapted from* Bradley and Phillipson [21]; with permission.)

HISTORY AND PHYSICAL EXAMINATION

History	Physical examination	Cardiac examination
Shortness of breath on exertion	Peripheral cyanosis	Right ventricular lift
Chest pain similar to the angina of coronary insufficiency	Acrocyanosis	Palpable P_2
	Digital clubbing	Widely split S_2 with increased P_2 intensity
Diminished appetite	Distended and elevated neck veins	Right-sided S_3
Weight gain	Abdominal ascites	Holosystolic murmur (tricuspid regurgitation)
Abdominal distention	Hepatic congestion with right upper quadrant tenderness	Early diastolic blow (pulmonic insufficiency)
Palpitations		
Syncopal symptoms	Presence of hepatojugular reflex	

FIGURE 1-24. Features of the history and physical examination in cor pulmonale. No symptom is specific for pulmonary hypertension or cor pulmonale [22]. The physical signs of pulmonary hypertension are similar regardless of the underlying etiology or pathophysiologic mechanism. Because of the large reverse-pressure gradient across the tricuspid valve in systole, the murmur produced is high-pitched and quite different from the usual low-pitched, blowing murmur associated with organic disease of the tricuspid valve. Furthermore, in cor pulmonale, increased intensity of the tricuspid systolic murmur during inspiration may not occur.

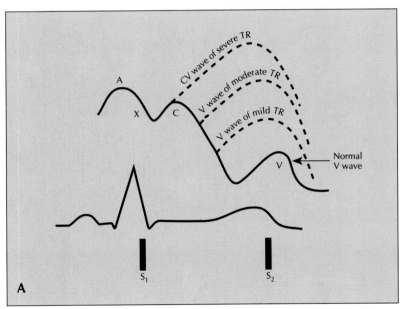

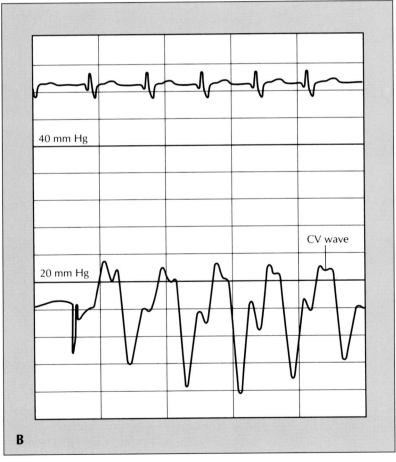

FIGURE 1-25. A, Jugular venous pulsation recording (*top*) with a simultaneous electrocardiogram (*middle*) and recording of the S_1 and S_2 heart sounds (*bottom*). The *interrupted lines* demonstrate increases in V waves with increasing tricuspid regurgitation (TR). With severe tricuspid regurgitation, the C and V waves merge to form a CV wave. This type of C wave morphology noted on recordings of jugular venous pulsation is typical of patients with advanced cor pulmonale. The slope of the *x descent*, which indicates atrial compliance properties, is marked *X*. **B,** Hemodynamic correlation of the physical finding of the CV wave shown on a phasic right atrial pressure recordings from a 63-year-old patient with cor pulmonale secondary to primary left ventricular failure. The recordings were taken with a pulmonary artery catheter located in the right atrium. Note the prominent elevation in the mean right atrial resting pressure (17 mm Hg) as well as the prominent CV wave. This pulse-wave contour represents chronic pressure and volume overload of the right ventricle with associated tricuspid regurgitation and is referred to as *ventricularization* of the right atrial pressure waveform. (Part A *adapted from* Constant [23]; with permission.)

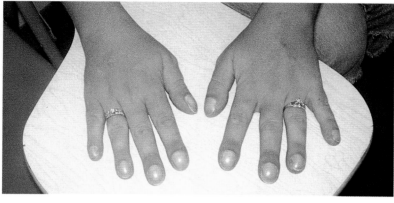

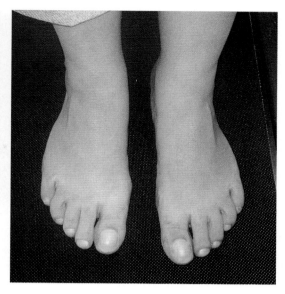

FIGURE 1-26. Severe clubbing and cyanosis of the fingertips of a 36-year-old woman with a complete atrioventricular canal defect and advanced pulmonary hypertension. Cyanosis is more likely to develop in the complete forms of endocardial cushion defects because pulmonary hypertension occurs more frequently than in the partial forms with an intact ventricular septum. As the pulmonary vascular resistance increases to systemic levels, the patient's left-to-right shunting decreases, with increased right-to-left-shunting accompanied by a marked decrement in systemic arterial oxygen saturation. The resulting hypoxemia accounts for her cyanosis. Patients with cyanotic heart disease often manifest clubbing, which is defined as bullous enlargement of the soft tissue of the distal segment of a finger or toe. Bony changes can occur in the more severe forms of clubbing.

FIGURE 1-27. Advanced clubbing and cyanosis of the toes of the same patient in Fig. 1-26.

ASSESSMENT

DIAGNOSTIC WORK-UP

DIAGNOSTIC TEST	GOALS
Oximetry	Need for continuous oxygen
Chest roentgenogram	RO infiltrative process RO connective tissue process RO vascular abnormalities
Electrocardiogram	Help assess severity of RV hypertrophy
Echocardiogram	Assess LV and RV function and thickness RO mitral stenosis RO intracardiac shunt RO congenital malformation
Radionuclide ventriculography	Assess LV function Assess RV function
Pulmonary function testing	Establish whether restrictive or obstructive lung physiology is present and the response to bronchodilator therapy
Lung scintigraphy	RO pulmonary embolism
Pulmonary angiography	RO pulmonary embolism RO peripheral pulmonic stenosis
Cardiac catheterization	Establish baseline hemodynamics Determine hemodynamic response to vasodilators RO coronary artery stenosis or malformation

FIGURE 1-28. Various diagnostic tests that are indicated in the work-up of a patient with cor pulmonale. The tests are listed in the left column; the right column contains the specific goals and, where applicable, the pathophysiologic entities that are to be ruled out after evaluation of the results. Given the risks of angiography in patients with pulmonary hypertension, pulmonary angiography is indicated only when the presenting history, results of the electrocardiogram and ventilation-perfusion scan, and a high probability of pulmonary embolism justify proceeding with this particular procedure. LV—left ventricular; RO—rule out; RV—right ventricular.

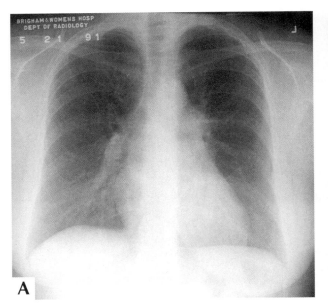
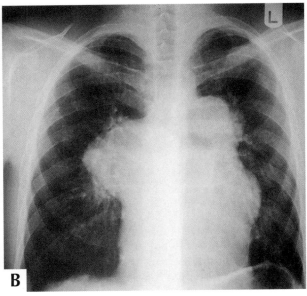

A

B

FIGURE 1-29. Chest radiographs demonstrating features of patients with advanced cor pulmonale secondary to primary pulmonary hypertension. **A,** Typical radiograph of a patient with primary pulmonary hypertension. Note the peripheral oligemia of the pulmonary vessels with mild bilateral enlargement of the main pulmonary arteries. The cardiothoracic ratio is within normal limits. **B,** Radiograph of a 45-year-old man who presented with a history of advanced shortness of breath with atypical chest discomfort. Note the enormous bilateral pulmonary artery aneurysms, consistent with the diagnosis of primary pulmonary hypertension.

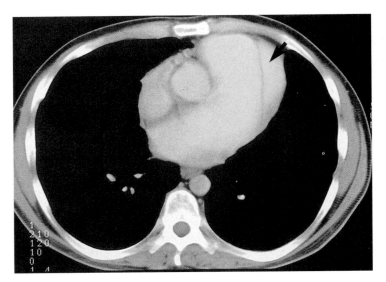

FIGURE 1-30. Pulmonary artery dissection as shown on a computed tomographic scan with contrast of the patient in Fig. 1-29B. The goal of the computed tomographic scan was to determine the etiology of the patient's presenting chest pain. The measurement of the aneurysm of this pulmonary artery was 9 cm on the right and 11 cm on the left. A dissection of the left pulmonary artery can be seen after injection of the contrast agent (*arrrow*). This patient eventually underwent successful bilateral sequential lung transplantation.

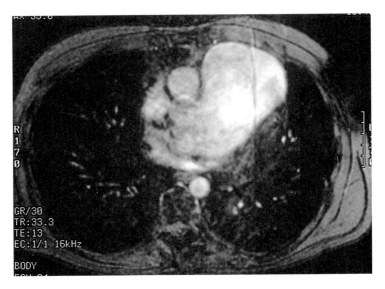

FIGURE 1-31. A magnetic resonance image of the pulmonary artery aneurysm complicated by dissection as seen in Figs. 1-29B and 1-30. Figs. 1-29, 1-30, and 1-31 demonstrate the specific use of three imaging modalities for patients who carry the diagnosis of primary pulmonary hypertension and cor pulmonale.

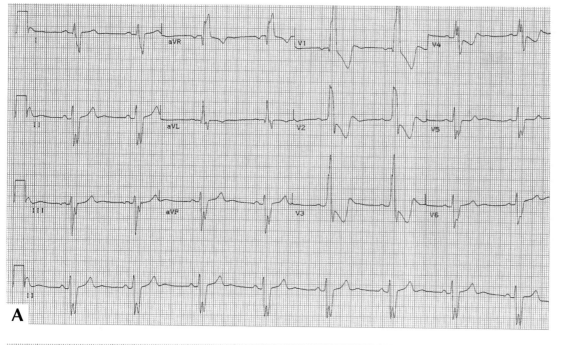

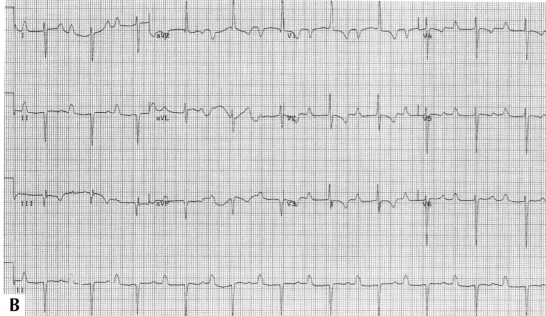

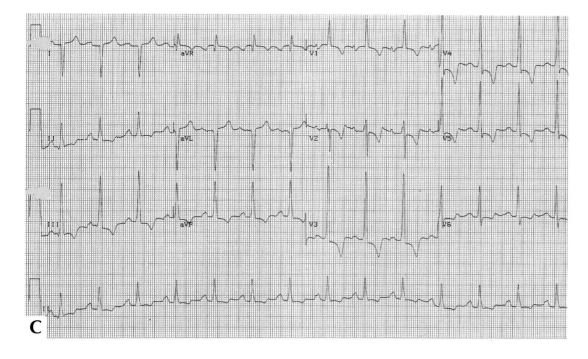

FIGURE 1-32. Electrocardiographic finding in patients with advanced cor pulmonale.

A, A 50-year-old man with classic Eisenmenger's physiology secondary to a muscular ventricular septal defect. Note the complete right bundle branch pattern with an RR'in lead V_1. This tracing demonstrates pressure and volume overload of the right ventricle, consistent with cor pulmonale.

B, A 35-year-old woman who presented with shortness of breath, cyanosis, and light-headedness secondary to a complete atrioventricular canal defect. Note the prominent S wave in V_5 and V_6 and first-degree atrioventricular block.

C, A 50-year-old woman with pulmonary hypertension and cor pulmonale secondary to a secundum atrial septal defect complicated by Eisenmenger's physiology. Note the prominent R wave in V_1, right axis deviation, and nonspecific ST- and T-wave abnormalities consistent with right ventricular hyper-trophy with strain.

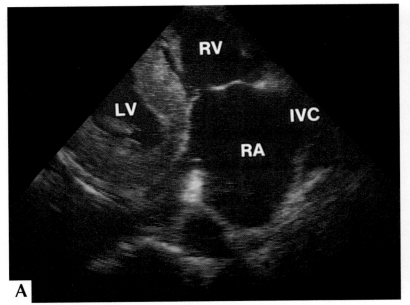

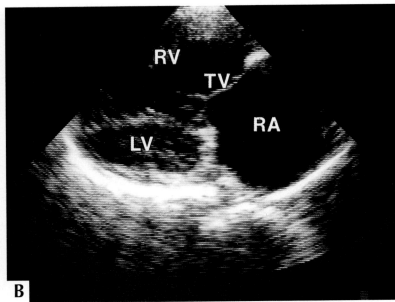

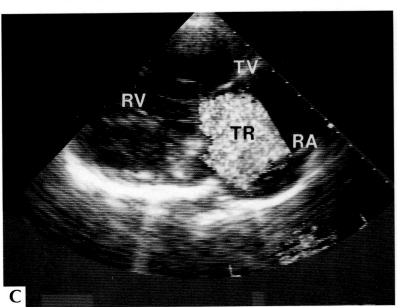

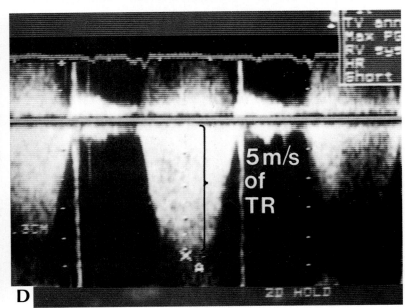

FIGURE 1-33. Echocardiographic evaluation of pulmonary hypertension in a patient with cor pulmonale.

A, Normal relationship of the left ventricle (LV), right ventricle (RV), tricuspid valve (TV), and right atrium (RA) in a normal heart.

B, Distorted anatomy of the interventricular septum secondary to enlargement of the RV and the RA in a patient with advanced cor pulmonale secondary to primary pulmonary hypertension.

C, Doppler images of advanced tricuspid regurgitation (TR).

D, Continuous-wave Doppler analysis of the peak flow associated with the tricuspid regurgitation seen in C. The continuity equation allows for an approximation of the peak pulmonary artery systolic pressure using the formula $4v^2$, where v is the peak instantaneous velocity, as indicated in the figure. This number added to the RA pressure gives an approximation of pulmonary artery systolic pressure. In this patient the calculation estimates a pulmonary artery pressure of 100 mm Hg plus the RA pressure, which is estimated by examination of the jugular venous pulsation. IVC—inferior vena cava.

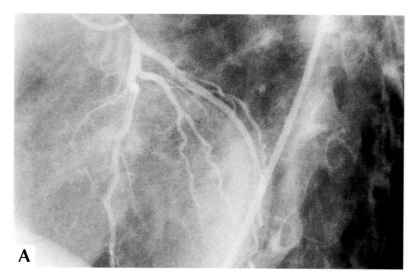

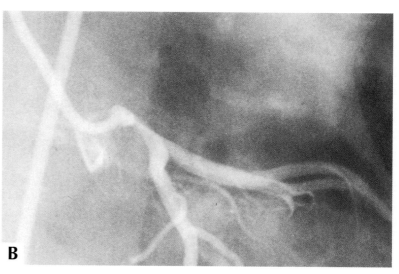

FIGURE 1-34. Coronary angiograms in a 36-year-old woman with pulmonary hypertension secondary to patent ductus arteriosus. This patient suffered an anterior myocardial infarction caused by compression of the left main coronary artery by a dilated main pulmonary artery. **A,** Left anterior oblique view. **B,** Right anterior oblique view.

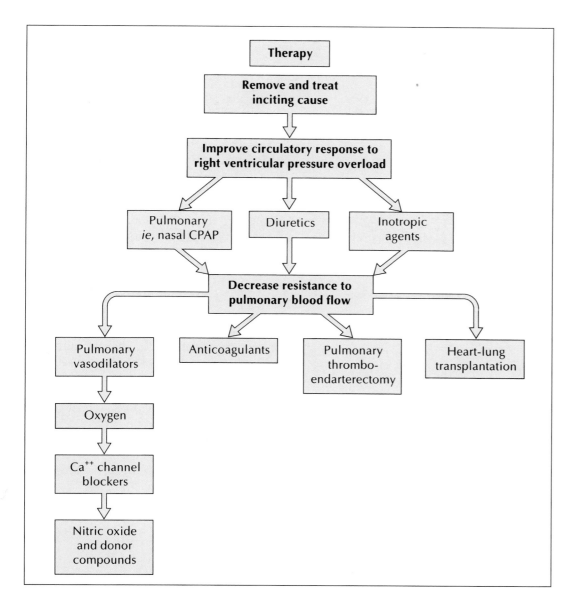

FIGURE 1-35. Therapy for patients with advanced cor pulmonale. It is important to establish the underlying cause of the disease in order to direct therapy appropriately. General goals of therapy include improving the circulatory response to right ventricular overload and/or decreasing resistance to pulmonary blood flow by various means, such as the administration of pulmonary vasodilators, anticoagulation therapy, pulmonary thromboendarterectomy, and also heart-lung transplantation as indicated. CPAP—continuous positive airway pressure.

DIURETIC THERAPY

AGENT	ROUTE	DOSE RANGE	ADVERSE EFFECTS
Furosemide	PO/IV	20–400 mg/d	Hypovolemia Hypokalemia
Metolazone	PO	2.5–20 mg/d	Hypovolemia Hypokalemia Hyponatremia
Bumetanide	PO/IV	0.5–4.0 mg/d	Hypovolemia Hypokalemia Hyperuricemia
Chlorothiazide	PO/IV	0.5–1.0 g/d	Hypovolemia Hypokalemia Hyponatremia Hypomagnesemia

FIGURE 1-36. Diuretic therapy for patients with fluid retention secondary to advanced cor pulmonale. The four most common pharmacologic agents are represented. Included also are the route, dose range, and typical side effects.

INOTROPIC AGENTS

AGENT	ROUTE	DOSE RANGE	ADVERSE EFFECTS
Digoxin	PO	0.125–0.375 mg/d	GI intolerance; PAT with block; VT
Dobutamine	IV	2.5–15 µg/kg/min	Sinus tachycardia; VT
Dopamine	IV	2.5–15 µg/kg/min	Sinus tachycardia; VT
Amrinone	IV	2.5–15 µg/kg/min	Sinus tachycardia; VT; thrombocytopenia
Milrinone	IV	0.5–0.75 µg/kg/min	Sinus tachycardia; VT

FIGURE 1-37. Inotropic agents used to treat advanced cor pulmonale patients who are refractory to conventional therapy. The initial agents of choice are digitalis preparations given at the oral dosing regimen listed in the table. Prominent adverse side effects include gastrointestinal intolerance, paroxysmal atrial tachycardia (PAT) with block, and ventricular tachycardia (VT). These disorders occur as dose ranging becomes more important with advancing cor pulmonale accompanied by decreased forward cardiac output and renal perfusion. The other agents listed are used primarily for hospitalized, moribund patients. Thrombocytopenia is associated with long-term use of amrinone.

VASODILATORS

α-Antagonists
  Tolazoline
  Phentolamine
  Phenoxybenzamine
  Prazosin
β-Agonists
  Isoproterenol
  Terbutaline
Direct-acting vasodilators
  Diazoxide
  Hydralazine
  Nitroprusside
  Isosorbide dinitrate
  Nitroglycerin

Calcium-channel blockers
  Nifedipine
  Diltiazem
  Verapamil
ACE inhibitors
  Captopril
Prostaglandins
  Prostaglandin E
  Prostacyclin
Cyclooxygenase inhibitors
  Indomethacin
Anticholinergics
  Acetylcholine
Oxygen

FIGURE 1-38. Vasodilators that have been used and studied in patients with primary pulmonary hypertension. The spectrum ranges from various oral agents to direct-acting vasodilators. Most of these preparations are available in oral form except for the prostaglandin derivatives, which are available only in intravenous form. The most promising data on long-term therapy with the goal of improving survival have been obtained with calcium channel blockers.

HISTOPATHOLOGY OF PULMONARY HYPERTENSION

CLASSIFICATION	HISTOPATHOLOGIC DESCRIPTION	VASODILATOR RESPONSE
Isolated medial hypertrophy (IMH)	Increased thickness of the medial smooth muscle and duplication of elastic laminae in muscular arteries	IMH is potentially reversible with vasodilator therapy; possibly, muscular atrophy accounts for failure of certain patients to respond
	Development of a well-formed smooth muscle layer (muscularization) in pulmonary arterioles; with long-standing disease, the medial smooth muscle may degenerate and be replaced by fibrous tissue	
Plexogenic pulmonary arteriopathy (PPA)	Variable admixture of medial hypertrophy, intimal lesions, and destructive lesions involving the entire arterial wall; concentric laminar intimal fibrosis is the most reliable and constant marker of PPA	Typified by rapidly progressive disease that is usually not responsive to vasodilators
Thrombotic pulmonary arteriopathy	Thrombi form because of in situ thrombosis of small muscular arteries; by definition, PPA lesions are absent	Almost never responsive to vasodilators

FIGURE 1-39. Histopathology of pulmonary hypertension and its relation to vasodilator response. The histopathology of lesions in patients with pulmonary hypertension provides a basis for evaluating and predicting the effects of various therapeutic endeavors. The three major types of hypertensive pulmonary arteriopathy are described. Other histopathologic types of pulmonary hypertension include hypertensive pulmonary venopathy (due to pulmonary veno-occlusive disease), chronic pulmonary venous hypertension, as well as the extremely rare pulmonary capillary hemangiomatosis [24]. For discussion of increased thickness of the medial smooth muscle and of the elastic laminae, concentric laminar intimal fibrosis, and in situ thrombosis of small muscular arteries, *see* Figs. 4-3*A*, 4-3*B*, and 4-3*D* in Chapter 4, respectively.

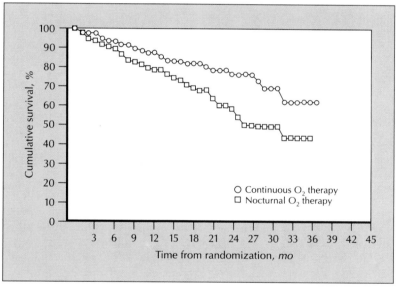

FIGURE 1-40. Oxygen therapy for hypoxemic chronic obstructive lung disease. When chronic bronchitis or emphysema is complicated by hypoxic cor pulmonale, the prognosis for surviving several years is poor. Therefore, the Medical Research Council sponsored a controlled clinical trial of administering nocturnal oxygen at home (15 hours per night of nasal prong oxygen; usually 2 L/min) versus no oxygen to determine whether oxygen therapy reduced the 3-year mortality rate [25]. The annual mortality rate was 29% among controls compared with 12% among those who received oxygen (*P*=0.04). Interestingly, no difference in the survival curves appeared until after approximately 500 days of oxygen therapy. It was not apparent whether continuous oxygen therapy would be superior to nocturnal oxygen. Therefore, the National Heart, Lung and Blood Institute initiated a trial at six centers in which 203 patients with hypoxemic chronic obstructive lung disease were allocated randomly either to continuous oxygen therapy or 12-hour nocturnal oxygen therapy and followed up for an average of 19 months [26]. The mortality rate was almost halved among patients who received continuous oxygen. The mechanism for this beneficial effect is not clear. Continuous oxygen reduced pulmonary vascular resistance more than nocturnal oxygen at 6 months after entry into the study; however, patients with larger decreases in pulmonary vascular resistance (>20 dynes/s × cm^5) paradoxically tended to have a greater mortality rate than patients with smaller decreases. Patients receiving continuous oxygen therapy had an average decrement of 11% in pulmonary vascular resistance, whereas patients receiving nocturnal oxygen therapy had an average increase of 6% in pulmonary vascular resistance (*P*=0.04). Thus, these data suggest that although continuous O$_2$ therapy reduced both mortality and pulmonary vascular resistance, the two phenomena appeared unrelated. (*Adapted from* Nocturnal Oxygen Therapy Trial Group [26]; with permission.)

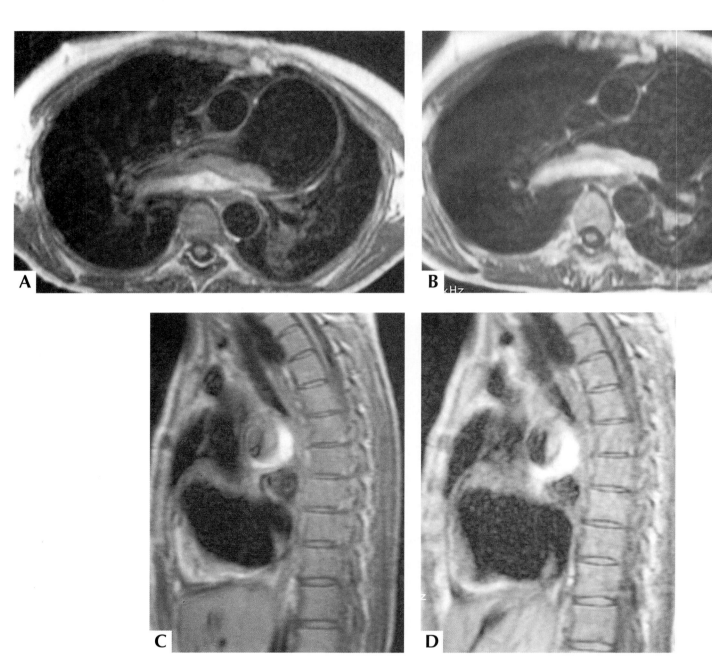

FIGURE 1-41. Magnetic resonance images demonstrating a rare complication of advanced pulmonary hypertension. The patient was a 60-year-old woman with Eisenmenger's complex (ventricular septal defect with systemic pulmonary artery pressure) who presented with a 2-month history of shortness of breath at rest, right-sided heart failure, and recent central cyanosis. She had not been treated prophylactically with systemic anticoagulation therapy. Panels A and C represent baseline study, and panels B and D represent repeat images obtained after a 24-hour infusion of systemic urokinase. The patient demonstrated symptomatic improvement after therapy.

A and **B,** Transverse images demonstrating an enormous, in situ pulmonary artery thrombus spanning the right and main pulmonary artery trunk with extension into the left main pulmonary artery. The right main pulmonary artery trunk is nearly occluded, and there is evidence of serpiginous recanalization channels. The two distinct T_2-weighted appearances of the thrombus most likely represent subacute and chronic in situ thrombi. The gray part of the thrombus most likely is more recent in origin and is the part of the clot that has diminished in size in response to thrombolytic therapy.

C and **D,** Sagittal images demonstrating the left main pulmonary artery in cross-section with a nearly totally occlusive thrombus pre-urokinase with some resolution after thrombolytic therapy.

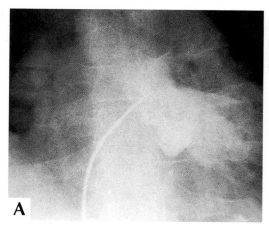
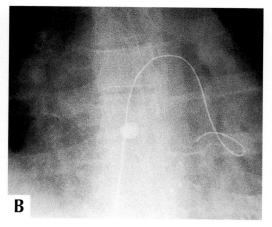
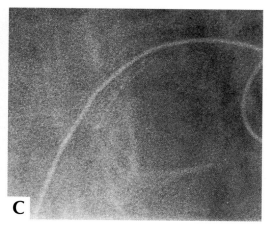

A **B** **C**

Figure 1-42. Percutaneous atrial septostomy. This patient underwent atrial septostomy to palliate advanced cor pulmonale due to primary pulmonary hypertension. (Please refer also to Fig. 4-32 in Chapter 4.)

A, Contrast agent delineates the interatrial septum after a controlled puncture of the septum with a Brockenbrough needle. A balloon pulmonary artery catheter is positioned through the interatrial septum to enlarge the initial puncture site. **B,** An expandable stent is then placed across the interatrial septum. After being anchored in position, the stent is expanded gradually to facilitate decompression of the right atrium and right ventricle. **C,** The final size of the stent is determined by assessing the degree of right-to-left shunting needed to reduce the elevated pressures in the right side of the heart and to augment forward cardiac output.

REFERENCES

1. Harvey W: *Exercitatio anatomica de motu cordis et sanguinis in animalibus*. Francofurti Guilielmi Fitzeri, 1628 [translated by Leake CD]. Springfield, IL: Charles C. Thomas; 1928:49–56.

2. McGinn S, White PD: Acute cor pulmonale resulting from pulmonary embolism. *JAMA* 1935, 104:1473–1480.

3. Netter FH: *The CIBA Collection of Medical Illustrations: Heart*, vol 5, ed 6. New York: The Case-Hoyt Corp.; 1987:81.

4. Bishop JM: Hypoxia and pulmonary hypertension in chronic bronchitis. *Prog Respir Res* 1975, 9:10.

5. Fowler NO: The normal pulmonary circulation. In *Textbook of Pulmonary Disease*, ed 2. Edited by Baum GL. Boston: Little, Brown and Co.; 1974:689–699.

6. Butler J: Cor Pulmonale. In *Textbook of Respiratory Medicine*. Edited by Murray JF, Nadel JA. Philadelphia: WB Saunders; 1988:1410–1453.

7. Tartulier M, Bourret M, Deyrieux F: Les Pressions arterielles pulmonaires chez l'homme normal: effets de l'age et de l'exercise musculaire. *Bull Physiopathol Resp* 1976, 12:637–650.

8. Weber KT, Janicki JS, Shroff S, Fishman AP: Contractile mechanisms and interaction of the right and left ventricles. *Am J Cardiol* 1981, 47:686–695.

9. McFadden ER, Braunwald E: Cor pulmonale. In *Heart Disease: A Textbook of Cardiovascular Medicine*, ed 4. Edited by Braunwald E. Philadelphia, WB Saunders, 1992:1581–1601.

10. Snyder SH, Bredt DS: Biological roles of nitric oxide. *Sci Am* 1992:266:68–71, 74–77..

11. Fineman JF, Chang R, Soifer SJ: EDRF inhibition augments pulmonary hypertension in intact newborn lambs. *Am J Physiol* 1992, 262:H1365–H1371.

12. Dinh-Xuan AT, Higenbottam TW, Clelland CA, *et al.*: Impairment of endothelium-dependent pulmonary-artery relaxation in chronic obstruction lung disease. *N Engl J Med* 1991, 324:1539–1547.

13. Stewart DJ, Levy RD, Cernacek P, Langleben D: Increased plasma endothelin-1 in pulmonary hypertension: marker or mediator of disease? *Ann Intern Med* 1991, 114:464–469.

14. Giaid A, Yanagisawa M, Langleben D, *et al.*: Expression of endothelin-1 in the lungs of patients with pulmonary hypertension. *N Engl J Med* 1993, 328: 1732–1739.

15. Christman BW, McPherson CD, Newman JH, *et al.*: An imbalance between the excretion of thromboxane and prostacyclin metabolites in pulmonary hypertension. *N Engl J Med* 1992, 327:70–75.

16. Higenbottam T: Pathophysiology of pulmonary hypertension: a role for endothelial dysfunction. *Chest* 1994, 105:7S–12S.

17. Enson Y, Giuntini C, Lewis ML, *et al.*: The influence of hydrogen ion concentration and hypoxia on the pulmonary circulation. *J Clin Invest* 1964, 43:1146–1162.

18. Kislo J: *Echocardiography—A Slide Atlas*. New York: Medi Cine Productions; 1988 [code 0996882].

19. Loscalzo J: Endothelial dysfunction in pulmonary hypertension. *N Engl J Med* 1992, 327:117–119.

20. Harris P, Heath D: Unexplained pulmonary hypertension. In *The Human Pulmonary Circulation*, ed 2. Edited by Harris P, Heath D. Edinburgh: Churchill-Livingston; 1977:418–440.

21. Bradley TD, Phillipson EA: Pathogenesis and pathophysiology of the obstructive sleep apnea syndrome. *Med Clin North Am* 1985, 69:1169–1185.

22. Palevsky HI, Fishman AP: Chronic cor pulmonale: etiology and management. *JAMA* 1990, 263:2347–2353.

23. Constant J: Jugular pressure and pulsations. In *Beside Cardiology*, ed IV. Edited by Constant J. Boston: Little Brown and Co.; 1993:69–95.

24. Pietra GG: Histopathology of primary pulmonary hypertension. *Chest* 1994, 105:2S–6S.

25. Report of the Medical Research Council Working Party: Long term domiciliary oxygen therapy in chronic hypoxic cor pulmonale complicating chronic bronchitis and emphysema. *Lancet* 1981, 1:681–686.

26. Nocturnal Oxygen Therapy Trial Group: Continuous or nocturnal oxygen therapy in hypoxemic chronic obstructive lung disease: a clinical trial. *Ann Intern Med* 1980, 93:391–398.

DIAGNOSIS OF ACUTE PULMONARY EMBOLISM

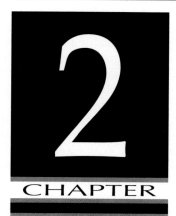

CHAPTER 2

Lorraine Skibo and Samuel Z. Goldhaber

Pulmonary embolism is the third most common cardiovascular disease, following acute myocardial ischemic syndromes and stroke. Pulmonary embolism and deep venous thrombosis together account for more than 250,000 hospitalizations per year in the United States. Pulmonary embolism causes or contributes to approximately 50,000 deaths per year in the United States, and is the most common cause of maternal mortality associated with live births. Despite advances in medical care, the mortality rate for pulmonary embolism has not declined in the past few decades [1].

Investigation of patients with idiopathic pulmonary embolism has a high yield for detecting underlying hypercoagulable disorders. Deficiencies of antithrombin-III, protein C, and protein S predispose to recurrent thrombosis and thromboembolism. Lupus anticoagulant and antiphospholipid antibodies are acquired hypercoagulable states that often occur in patients who do *not* have collagen vascular disease. Although lupus anticoagulant can prolong the partial thromboplastin time, it paradoxically increases the risk of venous thrombosis.

Acquired hypercoagulable states may be recognizable clinically. Recent surgical procedures and neoplasms are well-established risk factors, especially in hospitalized patients. Indwelling central venous catheters and inferior vena caval filters may also serve as a nidus for thrombus formation and possible embolization.

Pulmonary embolism is more common in older age groups and affects men more often than women. The death rate is relatively high even among young patients. Actual episodes of pulmonary embolism (determined from postmortem studies) exceed recognized cases because the clinical diagnosis remains elusive. Despite advances in medical imaging, pulmonary embolism often remains undetected until postmortem examination. Prompt and accurate diagnosis is the critical first step to reduce the morbidity and mortality of pulmonary embolism.

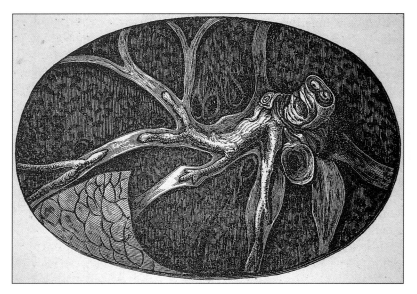

FIGURE 2-1. German pathologist Rudolf Virchow was the first to link deep vein thrombosis to pulmonary infarction and published this illustration of a thromboembolus in the pulmonary arteries in 1856 [2]. He had, in 1846, proven that thrombosis could occur in the low-flow, low-pressure venous system. He established the doctrine of embolism to the lungs from the deep leg veins. His classic triad of local trauma to the vessel wall, hypercoagulability, and stasis leading to intravascular coagulation remains a useful aid to the clinician thinking about risk factors for pulmonary embolism. In 1935, White [3] described the clinical diagnosis of pulmonary embolism based on its physiologic manifestations. White was so clinically astute that he was able to link the clinical signs of right heart failure with massive pulmonary embolism. At about the same time, Homans [4] clinically and Rossle [5] pathologically called attention to the frequent occurrence of deep venous thrombosis. With Hampton and Castleman's description of the radiologic appearance of pulmonary infarcts in 1940 [6], emphasis on the diagnosis of pulmonary embolism finally shifted from the autopsy table to the clinical arena.

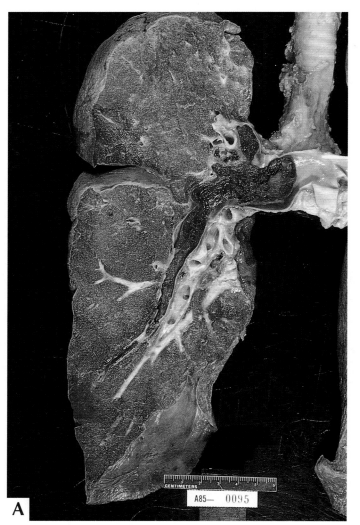

A

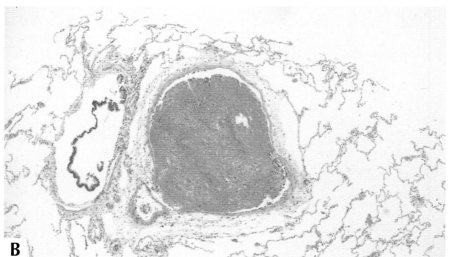

B

FIGURE 2-2. A, Gross specimen of the right lung, sectioned in a coronal plane at the vascular pedicle, showing a recent thromboembolus lodged in the right main pulmonary artery. Tails of clot extend into the right upper lobe pulmonary artery, the interlobar pulmonary artery, and some of the lower lobe segmental branches. Hemorrhage is seen in the lower lateral portion of the sectioned lung. The morphologic consequences of embolic occlusion depend upon the size of emboli, the presence of underlying lung disease, and circulatory physiology. Infarction occurs in 10% to 15% of emboli, and is most frequently seen with small thrombi that lodge distally. Experiments in laboratory animals have demonstrated that chest wall compression and pleural effusion predispose to infarction [7].

B, Histologic section of a medium-sized artery containing recent thromboembolus. (*continued*)

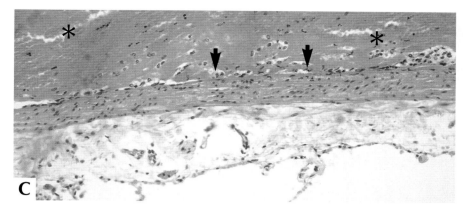

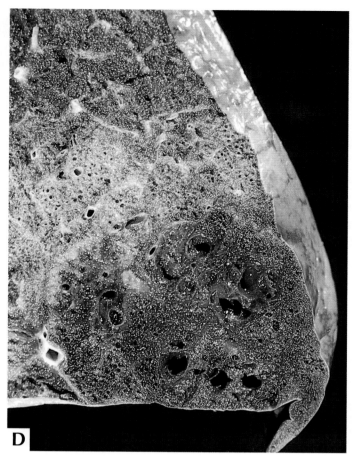

FIGURE 2-2. (*continued*) **C,** Initially, the thromboembolus (*asterisks*) fills the pulmonary artery; adherence of the thrombus to the wall causes fibroplastic ingrowth (*arrows*), as is seen at higher power. Fibrinoid necrosis with an acute inflammatory infiltrate is seen in an occasional arterial wall.

D, Within 1 to 2 days of embolization, pulmonary infarction (coagulative necrosis) can be recognized pathologically as a firm, wedge-shaped area of hemorrhagic consolidation with apposed fibrinous pleuritis. After red blood cells lyse, an influx of polymorphonuclear leukocytes causes the infarct to pale. A zone of vascular organization tissue at the periphery of the infarct may be present. Eventually, the infarcted alveolar walls, bronchioles, and vessels are replaced by fibrous tissue; this leads to a contracted scar with puckered overlying pleura. Airways within the fibrotic region may remain viable and patent because of their bronchial artery vascular supply. Rarely, fibrosis is followed by cavitation. In these circumstances a prominent leukocytic infiltrate is usually present [7]. (Courtesy of John J. Godleski, MD, Brigham and Women's Hospital, Boston, MA.)

PATHOPHYSIOLOGY

PULMONARY AND CARDIAC PHYSIOLOGIC ALTERATIONS

PHYSIOLOGY	EFFECT OF PULMONARY EMBOLUS	RESULT	CLINICAL MANIFESTATION
Hemodynamic	Vascular obstruction; vasoconstriction from vasoactive amines; vasoconstriction from baroreflex	Increased PA pressure	Left sternal border parasternal lift or heave
PA	Presence of thromboembolus	Increased PA size	Palpable pulmonic component of S_2
RV	Increased outflow pressure	Increased pressure, then dilatation and hypokinesis	RV failure
LV	Interventricular septum deviates to left; increased pericardial restraint from RV dilatation	Decreased preload	LV failure
PULMONARY			
Gas exchange	Vascular obstruction; hypoventilation R to L shunt; loss of exchange surfaces	Increased dead space; increased A-a O_2 gradient; impaired CO transfer	Hypoxemia; impaired CO_2 elimination
Ventilatory control	Stimulation of irritant receptors	Alveolar hyperventilation	Hypocapnia, respiratory alkalosis

FIGURE 2-3. Pulmonary and cardiac physiologic alterations are important indicators of the presence and severity of acute pulmonary thromboembolism [8]. The clinical manifestations of these changes may be the only clue that pulmonary embolism has occurred. LV—left ventricular; PA—pulmonary artery; RV—right ventricular.

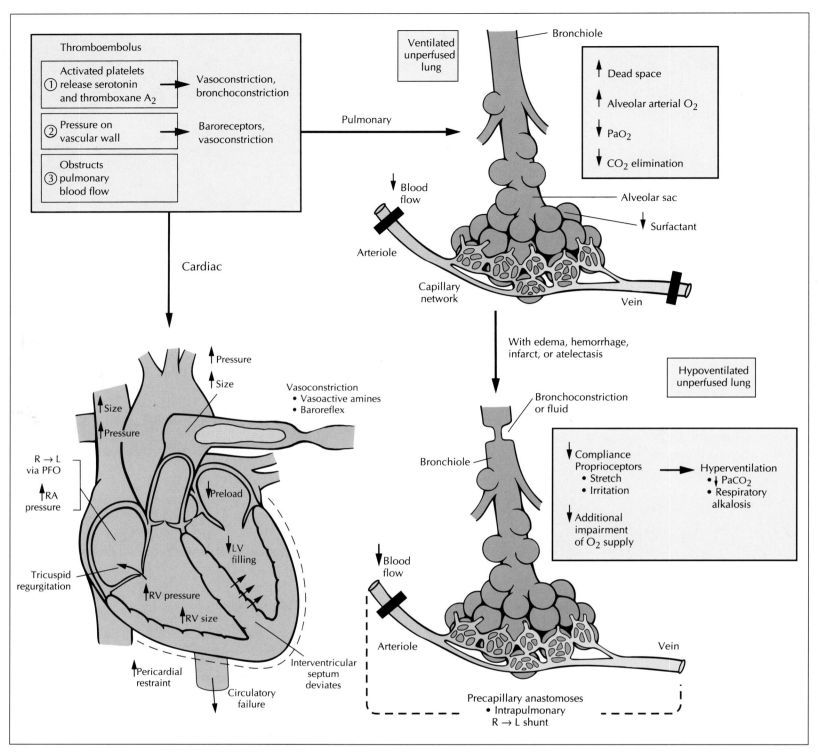

FIGURE 2-4. Following pulmonary thromboembolism, vascular obstruction causes a series of reactions that result in increased pulmonary vascular resistance. The media of large elastic pulmonary arteries (larger than 1000 μm in diameter, including lobar, segmental, and subsegmental branches) contain elastic fibrils (with some smooth muscle fibers) that can accommodate substantial increases in blood flow without increasing pulmonary artery pressures. This is well illustrated in postpneumonectomy patients in whom pulmonary arterial pressures usually remain normal despite doubling of arterial flow through the remaining lung. Pressures may not rise until the thromboembolic load is large, unless preexisting pulmonary or cardiac disease is present. The release of vasoactive amines or the baroreceptor reflex may cause vasoconstriction of pulmonary arteries. Aggregated platelets adherent to the surface of thromboemboli are sources of serotonin, which can cause smooth muscle contraction in pulmonary arteries. Baroreceptors present in pulmonary arteries may be activated by the pressure exerted against the arterial wall by the embolus itself, or by blood flowing past an embolus. The right ventricle responds to increased pulmonary arterial pressure by dilating and by causing the interventricular septum to impinge upon an intrinsically normal left ventricle, thereby potentially decreasing forward cardiac output. Diminished or absent perfusion of aerated lung units causes an increase in dead space. True right-to-left shunting of mixed venous blood can occur at the atrial level through a patent foramen ovale (when right heart pressures exceed left). Increased airway resistance and decreased pulmonary compliance may also accompany pulmonary embolism. Pulmonary infarction usually results from additional impairment of the oxygen supply to the parenchyma such as in concomitant left ventricular failure.

CLINICAL FINDINGS

SYMPTOMS OF PULMONARY THROMBOEMBOLISM

Dyspnea	Palpitations
Syncope	Wheezing
Pleuritic pain	Anginalike pain
Hemoptysis	Apprehension
Cough	Diaphoresis

FIGURE 2-5. Pulmonary thromboembolism has diverse manifestations because of its potential to affect the entire cardiopulmonary system. A high degree of clinical suspicion is warranted because pulmonary embolism can masquerade as many other diseases. Dyspnea and syncope are associated with massive pulmonary embolism.

A. PHYSICAL FINDINGS

Tachypnea (>20/min)	Wheezing
Rales	Homans' sign
Tachycardia (>100 bpm)	Right ventricular lift
Fourth heart sound	Pleural friction rub
Increased pulmonic component of second heart sound	Third heart sound
	Cyanosis
Diaphoresis	Evidence of paradoxic
Fever	arterial embolism, *eg*, stroke

B. CLINICAL SYNDROMES

Massive pulmonary embolism
  Syncope, profound dyspnea, cor pulmonale, cardiogenic shock, cardiac arrest, disseminated intravascular coagulation, paradoxic arterial emboli

Submassive pulmonary embolism
  Chest pain, dyspnea

Pulmonary infarction
  Hemoptysis, chest pain, dyspnea

FIGURE 2-6. A, The physical findings in acute pulmonary thromboembolism are nonspecific and reflect the physiologic effects of the embolus. Right ventricular lift and cyanosis are associated with massive pulmonary embolism. **B,** Patients suffering acute pulmonary embolism can often be described with various clinical syndromes that have differing prognoses.

LABORATORY AND ELECTROCARDIOGRAPHIC FINDINGS

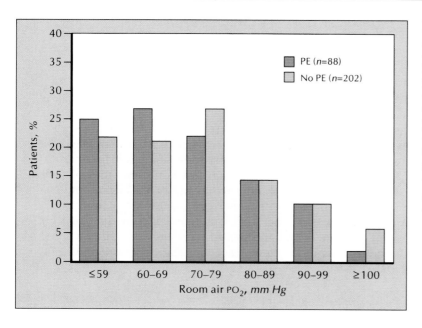

FIGURE 2-7. Distribution of the partial pressure of oxygen in arterial blood (PO_2) among 88 patients with angiographically proven pulmonary embolus and no preexisting cardiac or pulmonary disease compared with 202 similar patients in whom pulmonary embolism was suspected but excluded angiographically. Room air PO_2 can be normal in patients even with anatomically massive or submassive pulmonary embolus who have no previous cardiac or pulmonary disease [9]. In summary, arterial PO_2 cannot be used to exclude the diagnosis of pulmonary embolism. Measurement of arterial PO_2 remains useful in guiding the management of the oxygen requirement of patients with chronic CO_2 retention. (*Adapted from* Stein and coworkers [9]; with permission.)

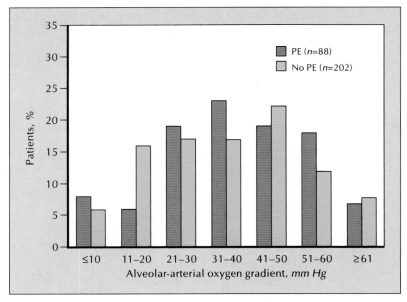

FIGURE 2-8. Distribution of the alveolar-arterial oxygen gradient among 88 patients with angiographically proven pulmonary embolus and no preexisting cardiac or pulmonary disease compared with 202 such patients in whom pulmonary embolus was suspected but excluded angiographically. Calculation of the alveolar-arterial oxygen gradient is shown in this study to be ineffective in excluding pulmonary embolism [9]. (*Adapted from Stein and coworkers [9]; with permission.*)

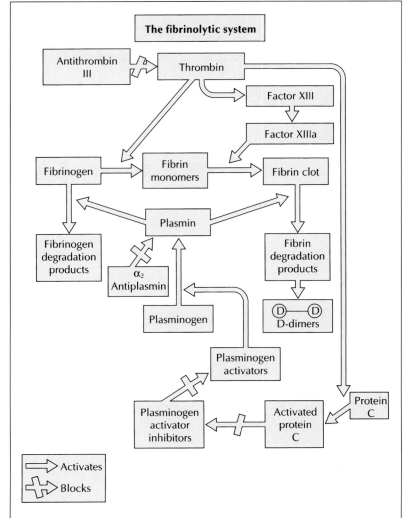

FIGURE 2-9. The fibrinolytic system. D-dimers are fibrin-specific degradation products of endogenous lysis of a fibrin clot. Elevated levels are not specific for pulmonary embolus since they are also found in disseminated intravascular coagulation, hemorrhage, surgery, cancer, and cirrhosis. However, a normal level of enzyme-linked immunosorbent assay (ELISA) quantitatively measured plasma D-dimer has a high negative predictive value in excluding pulmonary embolus. With an ELISA from STAGO (Asnieres-sur-seine, France), a plasma D-dimer ELISA level less than 500 ng/mL is associated with a greater than 90% likelihood of not having pulmonary embolism at angiography [10].

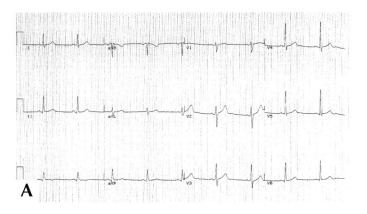

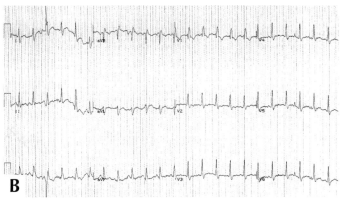

FIGURE 2-10. A, Normal preoperative electrocardiogram of a 49-year-old man. **B,** Electrocardiogram suggesting massive pulmonary embolus, which the patient suffered postoperatively. A sinus tachycardia is present with a heart rate of 139 bpm. The axis has shifted rightward. An incomplete right bundle branch block can be seen. Classic electrocardiographic findings described in pulmonary embolism are usually seen only after massive emboli, and represent the right heart strain imposed by the increased pulmonary vascular resistance. Findings may include right axis deviation, the $S_1Q_3T_3$ complex, right bundle branch block, and P pulmonale (peaked P waves) in the inferior leads [1]. Rhythm disturbances, most commonly premature ventricular contractions and less commonly new-onset atrial flutter or fibrillation, may also be observed.

RADIOGRAPHIC FINDINGS

FINDING	PATIENTS WITH PULMONARY EMBOLISM, n(%) (n=117)	PATIENTS WITHOUT PULMONARY EMBOLISM, n(%) (n=247)	P VALUE
Parenchymal consolidation or atelectasis	79(68)	119(48)	<0.001
Pleural effusion	56(48)	77(31)	<0.01
Subpleural consolidation	41(35)	53(21)	<0.01
Elevated hemidiaphragm	28(24)	46(19)	NS
Decreased pulmonary vascularity	25(21)	30(12)	<0.05
Enlarged central pulmonary artery	17(15)	28(11)	NS
Cardiomegaly	14(12)	27(11)	NS
Enlarged central artery and oligemia	8(7)	6(2)	NS
Pulmonary edema	5(4)	31(13)	<0.05

FIGURE 2-11. Specificity of chest radiographic findings in patients suspected of pulmonary embolism without previous cardiac or pulmonary disease. Only a minority of patients with pulmonary embolism have a completely normal chest radiograph, despite the contrary classical teaching. Among pulmonary embolism patients, effusions, lung consolidation, and atelectasis are quite common. (*Adapted from* Stein and coworkers [9]; with permission.)

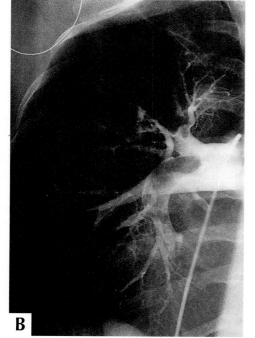

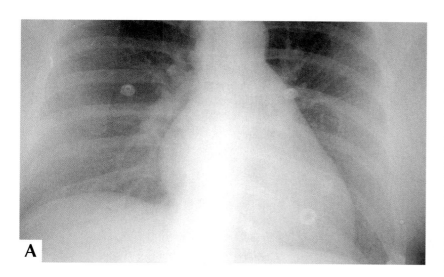

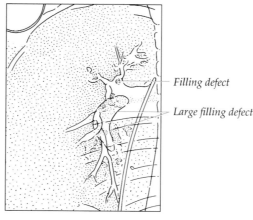

Filling defect

Large filling defect

FIGURE 2-12. Normal chest radiographs. **A,** In this patient who presented with severe shortness of breath and chest pain, the frontal chest radiograph was normal. The pulmonary angiogram demonstrated multiple thromboemboli. **B,** In the right posterior oblique view of the right pulmonary angiogram, a filling defect is present in the apical segmental artery of the right upper lobe, and a large filling defect can be seen in the interlobar pulmonary artery. The chest radiograph is usually the first imaging study obtained in the assessment of a patient with symptoms or signs of pulmonary embolism. Positive findings are nonspecific because the lung has a limited response to injury. Although more than half of the patients with pulmonary embolism have an abnormal chest radiograph, a near-normal chest radiograph in the setting of severe respiratory compromise is highly suggestive of massive pulmonary embolism. If clinically stable, patients should have upright posteroanterior and lateral chest radiographs with a 72-inch focus film distance and high kVp technique. Bedside radiography will result in suboptimal films. The supine position can make pleural effusions and pneumothoraces difficult to see. Chest radiographs used for comparison and interpretation of the lung scan should be obtained within 6 hours of scintigraphy because conditions can change rapidly in the unstable patient, and mucous plugs may cause only transient atelectasis.

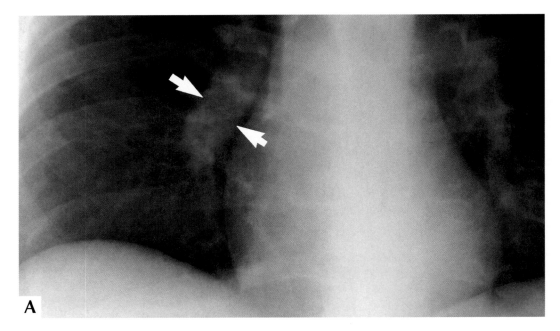

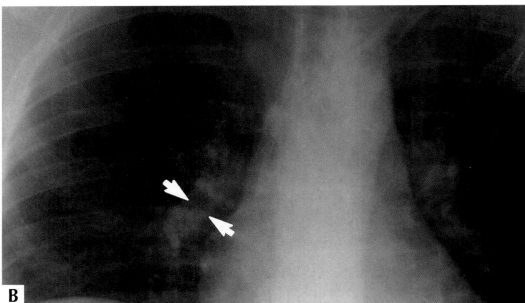

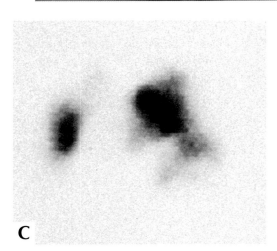

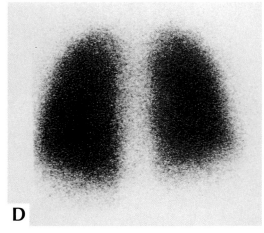

FIGURE 2-13. A 37-year-old man with anaplastic oligodendroglioma presented with dyspnea. **A,** Chest radiograph shows enlarged central pulmonary arteries (*arrows*). **B,** Film obtained 3 months previously shows normal size pulmonary arteries (*arrows*). Perfusion lung scannning shows multiple segmental areas of absent perfusion (**C**) with normal ventilation (**D**) and indicates a high probability for pulmonary embolism. Enlargement of a central pulmonary artery, especially with progressive enlargement on serial radiographs, is a cardinal sign of pulmonary embolism on plain chest radiography. The right pulmonary artery is best measured at its transition to the right interlobar pulmonary artery, at the level of the bronchus intermedius on the frontal chest film. When the artery measures more than 15 or 16 mm in diameter for women and men, respectively, it is considered enlarged [7]. The left pulmonary artery is difficult to measure on the frontal radiograph. On the lateral radiograph, the diameter should not exceed 18 mm measured posterior to the left upper lobe bronchus.

Central pulmonary arterial enlargement is usually caused by the physical presence of the thromboembolus rather than as a result of pulmonary hypertension. The dilatation will usually diminish within days, concurrent with lysis and fragmentation of the thromboembolus. When the vessel tapers rapidly after the enlarged portion, the finding may be referred to as the "knuckle sign." In the left pulmonary artery, this finding has also been referred to as the " seal sign" and, on the right, as the "sausage sign." Radiographic findings of cor pulmonale are not common in pulmonary embolism, and occur most frequently in patients with widespread peripheral emboli or massive central embolization. Manifestations include right ventricular enlargement, enlarged main pulmonary artery segment, and proximal dilatation of pulmonary arteries with rapid tapering. Right heart failure leads to central venous hypertension with distention of the azygos vein and superior vena cava. The central venous findings will be absent if a right-to-left shunt through a patent foramen ovale occurs following massive pulmonary embolism. (Courtesy of Kitt Shaffer, MD, Dana Farber Cancer Institute, Boston, MA.)

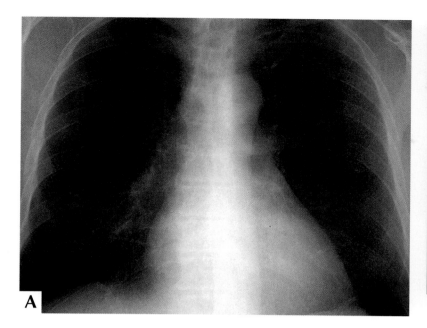

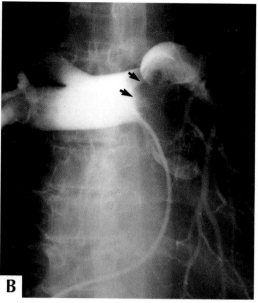

FIGURE 2-14. Local oligemia (Westermark's sign). **A**, Frontal chest radiograph shows a hyperlucent left lung compared with the right. The left pulmonary vessels are barely discernible.

B, Left pulmonary arteriogram reveals large intraluminal thromboembolus in the main and left pulmonary arteries (*arrows*) obstructing flow to both the left upper and lower lobe pulmonary arteries. Reduced blood volume in the pulmonary vessels in an embolized segment or lobe has been confirmed in animal experiments [7]. It may be caused by reduced flow distal to a large embolus from obstruction, vasospasm, or small vessel emboli. On chest radiography, the affected lung will appear relatively hyperlucent. Detection of oligemia on chest radiographs is difficult unless high-quality images, comparison films, and a high index of suspicion are present. There may be hyperinflation in the affected area as well, which can be highlighted with expiration films. This finding is not specific for pulmonary embolism, since a hyperlucent segment or lobe may also be seen in patients with emphysema, previous infections, or a hilar mass compressing the pulmonary artery.

Westermark [11] first described local oligemia from pulmonary embolus in 1938. Computed tomography of the chest may display this finding even more clearly than chest radiography, but is not necessary for confirmation. (Courtesy of Robert Pugatch, MD, Brigham and Women's Hospital, Boston, MA.)

PULMONARY PARENCHYMAL CHANGES

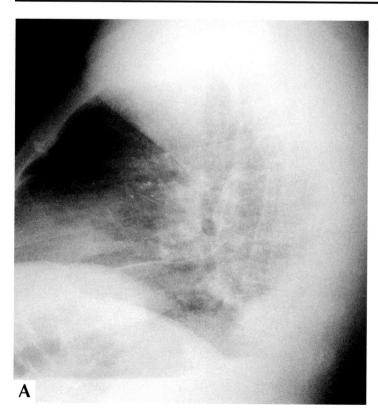

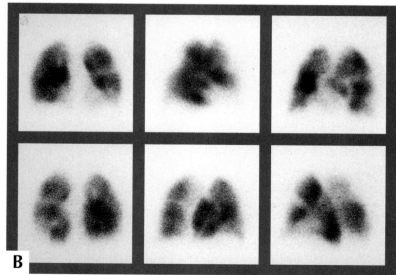

FIGURE 2-15. Consolidation (Hampton's hump). Lateral chest radiograph (**A**) reveals an approximately wedge-shaped homogeneous pulmonary opacity in the left posterior costophrenic sulcus. The base of the wedge rests on the adjacent pleural surface, and its apex is directed toward the hilum. Perfusion lung scan (**B**) reveals multiple segmental areas of reduced and absent perfusion, (*continued*)

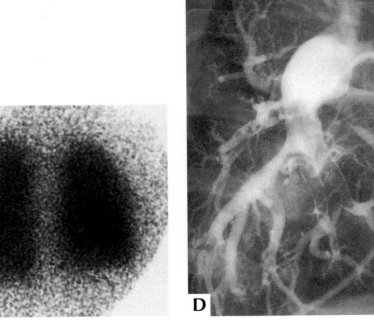

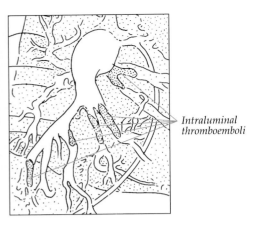

Intraluminal thromboemboli

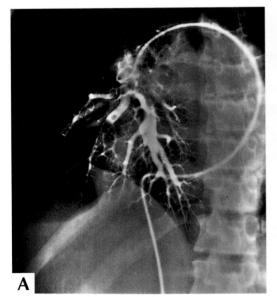

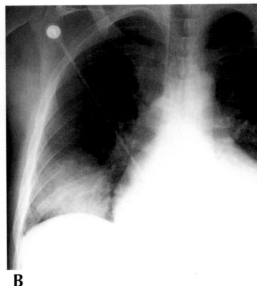

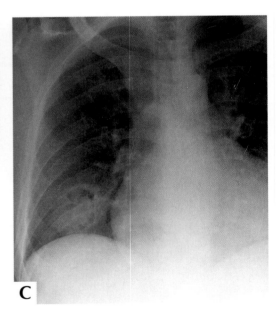

FIGURE 2-15. (*continued*) with normal ventilation (**C**). Angiogram (**D**) confirms multiple intraluminal thromboemboli in the lingular and all basilar lower lobe branches. Opacities in pulmonary embolism may represent either hemorrhage and edema alone, or superimposed infarction (tissue necrosis). Infarcts occur infrequently in pulmonary embolism, and have a predilection for the lower lobes, where there is greater blood flow in the upright patient. The radiographic appearance of infarcts was initially described by Hampton and Castleman in 1940 [6]. However, Heitzman *et al.* [12] have argued that infarcts have no predictable configuration because even though they may be subpleural, so are most pneumonias. Opacities may appear from 10 hours to several days after occlusion. If infarction occurs, it is usually confined to one or two segments. Rarely it can involve the whole lung. Air bronchograms are usually absent. Central emboli rarely result in infarction except in the presence of superimposed cardiac or pulmonary disease. In the normal lung, small emboli occluding small vessels typically cause infarction.

FIGURE 2-16. Infarction. **A**, Right interlobar pulmonary arteriogram shows multiple intraluminal filling defects in the basal segmental arteries of the right lower lobe, compatible with thromboemboli. **B**, Frontal chest radiograph demonstrates a rounded homogeneous opacity in the right lower lobe. On a single film, it is difficult to differentiate between infarct and hemorrhage. **C**, Follow-up chest radiograph reveals a decrease in the size of the right lower lobe opacity with sharp margins and no change in its shape.

Gas is present within the opacity as evidence of necrosis. Hemorrhage and edema in the lung secondary to pulmonary embolism usually resolve in 4 to 7 days, while infarction with necrosis may require 3 to 5 weeks to resolve [7]. Cavitation is indicative of necrosis, but is unusual in sterile pulmonary emboli. Pneumonias resolve by patchy clearing and seem to fade away. In contrast, the margins of an infarct will first become distinct, then will diminish gradually in size, without changing shape or homogeneity; Woesner *et al.* [13] coined the term "the melting sign" because the radiographic appearance of resolving pulmonary infarction reminded them of a melting ice cube. (Courtesy of Paul Stark, MD, Brigham and Women's Hospital, Boston, MA.)

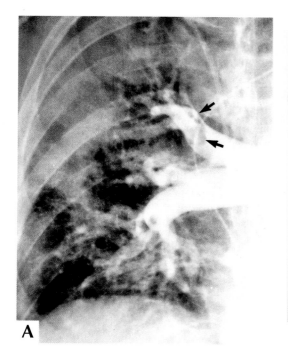
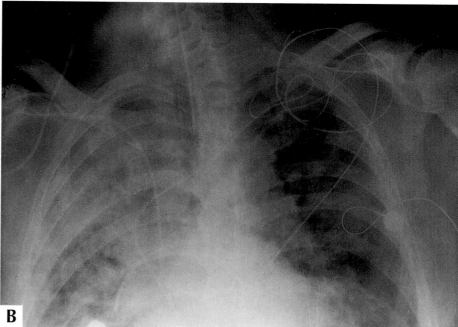

A

B

FIGURE 2-17. Pulmonary edema in pulmonary embolism. **A,** A right main pulmonary artery injection reveals emboli (*arrows*) in the upper lobe pulmonary artery and several basal segmental arteries. **B,** Frontal chest radiograph shows diffuse air space opacification, more severe on the right, in a patient with no preexisting cardiac or pulmonary disease. Diffuse pulmonary edema can develop after an episode of pulmonary embolism, although it is seen most frequently in patients with underlying cardiac disease. Neurogenic or humoral factors may account for pulmonary edema occurring bilaterally despite only unilateral emboli. Alternatively, pulmonary hypertension causing increased pulmonary capillary hydrostatic pressure can lead to pulmonary edema in the hyperperfused nonembolized lung (as in high altitude pulmonary edema). Unilateral pulmonary edema can be caused by massive contralateral pulmonary embolism. (Courtesy of Paul Stark, MD, Brigham and Women's Hospital, Boston, MA.)

VOLUME LOSS

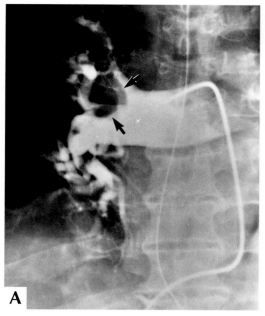
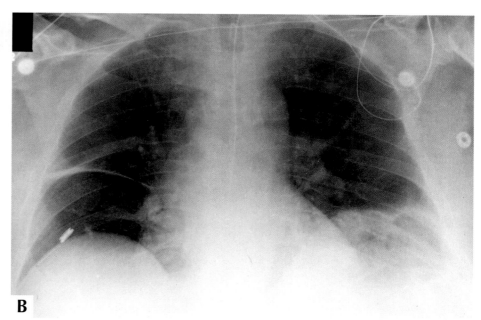

A

B

FIGURE 2-18. **A,** Right pulmonary arteriogram demonstrates a large intraluminal filling defect (*arrows*) straddling the right upper lobe and right intralobar pulmonary arteries. **B,** In this otherwise healthy patient, the lung volumes seen on chest radiography are low, as is manifested by elevation of both hemidiaphragms. Also present is a small amount of pleural fluid in the right minor fissure and the left costophrenic sulcus. The loss of lung volume in pulmonary embolism is caused by loss of surfactant or bronchoconstriction. Low lung volumes are manifested by elevation of the hemidiaphragm or downward displacement of the major fissures in both embolized and nonembolized lobes, thereby suggesting a humoral etiology. Low lung volumes are seen typically with infarction. (Courtesy of Paul Stark, MD, Brigham and Women's Hospital, Boston, MA.)

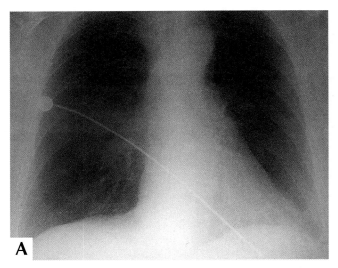

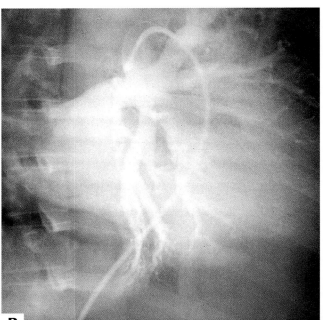

A

B

FIGURE 2-19. Atelectasis. **A,** In this patient with multiple pulmonary emboli demonstrated at angiography, chest radiography reveals horizontal linear opacities abutting the pleura in the left lower lobe. **B,** Another patient with multiple left pulmonary artery emboli (in the lingular and anteromedial basal segments) demonstrates angiographic evidence of atelectasis with crowding of the basal segmental pulmonary vessels, delayed but intense opacification of the atelectatic lung, and delayed venous return from the atelectatic segment. There is normal venous return from the uninvolved lung, while perfusion of the atelectatic lung remains in the arterial phase.

Platelike atelectasis (A) occurs mostly in the lung bases. Pathologic studies have shown that these linear opacities represent peripheral subpleural areas of atelectasis with invagination of the overlying pleura. They resolve or change rapidly. Other linear opacities that can be seen in pulmonary embolism include parenchymal scarring caused by previous pulmonary infarction. These opacities are oriented randomly and are permanent. Thrombosed arteries and veins with or without adjacent fibrosis may appear as linear opacities in the expected trajectory of vessels. They often point toward the left atrium and may not be obvious on the lateral projection [7]. Segmental or lobar atelectasis (B) may occur because of bronchospasm or loss of surfactant in the embolized lung. Visualization of atelectasis in nonembolized segments is probably due to vasoactive amines.

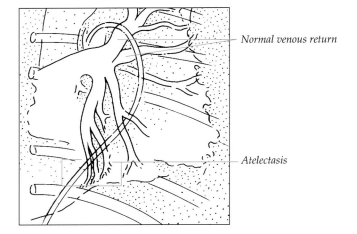

Normal venous return

Atelectasis

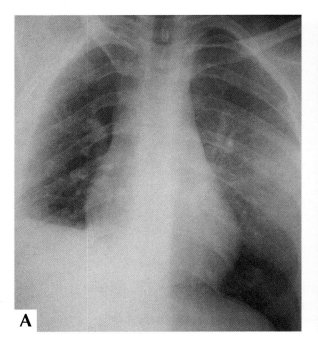

A

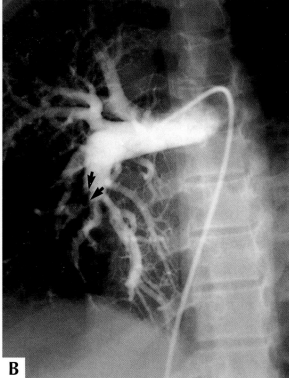

B

FIGURE 2-20. Compressive atelectasis. Right lateral decubitus chest radiograph (**A**) shows a free-layering right pleural effusion. Subsequent angiogram with selective injection of the right main pulmonary artery in the right posterior oblique position (**B**) shows thromboembolus in the basal segmental pulmonary arteries (*arrows*). Pleural effusions caused by pulmonary embolism are common. They are frequently unilateral and indicate that infarction is likely [7]. Effusions tend to be larger and more persistent when infarction has occurred, and reach maximal size within several days after embolization. Thoracentesis should be performed only if infection is strongly suspected because this procedure will preclude thrombolysis administration for up to 10 days.

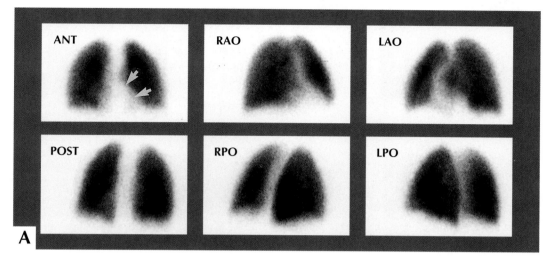

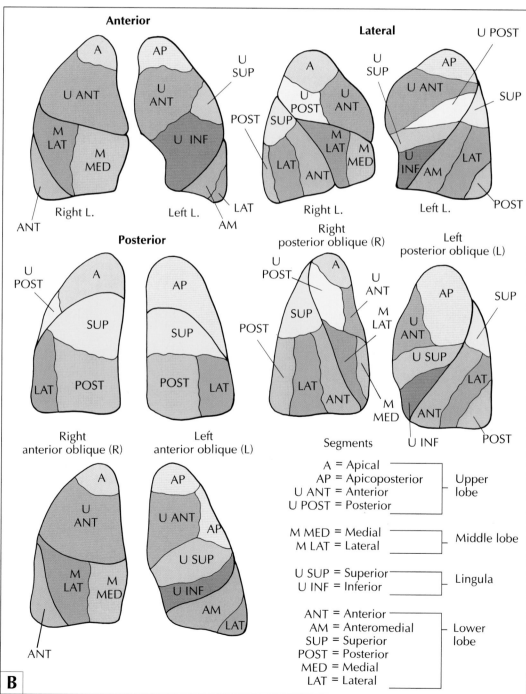

FIGURE 2-21. A, Six-view scan using the anterior and posterior oblique views in addition to anterior and posterior. Many centers use both lateral and oblique projections to complement the anterior and posterior views. The anterior view should correlate roughly with the chest radiograph. No perfusion is expected in the region of the cardiac silhouette (*arrows*). The aortic knob is often visualized as well. On the posterior view, the activity should taper toward the bases as the lungs become thinner in the posterior sulci. On lateral views (not shown), about one third of the activity comes from the contralateral lung (shine-through), so that areas of actual absent perfusion may be displayed as only decreased perfusion. On the left lateral and left anterior oblique views, the heart is evident as a large defect anteriorly. Most patients with pulmonary embolism have full segmental defects, although the wide normal variation in the size and shape of segments must be taken into account. Most patients with pulmonary embolism have multiple and bilateral emboli. More perfusion defects from emboli are seen in the lower lobes in comparison with the upper lobes, and more are seen in the right lung than the left lung.

B, The segmental lung anatomy is illustrated [14,15].

Segments

A = Apical		Upper lobe
AP = Apicoposterior		
U ANT = Anterior		
U POST = Posterior		
M MED = Medial		Middle lobe
M LAT = Lateral		
U SUP = Superior		Lingula
U INF = Inferior		
ANT = Anterior		Lower lobe
AM = Anteromedial		
SUP = Superior		
POST = Posterior		
MED = Medial		
LAT = Lateral		

VENTILATION AND PERFUSION SCANS

AGENT	AMOUNT	MECHANISM OF LOCALIZATION	RELATIVE CONTRAINDICATIONS	ELIMINATION	ADVANTAGES AND DISADVANTAGES
Perfusion					
Technetium 99m—labelled macroaggregated albumin (20–40 μm) 140 keV	200,000–500,000 particles, 2–4 mCi IV	0.1% Capillary blockade of perfused lung	Severe pulmonary hypertension, right-to-left shunts	Liver, spleen, half-time 2–9 h	—
Technetium 99m–labelled microspheres, 140 keV	100,000 particles IV	Capillary blockade of perfused lung	Severe pulmonary hypertension, right-to-left shunts	Liver, spleen, half-time 2–9 h	More uniform particle size, more expensive
Ventilation					
Xenon-133, insoluble and inert gas, 81 keV	8–15 mCi inhaled via closed system with oxygen	Ventilated lung segments	—	Exhalation, lung half-time 30 s	Interference from perfusion agent, no portable studies, needs trapping outlet
Technetium 99m aerosolized DTPA (0.25–2.0 μm), 140 keV	Single breath, 10–20 mCi	Particles deposited in ventilated segmental airways	Critically ill	Blood to kidneys, half-time 1.5 h	Washout phase not available, difficult in COPD, interference from perfusion agent

FIGURE 2-22. Agents for ventilation and perfusion scans [14]. Perfusion lung scintigraphy is a sensitive but nonspecific method for detecting pulmonary perfusion abnormalities. Small particulate aggregates of albumin or microspheres labelled with a gamma-emitting radionuclide are injected intravenously. The particles are trapped in the pulmonary capillary bed, reflecting pulmonary blood flow at the time of injection. Six to eight planar views of the chest are then obtained. Ventilation scans improve the specificity of the perfusion scan by indicating abnormal nonventilated lung, which could be an explanation for absent perfusion other than acute pulmonary embolism. COPD—chronic obstructive pulmonary disease.

INTERPRETATION OF VENTILATION-PERFUSION SCANS ACCORDING TO THE PIOPED CRITERIA

CATEGORY	FINDINGS
Normal	1. Normal perfusion 2. Perfusion outlines exactly the shape of the lungs as seen on the chest radiograph (hilar and aortic impressions may be seen; chest film or ventilation study may be abnormal)
Very low probability	1. One to three small (≤25% segment) perfusion defects; normal chest radiograph; ventilation irrelevant
Low probability	1. Nonsegmental perfusion defects (very small effusion, cardiomegaly, large aorta, hila, or mediastinum, and elevated hemidiaphragm) 2. Single moderate (>25% and <75% of a segment) perfusion defect; chest radiograph normal; ventilation irrelevant 3. Any perfusion defect substantially smaller than chest film defect; ventilation irrelevant 4. Large (>75% of a segment) or moderate segmental perfusion defects involving one to four segments of one lung or one to three segments of one lung region (upper, middle, or lower zone) with matching ventilation defects the same size or larger; chest film normal or abnormalities smaller than perfusion defects 5. More than three small perfusion defects; chest film normal
Intermediate probability	1. Abnormality that is not defined clearly by other criteria 2. Borderline high or low 3. Difficult to categorize as low or high
High probability	1. Two or more large (>75% of a segment) perfusion defects; ventilation and chest film normal 2. Two or more moderate perfusion defects and one large perfusion defect; ventilation and chest film normal 3. Four or more moderate perfusion defects; ventilation and chest film normal

FIGURE 2-23. The sensitivity and specificity of ventilation-perfusion lung scans for acute pulmonary thromboembolism were determined by the Prospective Investigation of Pulmonary Embolism Diagnosis (PIOPED) investigators [16] in a prospective trial of 931 patients undergoing scintigraphy. High-probability scans usually indicate acute pulmonary embolism, but of patients with acute pulmonary embolism, fewer than half have a high-probability scan. The diagnosis of pulmonary embolism is very unlikely in patients with normal and near-normal scans. Patients in whom there is strong clinical suspicion of pulmonary embolus but who have low- or intermediate-probability scans should undergo further diagnostic testing. (*Adapted from* the PIOPED Investigators [16]; with permission.)

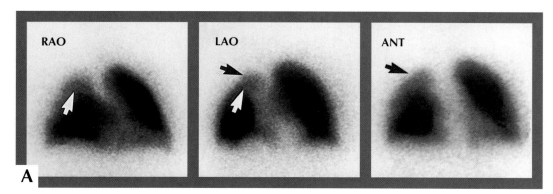

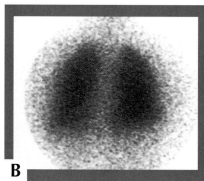

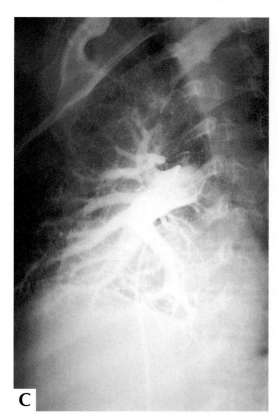

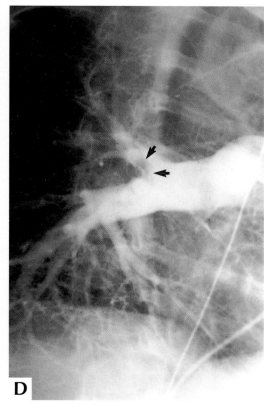

FIGURE 2-24. Three views of a low-probability perfusion lung scan. **A,** Decreased perfusion to the apical segment of the right upper lobe (*arrows*). **B,** The ventilation scan performed in the posterior position demonstrates no defects. Chest radiography was normal. Two views from the right pulmonary angiogram in right posterior oblique (**C**) and left posterior oblique (**D**) projections show a persistent intraluminal filling defect in the upper lobe pulmonary artery (*arrows in D*).

By the Prospective Investigation of Pulmonary Embolism Diagnosis (PIOPED) criteria [16], the scan depicted here is of low probability for pulmonary embolus. The positive predictive value of a low-probability lung scan for pulmonary embolus at angiography was 16% in the PIOPED study. When a low-probability scan was combined with a low clinical suspicion for embolus, the likelihood of pulmonary embolus at angiography was only 4%. However, nearly half the patients with the combination of low-probability lung scans and a high clinical suspicion of pulmonary embolism were found to have pulmonary embolism at angiography.

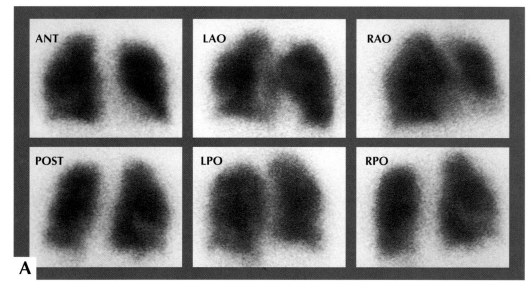

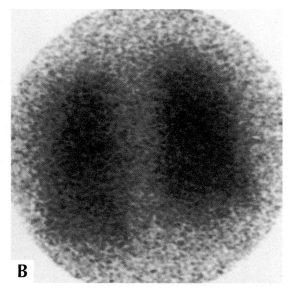

FIGURE 2-25. Intermediate-probability ventilation-perfusion lung scan. **A,** Six-view scan shows moderate-sized subsegmental defects in the left posterior and lateral basal segments and a moderate subsegmental defect in the right middle lobe. Perfusion is decreased in the right lower lobe lateral segment. **B,** Ventilation scan is normal as is the chest radiograph (not shown). (*continued*)

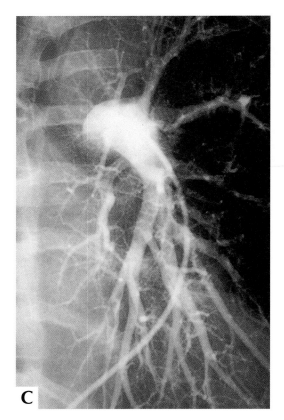

C

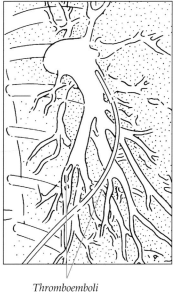

Thromboemboli

FIGURE 2-25. (*continued*) **C,** Left posterior oblique projection of the left pulmonary angiogram reveals thromboemboli in the left posterior and anteromedial basal segmental arteries. An intermediate-probability lung scan by PIOPED criteria [16] has about a one third likelihood of pulmonary embolus at angiography. Most patients with suspected pulmonary embolism who have intermediate-probability lung scans should be considered for angiography, especially if there is high clinical suspicion for pulmonary embolism, even though leg ultrasonography shows no evidence of deep vein thrombosis.

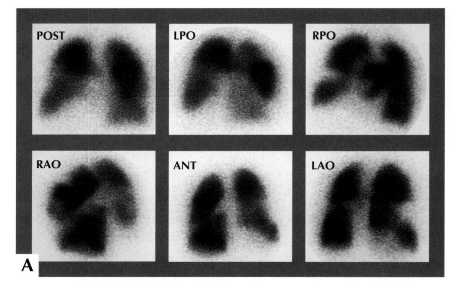

A

| POST | LPO | RPO |
| RAO | ANT | LAO |

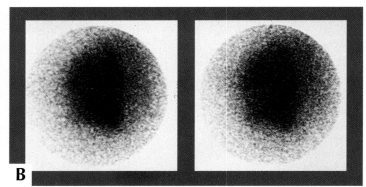

B

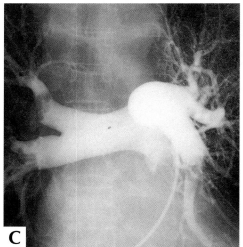

C

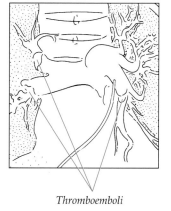

Thromboemboli

FIGURE 2-26. High-probability ventilation-perfusion lung scan. A clinical and diagnostic pearl is that high-probability lung scans are almost always abnormal bilaterally. Only extremely rarely is perfusion to one lung entirely normal in a patient with scintigraphic evidence of pulmonary embolism. **A,** Six-view scan shows absent perfusion in the right middle lobe and the superior segment of the left lower lobe. A moderate subsegmental defect is present in the apical-posterior segment of the left upper lobe. A nonsegmental defect is present in the right base. **B,** Ventilation scan obtained in the left posterior oblique projection was normal, as was the chest radiograph (not shown). **C,** Pulmonary angiogram with main pulmonary artery injection shows thromboemboli in the right upper lobe, right interlobar, and left interlobar pulmonary arteries. In the Prospective Investigation of Pulmonary Embolism Diagnosis (PIOPED) study [16], most patients with high-probability lung scans had angiographic evidence of pulmonary embolism (102 of 116 patients), yielding a positive predictive value of 88%. High-probability scans were shown to be 97% specific but, surprisingly, only 41% sensitive. Relying only on high-probability lung scans for diagnosis of pulmonary embolism would allow more than half (59%) of the pulmonary emboli to go unrecognized.

NONEMBOLIC CAUSES OF ABNORMALITIES OF LUNG PERFUSION

LUNG ABNORMALITIES

Emphysema
Inflammatory diseases
  Pneumonia
  Abscess
  Bronchiectasis
Pulmonary fibrosis
  Idiopathic
  Collagen vascular diseases
  Postradiotherapy
Bronchial obstruction
  (atelectasis or air-trapping)
  Infection
  Neoplasm
  Asthma
Reduced lung excursion
  Rib fractures
  Pleural effusions
  Pneumothorax
  Elevated hemidiaphragm
Surgery

PULMONARY VESSEL ABNORMALITIES

Congenital hypoplasia, absence
  of the pulmonary arteries
Peripheral pulmonary artery stenosis
Extrinsic vessel compression
  Neoplastic, primary, or metastatic
  Inflammatory
  Fibrosing mediastinitis
Intrinsic vessel abnormality
  Primary tumor
  Arteritis
Postcapillary venous hypertension
  Left ventricular failure
  Mitral valve disease
  Pulmonary veno-occlusive disease
Surgery

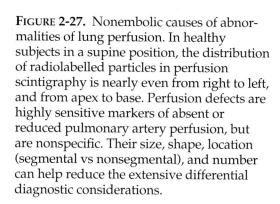

FIGURE 2-27. Nonembolic causes of abnormalities of lung perfusion. In healthy subjects in a supine position, the distribution of radiolabelled particles in perfusion scintigraphy is nearly even from right to left, and from apex to base. Perfusion defects are highly sensitive markers of absent or reduced pulmonary artery perfusion, but are nonspecific. Their size, shape, location (segmental vs nonsegmental), and number can help reduce the extensive differential diagnostic considerations.

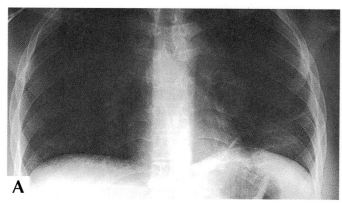

A

FIGURE 2-28. The combination of deep venous thrombosis of the leg plus pleuritic chest pain does not necessarily establish the diagnosis of acute pulmonary embolism. This 25-year-old black woman was 2 weeks postpartum and presented with left leg swelling and bilateral lower chest pleuritic pain. **A,** Chest radiograph shows an ill-defined opacity in the left lower lobe, and a hilar mass, suggesting lymph node enlargement. **B,** Left leg contrast venogram shows a central filling defect within the left popliteal vein, which is outlined by injected contrast along both edges. This is diagnostic of acute deep venous thrombosis. **C,** Pulmonary angiogram shows narrowing of the major branches of the pulmonary arteries, especially to the left lower lobe (*arrows*). (*continued*)

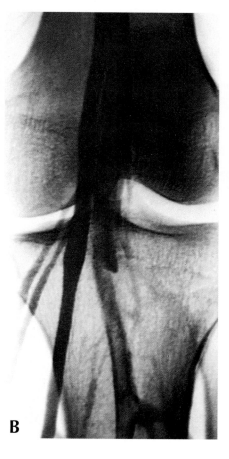

B

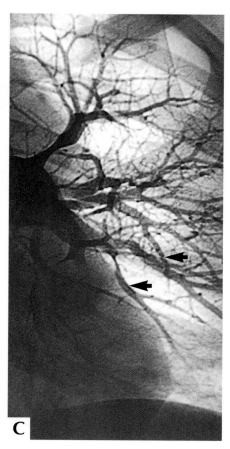

C

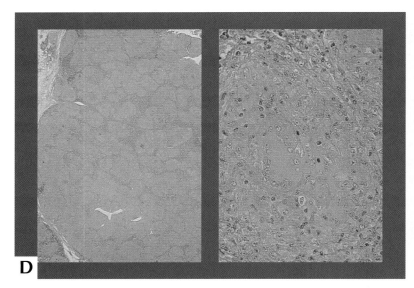

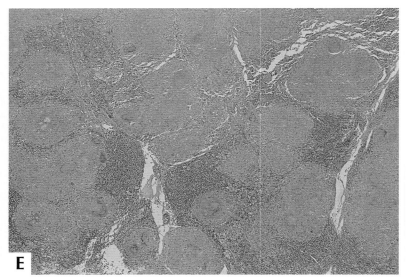

FIGURE 2-28. (continued) There is no evidence of pulmonary embolism. **D,** Low-power view of lymph node biopsy shows complete effacement of the nodal architecture by multiple non-necrotizing epithelioid granulomas (*left panel*). High-power view of biopsy shows a close-up of one of the granulomas with epithelioid cells and a multinucleated giant cell (in the middle of the *right panel*). These findings are consistent with sarcoid in the absence of infec-

tious etiologies. **E,** Medium-power lymph node biopsy emphasizes the presence of lymphoid infiltrate with small round lymphoid cells (*blue areas*) surrounding the epithelioid granulomas. (Part C courtesy of B. Bentley Faitelson, MD, Brigham and Women's Hospital, Boston, MA; parts D and E courtesy of Ramon Blanco, MD; Brigham and Women's Hospital.)

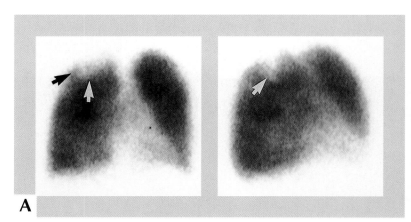

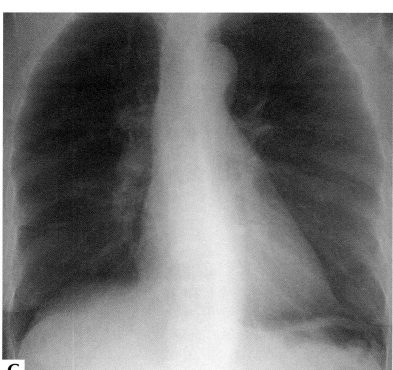

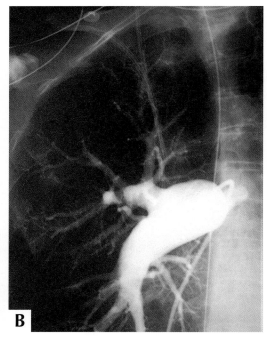

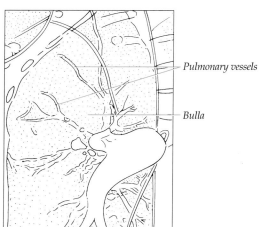

Pulmonary vessels

Bulla

FIGURE 2-29. Pulmonary disease and perfusion defects in emphysema. **A,** Anterior and right anterior oblique views from a six-view perfusion scan show a segmental defect in the apical portion of the right upper lobe (*arrows*). **B,** Corresponding angiogram reveals a bulla in the right upper lobe corresponding to the perfusion defect. Pulmonary vessels appear draped around the bullae. No evidence of pulmonary embolism was seen. **C,** In another patient, a frontal chest radiograph reveals diminished vascularity in both lungs. (*continued*)

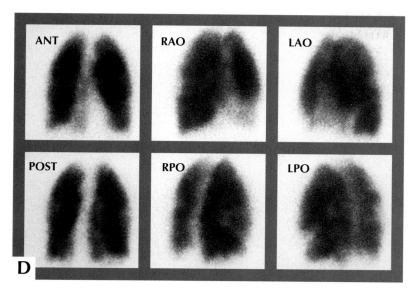

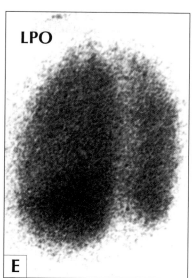

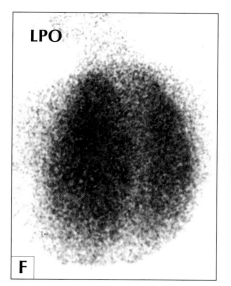

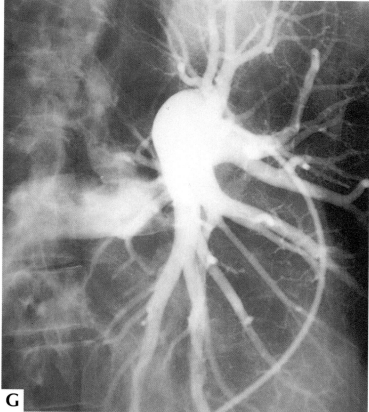

FIGURE 2-29. (*continued*)
D, Pulmonary perfusion scan has diffuse heterogeneous perfusion with several small subsegmental defects. On the ventilation scan, the steady state (**E**) and last washout image at 2 minutes (**F**) show diffuse air-trapping. **G,** A left pulmonary angiogram in the left posterior oblique projection was performed because of high clinical suspicion of pulmonary embolism, but demonstrates no evidence of pulmonary embolism.

In chronic bronchitis and emphysema, perfusion scans often demonstrate patchy, uneven tracer activity. Multiple nonsegmental perfusion defects may be present due to bullae or an unventilated lung distal to a mucous plug [14]. Ventilation scans are the key to interpretation of abnormalities seen at perfusion scanning in primary pulmonary disease. The initial breath images reflect regional ventilation rates if a maximum inspiratory effort is obtained. Equilibrium images display the aerated volume of lung. Washout images can only be obtained with the inert gases, and, normally, activity should be cleared within 2 to 3 minutes. The washout phase is most sensitive for air-trapping [14].

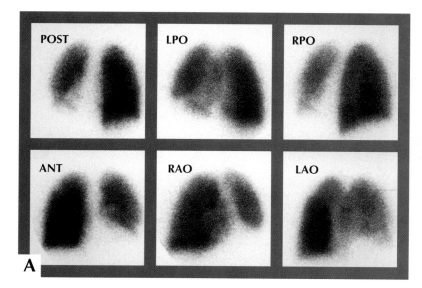

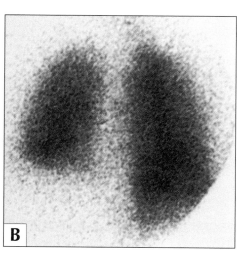

FIGURE 2-30. Pleural effusion and perfusion defects. Six-view perfusion (**A**) and posterior view ventilation (**B**) scans display matched, nonsegmental left lower lobe defects. (*continued*)

DIAGNOSIS OF ACUTE PULMONARY EMBOLISM
2.19

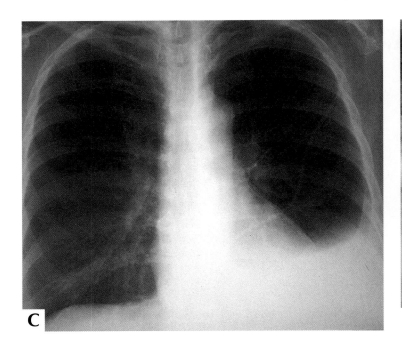

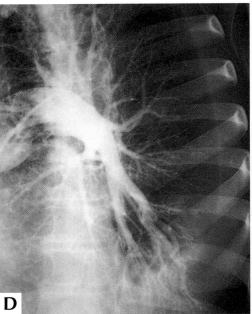

FIGURE 2-30. (*continued*) A chest radiograph (**C**) confirms the presence of a left pleural effusion. Because of high clinical suspicion, pulmonary angiography was performed. A single film in right posterior oblique projection (**D**) after left main pulmonary artery injection confirms the pleural effusion with the patient supine. No evidence of pulmonary embolism was seen on either side.

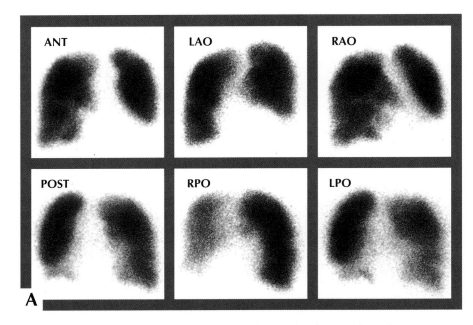

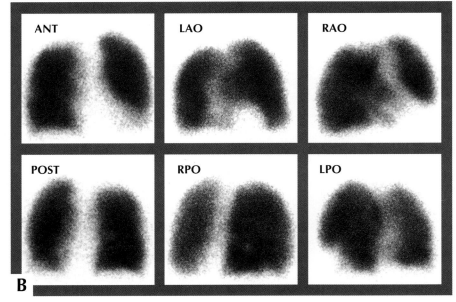

FIGURE 2-31. Left ventricular failure and perfusion defects. **A,** Six-view perfusion scan is of low probability for pulmonary embolus with heterogeneous perfusion in both lungs. Because of high clinical suspicion, pulmonary artery catheterization and angiography were performed; the pulmonary capillary wedge pressure was 28 mm Hg. No pulmonary embolus was seen. **B,** A repeat perfusion scan after treatment of left ventricular failure shows more uniform perfusion, with a persistent nonsegmental defect in the right base due to pleural effusion. Scintigraphic findings in congestive heart failure include an enlarged cardiac silhouette, thickened fissures, basilar defects due to pleural effusion, and redistribution of blood flow to the upper lobes. Interstitial edema may produce irregular perfusion, and air space edema will result in focal nonsegmental defects [14].

ECHOCARDIOGRAPHIC FINDINGS IN ACUTE PULMONARY EMBOLISM

<u>DIRECT</u>

Thromboemboli in right heart or pulmonary arteries

<u>INDIRECT</u>

Right ventricular dilatation

Right ventricular hypokinesis

Abnormal intraventricular septal position and paradoxic
  systolic motion

Reduced left ventricular size

Increased right:left ventricular diameter ratio

Pulmonary artery dilatation

Unusual degree of tricuspid or pulmonic valve regurgitation

Increased flow velocity within tricuspid and pulmonic valve
  insufficiency jets

Decreased mitral valve opening on M-mode echocardiography

FIGURE 2-32. Echocardiography with Doppler imaging can occasionally visualize directly acute pulmonary thromboemboli in the right heart chambers or pulmonary arteries. More often, assessment of right ventricular size and function and estimation of pulmonary arterial pressures reveal abnormalities consistent with acute pulmonary hypertension. In the proper clinical context, these findings reflect the hemodynamic consequences of pulmonary embolism. Echocardiography allows a noninvasive assessment and a means for following responses to therapeutic interventions in acute pulmonary embolism [17]. Importantly, echocardiography can help exclude life-threatening conditions that may mimic pulmonary embolism, such as dissection of the aorta, pericardial tamponade, or left ventricular infarction.

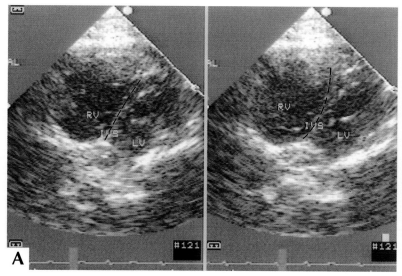

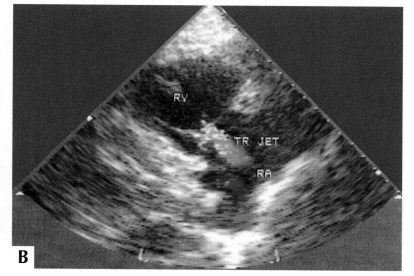

FIGURE 2-33. A 67-year-old woman with coronary artery disease presented with a 4-day history of dyspnea. On physical examination, her systolic blood pressure was 70 to 80 mm Hg. The chest radiograph was negative, and electrocardiographic findings suggested pulmonary embolism. Emergent portable transthoracic echocardiography was performed. **A,** Systolic (*left*) and diastolic (*right*) views of the heart in long axis. The right ventricle (RV) is moderately enlarged with decreased systolic function. Persistent septal flattening is present, compatible with RV pressure overload. Left ventricular (LV) function was intact, even though the LV volume was decreased because of the bowing of the intraventricular septum (IVS) into the LV (*dotted lines*). **B,** Doppler interrogation revealed tricuspid regurgitation (TR) with a peak jet velocity of 3 m/s compatible with a pulmonary artery systolic pressure of 45 to 50 mm Hg as calculated by a modified Bernoulli equation where pressure = $4 \times$ (peak velocity)^2 + right atrial (RA) pressure (**C**). (*continued*)

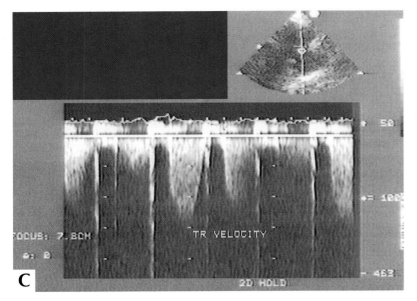

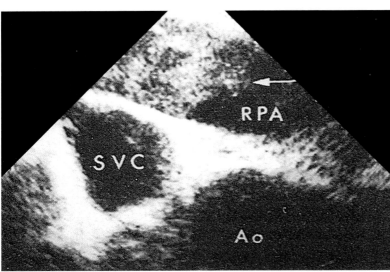

C

FIGURE 2-33. (*continued*) Following peripheral intravenous injection of 100 mg of recombinant tissue plasminogen activator as a continuous infusion over 2 hours, the patient's hemodynamic condition stabilized, and subsequent pulmonary scintigraphy and angiography revealed multiple bilateral pulmonary thromboemboli. Right heart catheterization demonstrated a mean RA pressure of 12 mm Hg, RV pressure of 32/15 mm Hg, and mean pulmonary artery pressure of 22 mm Hg. Transthoracic echocardiography is an excellent modality to assess the effects of pulmonary embolism on the right heart. Portable and noninvasive, it can be used in unstable patients too ill to transport to other locations for diagnostic imaging. Although direct visualization of thromboemboli in the RA, RV, or pulmonary arteries is unusual, indirect evidence of increased RV afterload is often observed. Underlying cardiopulmonary disease can alter the findings if there is preexisting RV hypertrophy, systolic dysfunction, or valvular abnormality. Response to either medical or surgical therapy in pulmonary embolism can also be assessed with serial echocardiography. (*Adapted from* Wolfe and coworkers [18]; with permission.)

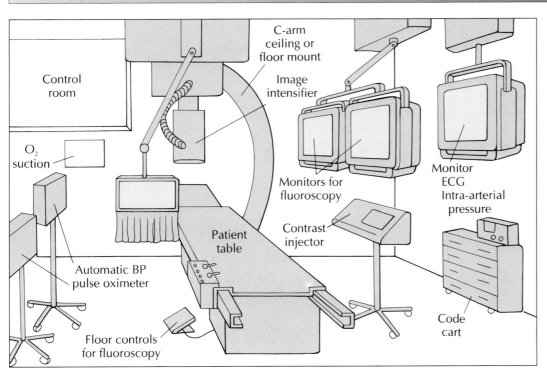

FIGURE 2-34. Large thromboembolus (*arrow*) in the right main pulmonary artery (RPA). Although transesophageal echocardiography requires esophageal intubation, it offers improved resolution and eliminates the problem of poor transthoracic imaging windows. Traumatic intubation of the esophagus may preclude thrombolytic therapy. Ao—ascending aorta; SVC—super vena cava. (*Adapted from* Gelernt and coworkers [19]; with permission.)

PULMONARY ANGIOGRAPHY

FIGURE 2-35. A contemporary angiography laboratory must be at least 60 m² and have a minimum ceiling height of 3 m. Most systems have a C-arm–mounted image intensifier and tube to facilitate movement. Patient tables should have ergonomically designed controls for patient positioning and digital fluoroscopy capability. Access to the patient in elective and emergent situations is another cardinal concern in design. The surrounding work area must include space for monitoring equipment such as the electrocardiograph, automated blood pressure recording, and pulse oximeter machines. A code cart with a defibrillator, emergency airway equipment, and medications should be labelled clearly and be within easy access. Space and equipment should be allocated for potential general anesthesia requirements. Transparent storage space for catheters, guidewires, and other angiographic necessities often consumes an entire wall of the room. Sufficient space for stretcher movement in and out of the suite is also essential.

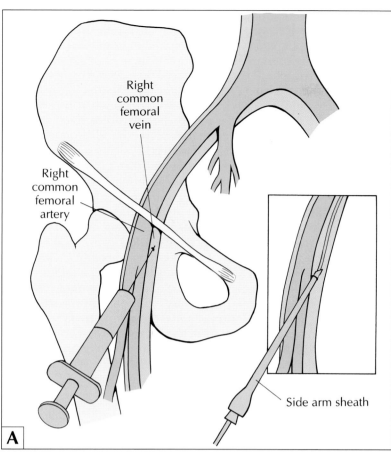

FIGURE 2-36. A, Vascular access for pulmonary angiography is usually gained via the right common femoral vein. After administering local anesthesia, a percutaneous Seldinger single-wall puncture technique over the femoral head is used to prevent inadvertent additional puncture of the adjacent femoral artery. (Alternative access sites include the left common femoral vein, the right internal jugular vein, or the superficial antecubital veins.) Once access has been obtained, a side arm sheath can be inserted for easy manipulation and exchange of catheters.

B, Catheters should be of a pigtail-type configuration as in the Grollman (right) or pigtail (left). Use of pigtail-type catheters prevents the rare complication of cardiac perforation, which can occur with end-hole catheters.

C, Pigtail catheter placement. The pigtail catheter is placed in the right atrium (1). A tip deflector guidewire is inserted into the catheter with the tip just proximal to the loop of the pigtail.

The guidewire is deflected using the external handle (**D**), so the catheter is directed toward the tricuspid valve (2). The guidewire is fixed and the catheter advanced into the right ventricle (3). Tip deflection is released, allowing the catheter to point toward the right ventricular outflow tract (4). Application of counterclockwise torque and simultaneous catheter advancement will take the catheter into the main pulmonary artery (5). Advancing the catheter further will usually direct it into the left main pulmonary artery. The tip deflector wire can be used to deflect the catheter into the right main pulmonary artery. Pressure measurements are obtained in each cardiac chamber and in the main pulmonary artery as the catheter is advanced. (*continued*)

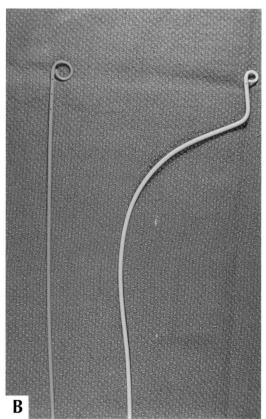

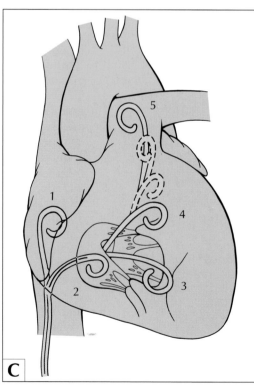

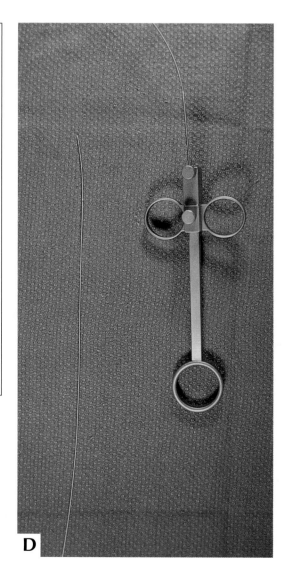

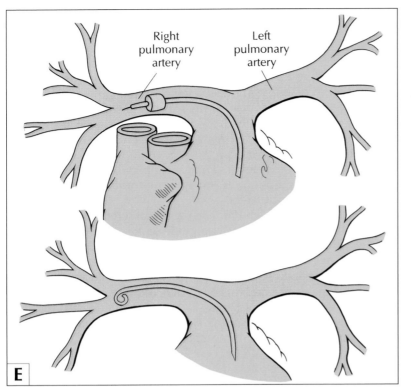

FIGURE 2-36. (*continued*) **E,** An alternative technique for pulmonary artery catheterization uses a double-lumen Swan-Ganz catheter, which is floated into position in the pulmonary artery after appropriate pressure measurements have been obtained in each cardiac chamber. It is then replaced by a pigtail catheter over a 0.035-inch exchange length guidewire. This method allows measurement of pulmonary capillary wedge pressure in patients with suspected left ventricular failure. For all catheterizations traversing the right heart in patients with left bundle branch block, ready access to a pacing catheter or external pacing device should be ensured because of the possibility of inducing third-degree heart block. Catheter positions should be checked with hand injections of contrast to ensure filling of the upper lobe arteries and to estimate flow rates. Contrast agent is then injected at 20 to 25 mL/s for a total of 40 to 50 mL in either the left or right main pulmonary arteries. Filming rates are usually 3 per second for 3 seconds, then 1 per second for 4 to 6 seconds. Flexibility with filming rates is increased with digital acquisition. The initial view obtained is either the posterior oblique of the lung of interest or the anteroposterior view. If pulmonary embolus is not seen, a second view is obtained. If no emboli are found on two views of the first lung injected (chosen from the lung perfusion scan as that most likely to contain embolus), then the contralateral pulmonary artery is catheterized and studied angiographically. (Part C *adapted from* Meyerovitz [20]; with permission.)

RADIOGRAPHIC CONTRAST AGENTS

PRODUCT	MOLECULE/ CATION	CHEMICAL STRUCTURE	TOTAL IODINE *mg/mL*	RELATIVE VISCOSITY 25°C/37°C	OSMOLALITY, *mOsm/kg H₂O*
Hexabrix	Ioxaglate/ meglumine and sodium	Ionic dimer	320	15.7/7.5	600
Optiray 320	Ioversol	Nonionic	320	9.9/5.8	702
Conray 325	Iothalamate/ sodium	Ionic	325	4.1/2.8	1797
Omnipaque 350	Iohexal	Nonionic	350	20.4/10.4	844
Hypaque-76	Diatrizoate/ meglumine and sodium	Ionic	370	13.3/8.3	2016
Renografin-76	Diatrizoate/ meglumine and sodium	Ionic	370	15.1/9.3	2188
Angiovist-370	Diatrizoate/ meglumine and sodium	Ionic	370	13.8/8.4	2076
MD-76	Diatrizoate/ meglumine and sodium	Ionic	370	14.7/9.0	2179
Isovue 370	Iopamidol	Nonionic	370	20.4/9.4	796

FIGURE 2-37. Intravascular contrast agents came into use shortly after the discovery of x-rays in 1895. Currently used agents were developed in the 1950s using a fully substituted benzene ring with three iodine atoms attached. Conventional high osmolality agents are made up of an anion (benzene component) and cation (sodium or methylglucamine). Low osmolality agents have two benzene rings linked with one cation, lowering the osmolality in solution. Nonionic contrast agents carry no charge and thus no counter-ion is needed, further reducing osmolality.

All intravascular contrast agents are hyperosmolar to blood (600–2188 mOsm/kg H_2O), are small molecules (with weights of approximately 800 D), and exhibit high viscosity. They are excreted nearly exclusively by glomerular filtration and have a half-life of about 1 hour. Clinical manifestations of the toxic effects of intravascular contrast are rarely serious, but minor transient effects are surprisingly common. Pain, discomfort, and heat sensation are the most common side effects and appear to have a threshold of osmolality above 400 to 500 mOsm/kg H_2O. Cardiac effects include decreased systemic arterial pressure, tachycardia, and dysrhythmias. Hematologic effects include aggregation and deformability of red blood cells, but the effects on fibrin polymerization are controversial.

Clinical reports of increased thrombogenicity of nonionic contrast agents are numerous, and although there is no direct evidence of a procoagulant effect, increased care must be taken with meticulous and frequent saline flushes after injection. Contrast-related nephrotoxicity occurs, especially in patients with preexisting renal dysfunction. Adequate hydration and restricting the volume of injected contrast material are the most effective ways to prevent renal toxicity.

The full range of anaphylactic reactions is possible with intravascular contrast agents. Corticosteroids are effective in preventing recurrent reactions and are usually administered orally 12 and again 2 hours prior to contrast injection. Toxicity of iodinated intravascular contrast agents is believed to be mostly related to hyperosmolality, and to a lesser degree to protein binding and lipophilicity. Chemical formulation differences are minor, although they may affect toxicity. Attempts to reduce toxicity have been directed primarily at lowering osmolality [21].

COMPLICATIONS OF PULMONARY ANGIOGRAPHY

COMPLICATION	OCCURRENCE RATE, %
Major complications	
Death	0.5
Respiratory distress: cardiopulmonary resuscitation or intubation	0.4
Renal failure: dialysis	0.3
Hematoma: two-unit transfusion	0.2
Minor complications	
Respiratory distress: prompt response to treatment	0.4
Renal dysfunction: response to drug and fluid therapy	0.9
Angina: coronary care unit monitoring	0.2
Hypotension: prompt response to drug and fluid therapy	0.2
Pulmonary congestion: prompt response to drugs	0.4
Urticaria, itching, or periorbital edema	1.4
Hematoma: no transfusion	0.8
Arrhythmia: spontaneous conversion or prompt response to drugs	0.5
Subintimal contrast stain	0.4
Narcotic overdose: treated with naloxone	0.09
Nausea and vomiting	0.09
Right bundle branch block	0.09
Nondiagnostic angiogram	3

FIGURE 2-38. Complications of pulmonary angiography. The listed complications occurred in 1111 patients [22] undergoing pulmonary angiography, with 14 major complications and 60 minor complications. Ionic, high osmolar contrast agents were used for all studies. Injection rates were 20 to 25 mL/s, with a total of 40 to 50 mL being injected over 2 seconds in the left and right pulmonary arteries. The morbidity and mortality of pulmonary angiography today are low, but the procedure remains invasive. The risk of complication is greatest in the most severely ill patients. Clinical judgment remains the best guide in patient selection.

PULMONARY ANGIOGRAPHIC FINDINGS IN THROMBOEMBOLISM

PRIMARY SIGNS

Filling defect

Persistent intraluminal radiolucency, central or marginal, without complete obstruction of blood flow

Proximal edge of an intraluminal radiolucency when there is complete obstruction of distal blood flow (convex meniscus)

SECONDARY SIGNS

Abrupt occlusion ("cut-off") of a pulmonary artery without visualization of an intraluminal filling defect

Perfusion defect (asymmetric filling)

Areas of oligemia or avascularity

Focal areas in which the arterial phase is prolonged (especially lower lobes); usually accompanied by slow filling and emptying of the pulmonary veins

FIGURE 2-39. Pulmonary angiography is the definitive test for acute pulmonary thromboembolism. The examination must be of high quality for accurate diagnosis. If areas are suspicious after two views have been obtained, balloon occlusion or superselective angiograms may clarify the area in question. (*Adapted from* Sagel and Greenspan [25]; with permission.)

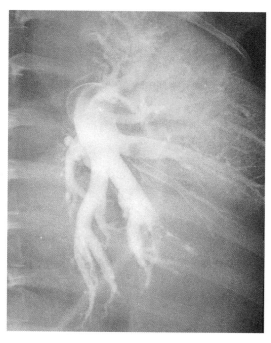

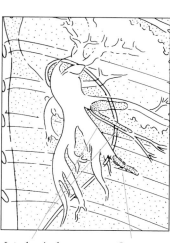

Intraluminal filling defect   *Convex lucent margin*

FIGURE 2-40. Left posterior oblique left main pulmonary arteriogram shows a long intraluminal filling defect in the contrast in the lingular segmental arteries of the left upper lobe. This finding is direct evidence of an embolus. Note the convex lucent margin at the proximal end of the embolus. If the embolus had obstructed flow completely, only this convex meniscus would still be visible, and would constitute a primary sign of embolus. Visualization of a meniscus indicates that the embolus is acute rather than chronic.

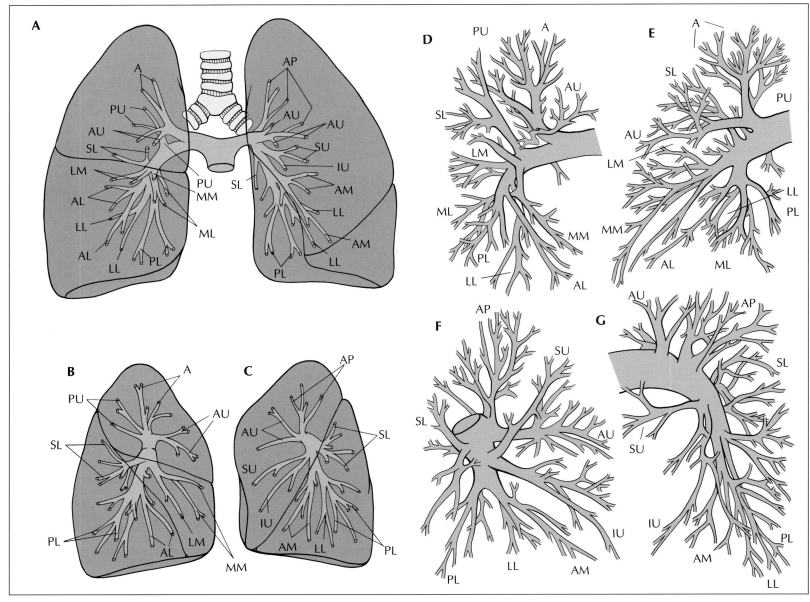

FIGURE 2-41. Pulmonary arterial anatomy. A, Frontal view.
B, Right lateral view (right lung). C, Left lateral view (left lung).
D, Right anterior oblique right lung. E, Left anterior oblique right
lung. F, Right anterior oblique left lung. G, Left anterior oblique
left lung. Segments: A—apical right upper lobe; AL—anterior
basal right lower lobe; AM—anteromedial basal right lower lobe;
AP—apical-posterior left upper lobe; AU—anterior upper lobe;

IU—inferior lingular lobe; LL—lateral basal lower lobe; LM—
lateral right middle lobe; ML—medial basal right lower lobe;
MM—medial right middle lobe; PL—posterior basal lower lobe;
PU—posterior right upper lobe; SL—superior lower lobe; SU—
superior lingular lobe. (Parts A–C *adapted from* Yamashita [23];
parts D–G *adapted from* Kandarpa [24]; with permission.)

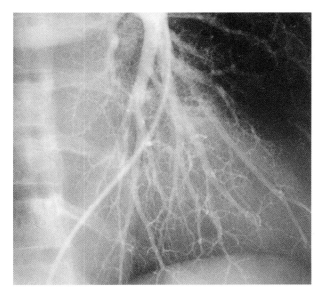

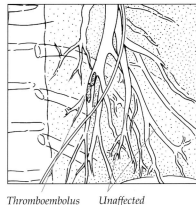

Thromboembolus *Unaffected
arteries*

FIGURE 2-42. In this example of oligemia, the
segmental arteries distal to a pulmonary embolus are smaller and more irregular than the
adjacent unaffected segmental pulmonary
arteries. The thromboembolus is in the posterior segmental branch of the left lobe pulmonary artery. Localized areas of decreased vascularity of the lung seen at angiography can indicate either pulmonary parenchymal or arterial
disease. Although focal oligemia does constitute a secondary sign of pulmonary embolus,
the finding is relatively nonspecific and is perhaps best used as a guide to help search for
intraluminal filling defects. In areas of focal
oligemia where the embolus cannot be seen,
subselective injections should be performed.

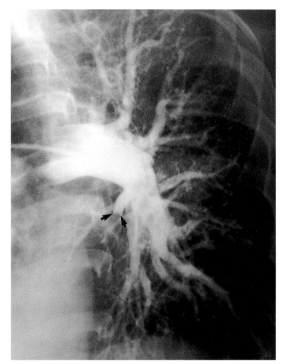

FIGURE 2-43. Right posterior oblique view of a left main pulmonary arteriogram reveals the inferior lingular segmental artery "cut off" (*arrows*). The embolus here is occlusive and, therefore, contrast cannot outline the entire embolus. Only the most proximal portion of the embolus is visualized. This is also considered a sign of pulmonary embolus.

OTHER IMAGING MODALITIES

COMPUTED TOMOGRAPHY

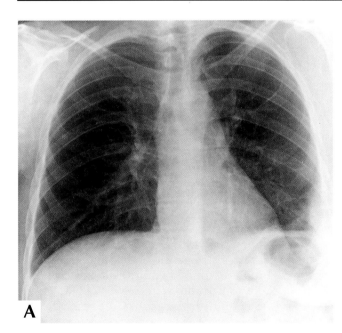

A

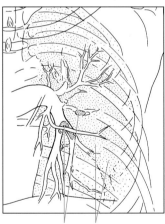

B

Thromboemboli   *Delayed opacification*

FIGURE 2-44. Pulmonary infarct. **A,** Frontal chest radiograph reveals a rounded area of homogeneous pulmonary opacity in the left lower lobe laterally and slight elevation of the left hemidiaphragm. **B,** Anteroposterior film from the left pulmonary arteriogram shows thromboemboli in the left anteromedial, lateral basal, and lingular pulmonary arteries. Note delayed opacification of the involved lung segments compared with the uninvolved upper lobe. (*continued*)

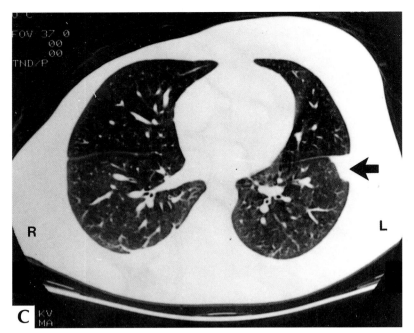

FIGURE 2-44. (*continued*) **C,** Computed tomographic (CT) image of the left lower lung confirms a homogeneous wedge-shaped opacity with its base abutting the pleura. No oligemia is evident. Chest CT provides high-contrast resolution and overlap-free cross-sectional images. A pulmonary artery branch can often be seen leading to triangular or wedge-shaped consolidation. Areas of infarction (*arrow*) and oligemia can be seen earlier and in greater numbers than on conventional chest radiographs. Good correlation exists between CT findings and perfusion defects seen at lung scintigraphy (unlike chest radiography), making it possible to use CT as effectively as scintigraphy in the diagnosis of pulmonary embolism. However, because of the greater cost of CT and the lack of ventilation data, it is not currently used as a primary imaging method in diagnosing pulmonary embolism. L—left; R—right. (Courtesy of Paul Stark, MD, Brigham and Women's Hospital, Boston, MA.)

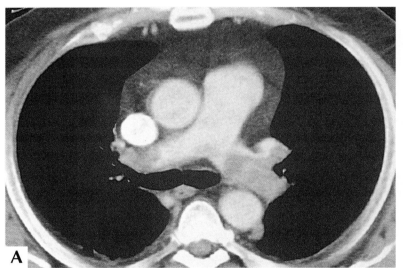

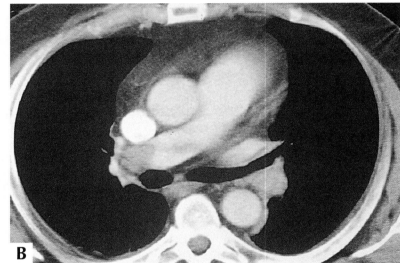

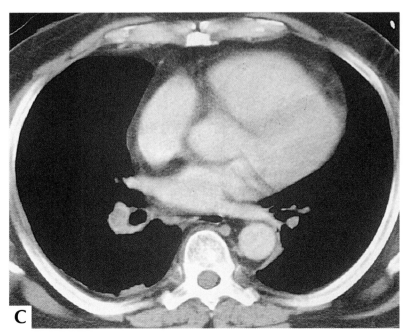

FIGURE 2-45. Dynamic contrast computed tomography (CT) displayed at mediastinal windows shows low attenuation thromboembolus in contrast-enhanced left (**A**) and right (**B**) pulmonary arteries. Thrombus is also evident in the right interlobar pulmonary artery (**C**).

Dynamic contrast-enhanced CT is an excellent modality to assess the central pulmonary vasculature. Cardiac motion does not degrade images substantially because of fast imaging times. Helical CT uses a new technique in which continuous scanning is performed while the patient is moved through the scanning plane. It allows for imaging of sections of the body during a single breath-hold (provided the patient can suspend respiration for 24 to 40 seconds), eliminating respiratory misregistration. The volume of contrast material can usually be reduced relative to conventional CT. With high injection rates (5 to 7 mL/s), the central pulmonary arteries can be displayed optimally. Electron-beam CT is another new CT modality that can perform axial scans in 100 ms, thereby eliminating the need for breath-holding. Potential exists to visualize the proximal segmental arteries using helical dynamic CT and electron-beam CT. Accuracy for pulmonary embolism using these methods appears to be high [26,27]. (Courtesy of James Fraser, MD, Victoria General Hospital, Halifax, Canada.)

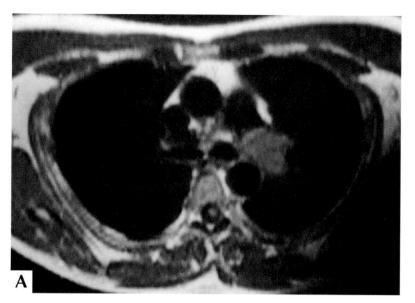

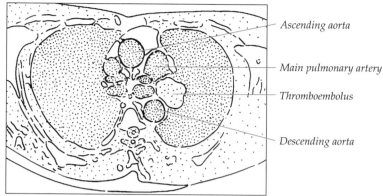

Ascending aorta

Main pulmonary artery

Thromboembolus

Descending aorta

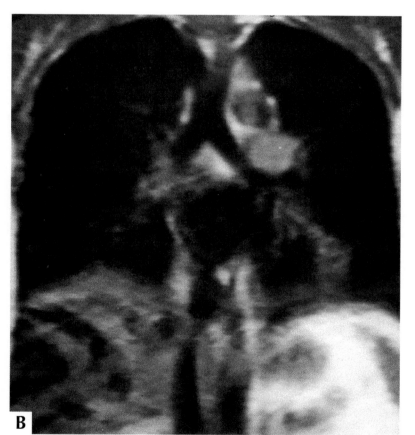

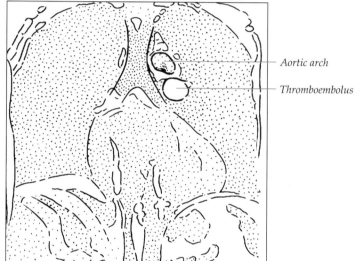

Aortic arch

Thromboembolus

FIGURE 2-46. A, Axial T_1-weighted spin-echo image of the thorax shows a large high-signal thromboembolus in the distal main and proximal left pulmonary arteries. Normally, flowing blood leaves a signal void as seen in the ascending aorta, descending aorta, and main pulmonary artery. Because slow flow or flow within the imaging plane can cause increased signal intensity in vessels, suspected thrombus in vessels should be confirmed by obtaining another pulse sequence or imaging plane. **B,** The coronal T_1-weighted image confirms the large left pulmonary artery thromboembolus expanding the artery to a size larger than the aortic arch directly above. (*continued*)

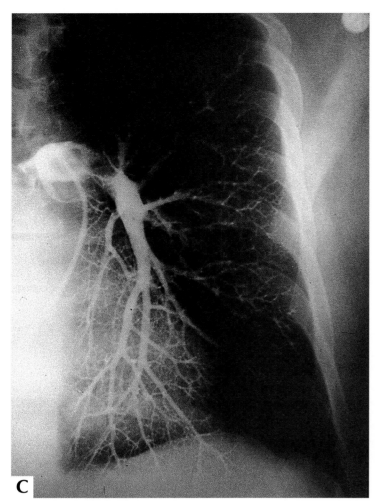

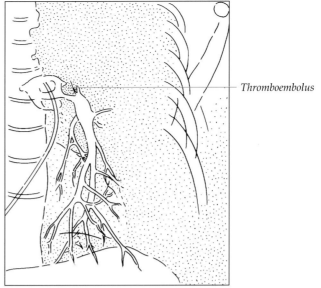

Thromboembolus

FIGURE 2-46. (*continued*) **C,** Angiography confirms the left pulmonary artery thromboembolus. Magnetic resonance (MR) imaging has potential to contribute to the diagnosis of pulmonary embolism. Although resolution has been limited by cardiac and respiratory motion, new pulse sequences and imaging techniques have allowed visualization of vessels less than 1 cm [28]. Disadvantages of MR imaging include its reduced availability compared with other imaging methods, expense, and difficulty monitoring unstable patients in the magnet. Potential advantages of MR imaging in the diagnosis of pulmonary embolism have not yet been fully explored. The intrinsic sensitivity of MR imaging to blood flow, its noninvasive nature, and the avoidance of contrast agents make it an extremely attractive imaging method. (Courtesy of E. Kent Yucel, MD, Boston University, Boston, MA.)

DIAGNOSIS

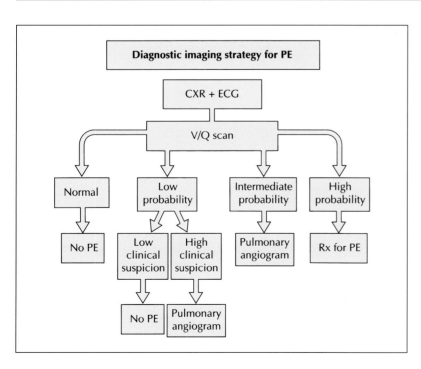

FIGURE 2-47. Diagnostic algorithm for pulmonary embolism (PE). In confirming the diagnosis of acute PE, a high degree of clinical suspicion must be maintained because it is more frequently underdiagnosed than overdiagnosed. CXR—chest x-ray; ECG—electrocardiogram; V/Q—ventilation-perfusion.

References

1. Goldhaber SZ, Braunwald E: Pulmonary embolism. In *Heart Disease*, 4th ed. Edited by Braunwald E. Philadelphia: WB Saunders; 1992:1558–1580.

2. Virchow R: *Gesammelte Abhandlungen*. Frankfurt: Verlag von Meidinger Sohn and Comp: 1856.

3. White PD: The acute cor pulmonale. Ann Intern Med 1935, 9:115–122.

4. Homans J: Thrombosis of deep veins of the lower leg, causing pulmonary embolism. *N Engl J Med* 1934, 211:993–997.

5. Rossle R: Uber die Bedeutung und die Entstehung der Wadenvenenthrombosen. *Virchows Arch* 1937, 300:180.

6. Hampton AO, Castleman B: Correlation of post-mortem chest tele-roentgenograms with autopsy findings: pulmonary embolism and infarction. *Am J Roentgenol* 1940, 43:305.

7. Fraser RG, Pare JAP, Pare PD, *et al.*: *Diagnosis of Diseases of the Chest*, 3rd ed. Philadelphia: WB Saunders; 1990.

8. Elliot CG: Pulmonary physiology during pulmonary embolism. *Chest* 1992, 101:163S–171S.

9. Stein PD, Terrin ML, Hales CA, *et al.*: Clinical, laboratory, roentgenographic, and electrocardiographic findings in patients with acute pulmonary embolism and no pre-existing cardiac or pulmonary disease. *Chest* 1991, 100:598–603.

10. Simons GR, Goldhaber SZ, Elliott CG, *et al.*: Quantitative plasma D-dimer levels among patients undergoing pulmonary angiography for suspected pulmonary embolism. *JAMA* 1993, 270:2819–2822.

11. Westermark N: On the roentgen diagnosis of lung embolism. *Acta Radiol* 1938, 19:357–372.

12. Heitzman ER, Markariam B, Dailey ET: Pulmonary thromboembolic disease: a lobular concept. *Radiology* 1972, 103:529–537.

13. Woesner ME, Sanders I, White GW: The melting sign in resolving transient pulmonary infarction. *AJR Am J Roentgenol* 1971, 111:782–790.

14. Mettler FA, Guiberteau MJ: *Essentials of Nuclear Medicine Imaging*, 3rd ed. Philadelphia: WB Saunders; 1991.

15. Fogelman I, Maisey M: *An Atlas of Clinical Nuclear Medicine*. St. Louis: Mosby; 1988.

16. The PIOPED Investigators: Value of the ventilation/perfusion scan in acute pulmonary embolism. *JAMA* 1990, 263:2753–2759.

17. Come PC: Echocardiographic evaluation of pulmonary embolism and its response to therapeutic interventions. *Chest* 1992, 101:151S–162S.

18. Wolfe MW, Skibo LK, Goldhaber SZ: Pulmonary embolic disease: diagnosis, pathophysiologic aspects, and treatment with thrombolytic therapy. *Curr Prob Cardiol* 1993, 18:585–636.

19. Gelernt MD, Mogtader A, Hahn RT: Transesophageal echocardiography to diagnose and demonstrate resolution of an acute massive pulmonary embolus. *Chest* 1992, 102:297–299.

20. Meyerovitz MF: How to maximize the safety of coronary and pulmonary angiography in patients receiving thrombolytic therapy. *Chest* 1990, 94:134S.

21. Bettmann MA: Contrast agents. In *Peripheral Vascular Imaging and Intervention*. Edited by Kim D, Orron DE. St. Louis: Mosby; 1992:75–82.

22. Stein PD, Athanasoulis C, Alavi A, *et al.*: Complications and validity of pulmonary angiography in acute pulmonary embolism. *Circulation* 1992, 85:462–468.

23. Yamashita H: *Roentgenologic Anatomy of the Lung*. Tokyo: Igaku-Shoin; 1978.

24. Kandarpa K, ed: *Handbook of Cardiovascular and Interventional Radiologic Procedures*, 1st ed. Boston: Little & Brown; 1989:222–225.

25. Sagel SS, Greenspan RH: Nonuniform pulmonary arterial perfusion. *Radiology* 1970, 99:541–548.

26. Remy-Jardin M, Remy J, Wattinne L, *et al.*: Central pulmonary thromboembolism: diagnosis with spiral volumetric CT with the single-breath-hold technique. Comparison with pulmonary angiography. *Radiology* 1992; 185:381–387.

27. Teigen CL, Maus TP, Sheedy II PF, *et al.*: Pulmonary embolism: diagnosis with electron beam CT. *Radiology* 1993, 188:839–845.

28. Schiebler ML, Holland GA, Hatabu H, *et al.*: Suspected pulmonary embolism: prospective evaluation with pulmonary MR angiography. *Radiology* 1993, 189:125–131.

TREATMENT OF ACUTE PULMONARY EMBOLISM

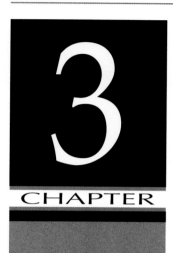

3

CHAPTER

Samuel Z. Goldhaber

During the past decade, there have been major advances in the understanding and treatment of pulmonary embolism. Recently, our ability to establish an accurate prognosis has been enhanced with echocardiography. We no longer rely exclusively on angiographic evaluation and invasive hemodynamic monitoring. Pulmonary emboli that occur in the setting of normal right ventricular function, as documented on echocardiogram, generally portend a favorable prognosis if treated with anticoagulation therapy alone. Patients can, however, appear to be hemodynamically stable, with normal systemic artery pressure, and yet have a pulmonary embolism that causes failure of the right ventricle. Often, such patients cannot be identified on physical examination; however, echocardiography can be very useful for risk stratification. Individuals with right ventricular hypokinesis appear to be at increased risk of recurrent pulmonary embolism, which may be fatal if treated with anticoagulation therapy alone. Such patients generally have more than 30% of the lung nonperfused on lung scanning. The guiding concept in treatment of pulmonary embolism is to manage patients more aggressively with contemporary interventional procedures if the prognosis appears to be poor with conservative measures. Thrombolysis and mechanical intervention can hasten recovery of the right ventricle.

Anticoagulation therapy remains the cornerstone of pulmonary embolism treatment. There is increased realization that inadequate doses of heparin must be avoided. Therefore, correct protocols for heparin use generally call for doses of at least 30,000 units during each 24-hour period. In the future, low molecular weight heparin, which can be injected subcutaneously, may permit outpatient treatment for a subset of low-risk patients with small pulmonary emboli.

Innovations in thrombolysis regimens are exciting, especially because they appear to reduce the risk of bleeding and increase the speed of clot dissolution compared with more traditional lytic regimens. Thrombolysis of pulmonary embolism has become more streamlined and economic than it was just a few years ago. Angiography is no longer mandatory if a lung scan or an echocardiogram (in the presence of hypotension) creates a high index of clinical suspicion. No coagulation blood tests are necessary during lytic infusion, which is given on a fixed-dose (*eg*, recombinant tissue-type plasminogen activator or streptokinase) or weight-adjusted (*eg*, urokinase) basis. There are important differences between thrombolytic therapy for pulmonary embolism and that for myocardial infarction. The most striking difference is that the time window for pulmonary embolism thrombolysis is at least 14 days after the most recent symptoms or signs have occurred.

The choice of mechanical interventions has expanded to include not only placement of a filter into the inferior vena cava but also embolectomy (transcatheter or surgical), clot fragmentation with a pulmonary artery catheter, and closure of a patent foramen ovale or other right-to-left shunt that may otherwise permit paradoxic embolization. For hypotensive patients, dobutamine is usually the most effective sympathomimetric agent. After recovery from the acute emergency, increasing emphasis is being placed on providing adequate emotional support for individuals who have been stricken with pulmonary embolism.

SYNDROMES OF PULMONARY EMBOLISM

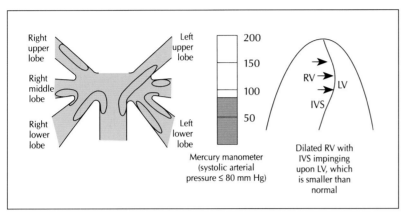

FIGURE 3-1. Massive pulmonary embolism. Patients with massive pulmonary embolism commonly have thrombosis evident in at least half of the pulmonary arterial vasculature. In this syndrome, clot is almost always present bilaterally. Patients most commonly present with breathlessness, and the most dramatic presentations are syncope or cyanosis; unremitting chest pain is only rarely part of this syndrome. The definitive clinical finding is persistent systemic artery hypotension despite a fluid challenge. Such patients ordinarily require pressor support while a definitive management strategy is being formulated. Treatment with thrombolytic agents is almost universally employed. If thrombolytic therapy fails or is contra-indicated, mechanical intervention either with surgical embolectomy or with catheter modalities, such as suction embolectomy or mechanical fragmentation of clot, is necessary. IVS—interventricular septum; LV—left ventricle; RV—right ventricle.

FIGURE 3-2. Moderate to large pulmonary emboli with associated right ventricular dysfunction. Pulmonary embolism most commonly presents as moderate in size. Right ventricular (RV) hypokinesis evident on echocardiography is evident in 50% of moderate size pulmonary embolisms, although such patients usually appear hemodynamically stable and have normal systemic artery pressure. Echocardiography may also reveal RV dilatation, moderate tricuspid regurgitation, and an interventricular septum (IVS) that is displaced toward the left ventricle (LV). As a result, the size of the LV cavity is reduced. A randomized controlled trial of thrombolytic therapy followed by heparin versus heparin alone indicated that patients with RV dysfunction appear to have fewer clinical adverse events (fatal or nonfatal recurrent pulmonary embolism) if treated with thrombolytic agents followed by heparin than do those treated with heparin alone [1]. Nearly all patients with right ventricular dysfunction have at least 30% of the lung appear nonperfused on perfusion lung scan [2].

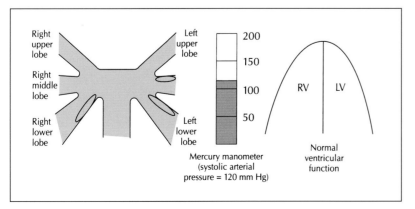

FIGURE 3-3. Small to moderate pulmonary emboli with normal right ventricular function. Individuals with this disorder have normal echocardiograms at baseline, although their clinical presentation may be identical to that of patients with right ventricular (RV) dysfunction and normal systemic artery pressure. If RV function is normal, anticoagulation therapy alone is associated with a good prognosis [1]. LV—left ventricle.

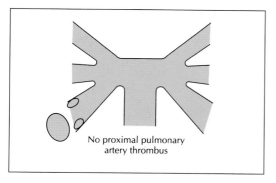

FIGURE 3-4. Pulmonary infarction. These patients often present with unremitting chest pain, which is occasionally accompanied by hemoptysis. The embolus often lodges in the peripheral pulmonary arterial tree, near the pleural lining and close to the diaphragm. Tissue infarction usually occurs 3 to 7 days after embolism. In this highly innervated peripheral location, exquisite pain is the paramount complaint. Physical examination often uncovers evidence of lung consolidation or a pleural rub. Despite the dramatic presentation and associated pain that is often unresponsive to narcotics, these patients rarely have life-threatening illness and can ordinarily be managed with anticoagulation therapy and nonsteroidal anti-inflammatory medication.

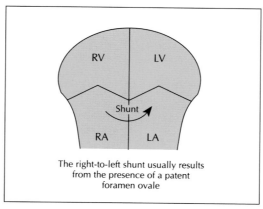

FIGURE 3-5. Paradoxic embolism. The most striking presentation of this type of embolism is a sudden and devastating stroke. Such patients usually suffer concomitant pulmonary embolism. Thrombi in this setting often embolize from leg veins to the right atrium and then gain access to the systemic arterial circulation through a patent foramen ovale, which is the most common cause of right-to-left shunting. The source of the stroke in patients with paradoxic embolism may often be occult isolated calf vein thrombosis [3]. LA—left atrium; RA—right atrium; RV—right ventricle.

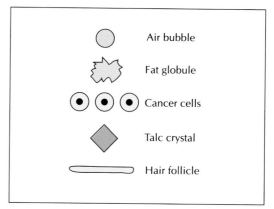

FIGURE 3-6. Nonthrombotic pulmonary embolism. Many types of pulmonary emboli can occur in addition to thrombus [4]. Air embolus from an improperly removed central venous catheter can be fatal, as can fat embolus in the setting of pelvic trauma or hip replacement and tumor embolus in patients with metastatic adenocarcinoma. Intravenous drug abusers tend to inject several substances that embolize to the lungs, including hair, talc, and cotton. These individuals are also susceptible to septic pulmonary embolism, which may be accompanied by endocarditis of the tricuspid or pulmonic valves.

PATHOPHYSIOLOGY

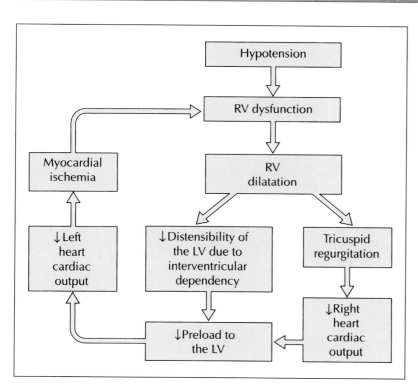

FIGURE 3-7. Pulmonary vascular obstruction leads to a spiraling cycle of heart failure in massive pulmonary embolism. Massive obstruction of the pulmonary artery causes systemic hypotension with ensuing right ventricular (RV) dysfunction. As the right ventricle dilates, the distensibility of the left ventricle (LV) decreases because of interventricular dependency. In turn, the left ventricular preload is decreased, which leads to diminished left ventricular output. As cardiac output falls, the coronary arteries are inadequately perfused and myocardial ischemia ensues. Reduced right coronary artery flow causes further right ventricular dysfunction, thereby renewing and worsening the cycle of heart failure.

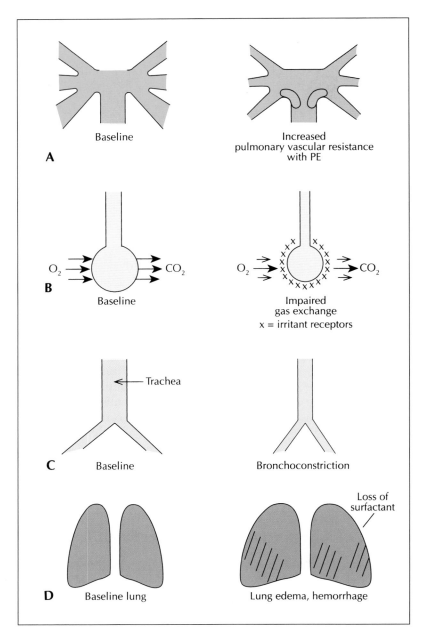

FIGURE 3-8. Pathophysiology of pulmonary embolism (PE). **A,** Increased pulmonary vascular resistance due to vascular obstruction, vasoconstriction by neurohumoral agents, vasoconstriction because of baroreceptors in the pulmonary arteries (which sense pressure exerted against the wall of the pulmonary artery by blood flowing past an obstructing blood clot), or increased pulmonary artery pressure. Baroreceptors may induce reflex pulmonary vasoconstriction. **B,** Impaired gas exchange due to irritant receptors, increased alveolar dead space (from vascular obstruction), hypoxemia (from alveolar hypoventilation), and right-to-left shunting; impaired carbon monoxide transfer due to loss of gas exchange surface also occurs. **C,** Increased airway resistance due to bronchoconstriction. **D,** Decreased pulmonary compliance due to lung edema and hemorrhage as well as loss of surfactant [5].

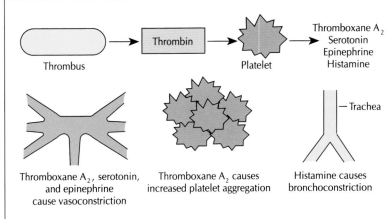

FIGURE 3-9. Neurohumoral pathophysiology. Thrombin contained in pulmonary emboli may cause platelet aggregation and degranulation, with subsequent release of such neurohumoral agents as thromboxane A_2, serotonin, epinephrine, and histamine. These vasoactive agents impair gas exchange, increase pulmonary vascular resistance, and increase airway resistance. Impairment of gas exchange occurs, in part, because neurohumoral substances cause a loss of surfactant, resulting in atelectasis, intrapulmonary shunting, and hypoxemia. (Local hypoxemia may also provoke regional pulmonary vasoconstriction.) Serotonin from platelets can cause direct constriction of pulmonary arteries. Thromboxane A_2 also causes increased platelet aggregation. Neurohumoral substances increase airway resistance by causing bronchoconstriction either directly (*eg*, serotonin) or via reflex mechanisms (*eg*, histamine stimulation of the vagus nerve which, in turn, may stimulate pulmonary bronchoconstrictive receptors in the airway or in the alveolar wall).

PULMONARY EMBOLISM TREATMENT OBJECTIVES

↓ Death rate (30,000–50,000/y in US)

↓ Recurrence of embolism during initial hospitalization (occurs in about 10% of patients)

↓ Time out of work

↓ Medical costs of therapy

↓ Pain and suffering

↓ Development of chronic pulmonary hypertension

FIGURE 3-10. Objectives of pulmonary embolism treatment. The goal of therapy is to reduce the frequency of all of these adverse outcomes.

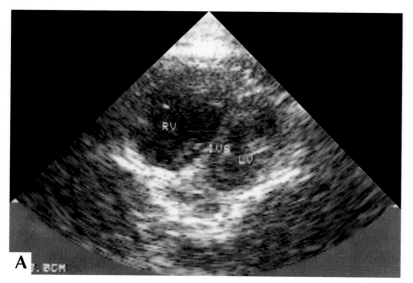

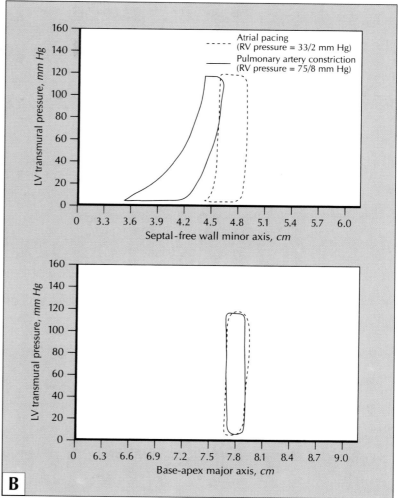

FIGURE 3-11. Ventricular interdependence and interaction. During massive pulmonary embolism, there are reciprocal changes in both dimensions and pressures between the right (RV) and left (LV) ventricles. **A,** Moderate RV enlargement, flattening of the interventricular septum, and diminished LV volume in a women aged 67 years with massive pulmonary embolism. RV systolic function was reduced, but LV systolic function was intact. An acute increase in RV afterload causes dilatation of the RV as well as marked reduction in LV preload, which results in a small LV chamber size (*see* Figs. 3-1 and 3-2). Volume expansion increases RV volume proportionately more than LV volume. Further elevation in RV preload will lead to additional deterioration of RV function and impairment of LV filling. Therefore, inotropic support with an agent, such as dobutamine, appears useful because RV systolic function is improved [6].

B, In an experimental canine model of acute right ventricular hypertension, induced by pulmonary artery constriction, both LV end-diastolic volume and stroke volume decreased [7]. Representative transmural pressure-dimension loops are shown for the LV septal–free-wall minor axis (*top*) and for the base-apex major axis (*bottom*). Data collected during pulmonary artery constriction appear as solid loops. The broken loops were constructed from data collected at a matched heart rate (140 beats/min) during atrial pacing. Most of the decrease in LV septal–free-wall dimension occurred during relaxation and early diastole rather than during ejection. The LV end-diastolic dimension and the systolic shortening in the base–apex major axis (*bottom*) did not change significantly. These findings suggest that during pulmonary embolism, impairment of LV systolic function and rearrangements in LV dynamic geometry are primarily the result of the anatomic contiguity of the RV and LV [7].

A ANTICOAGULANT

Heparin
  Unfractionated
  Low molecular weight
Warfarin
Dextran (use when heparin
  poses too great a risk
  of bleeding or
  thrombocytopenia)

B THROMBOLYTIC

Principles
  Administer through peripheral vein
    (not through a pulmonary artery catheter)
  Administer as a fixed or weight adjusted
    dose, without using laboratory
    parameters to adjust the dose
  Same contraindications as for acute
    myocardial infarction

Specific dosing recommendations (FDA
  approved)
rt-PA 100 mg/2 h (consider lower dose
  if weight <60 kg)
Urokinase 4400 U/kg as a loading dose
  followed by 4400 U/kg/h for 12–24 h
Streptokinase 250,000 U as a loading
  dose followed by 100,000 U/h for 24 h

C MECHANICAL

Inferior vena caval filter
Embolectomy
  Catheter suction
  Surgical
Fragmentation of clot
  Catheter
  Ultrasound (experimental)
Balloon angioplasty

D ADJUNCTIVE

Dobutamine (if hypotensive)
Oxygen
Mechanical ventilation (if persistently hypoxic)

Nonsteroidal anti-inflammatory agents (usually
  more effective for pain relief than narcotics)
Emotional support

FIGURE 3-12. Anticoagulant (**A**), thrombolytic (**B**), mechanical (**C**), and adjunctive (**D**) treatment modalities. A variety of pharmacologic and mechanical therapeutic modalities, often complementary, may be used to treat patients with acute pulmonary embolism.

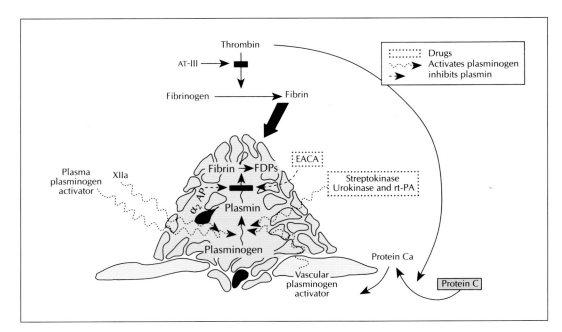

Figure 3-13. Anticoagulation versus thrombolysis. Heparin accelerates the action of antithrombin III (ATIII) about 1000-fold and prevents formation of additional fibrin clot [8]; however, heparin does not lyse existent thrombus. To dissolve existent thrombus, a thrombolytic agent must be used; such agents cause plasmin to lyse much of the thrombus. Thrombolytic therapy should, however, be considered adjunctive and must be followed by heparin anticoagulation therapy to prevent recurrent thrombosis. α_2 AP—α_2 antiplasmin; EACA—epsilon aminocaproic acid; FDPs—fibrin degradation products. (*Adapted from* Stead [8]; with permission.)

ANTICOAGULATION

EFFICACY OF HEPARIN IN PE TREATMENT

OUTCOME	HEPARIN (*n*=16)	NO HEPARIN (*n*=19)
Fatal PE	0	5
Nonfatal PE	0	5

Figure 3-14. Anticoagulation is the cornerstone of pulmonary embolism (PE) treatment. The only randomized trial of anticoagulation therapy versus no anticoagulation therapy in pulmonary embolism was published by Barritt and Jordan in 1960 [9]. Envelopes containing an equal number of cards marked *anticoagulant* or *no anticoagulant* were prepared. When a patient was enrolled, a card was drawn. Each individual selected for anticoagulation therapy received six doses of heparin of 10,000 units each every 6 hours, without laboratory control. Oral anticoagulation was started concomitantly with a target prothrombin time of two to three times the control value. After 35 patients were recruited, the results were reviewed. Of the 19 patients who did not receive anticoagulants, five died of recurrent PE. Another five had nonfatal recurrences of PE. Of the 16 patients who received anticoagulants, none died of PE, and none had recurrent PE. Therefore, the trial was discontinued.

UNFRACTIONATED HEPARIN DOSING RECOMMENDATIONS

Intravenous	5000–10,000 U as a bolus, followed immediately by: 20 U/kg/h or a fixed dose of 1250 U/h
Monitoring	Initial aPTT 4–6 h after bolus. Target aPTT 1.5–2.5 times upper limit of normal
Subcutaneous	500 U/kg/24 h subdivided into 2–3 (usually 3) injections
Monitoring	Obtain aPTT at the midpoint between injections (*eg*, 4 h after injection if receiving injections every 8 h) Target aPTT 1.5–2.5 times upper limit of normal

Figure 3-15. Guidelines for heparinization. Most patients with acute pulmonary embolism (PE) receive subtherapeutic doses of heparin during the first few critical days of hospitalization. This may be a result of poor understanding of heparin kinetics, overcautious behavior of physicians, or high heparin requirements [10]. Recurrent PE is associated with heparin doses that yield an activated partial thromboplastin time (aPTT) less than 1.5 times control values; however, bleeding induced by heparin is not closely associated with aPTT levels greater than 2.5 times control values [11]. Patients who suffer recurrent venous thrombosis tend to be individuals whose heparin requirements are high and who were not adequately heparinized when initially treated [12]. Furthermore, for patients who fail anticoagulation and have recurrent thrombosis, an alternative to placing an inferior vena caval filter is to administer a new course of high dose continuous infusion heparin in which a therapeutic aPTT is achieved rapidly. Thus, rapid and intensive anticoagulation appears to be even more important than previously realized. The illustration provides guidelines for intensive anticoagulation therapy with unfractionated heparin.

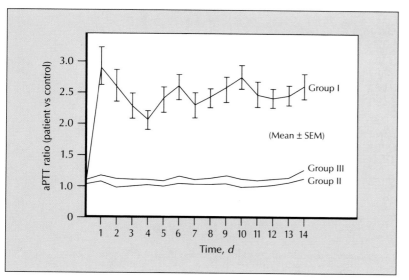

FIGURE 3-16. Low molecular weight heparin for pulmonary embolism treatment. Subcutaneous administration of low molecular weight heparin (LMWH) at a fixed dose offers several advantages over continuous intravenous infusion of unfractionated heparin adjusted according to the activated partial thromboplastin time (aPTT). Patients receiving LMWH might potentially: 1) be treated at home, 2) need less nursing time because no intravenous infusion equipment is required, and 3) need fewer laboratory tests because aPTTs are not used clinically with fixed-dose LMWH. In a randomized, controlled trial of 101 patients with sub-massive pulmonary embolism, unfractionated heparin administered by continuous intravenous infusion was compared with administration of two or three daily subcutaneous injections of Fraxiparine (Choay) at different concentrations. The Fraxiparine dose of 400 anti-Xa Institute Choay U/kg (Group II) was found to be as effective and safe as unfractionated heparin [13]. Among patients who received unfractionated heparin (Group I), aPTTs were two to three times control values during the 14 days of treatment; however, patients who received LMWH had virtually no elevation in aPTT. Group III patients received 600 anti-Xa Institute Choay U/kg. (*Adapted from* Théry and coworkers [13]; with permission.)

A. GUIDELINES FOR INITIATION OF WARFARIN

CLINICAL SCENARIO	SUGGESTED DOSE, mg
Age ≥80 y	2
Known liver disease or alcholism	2
Medical frailty or malnourishment	2
Amiodarone use	2
"The average patient"	5
Age ≤50y and weight 80–100 kg	7.5
Weight >100 kg	10

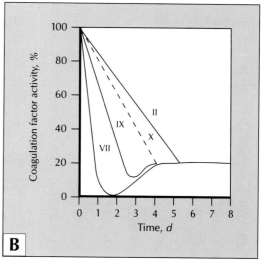

B

FIGURE 3-17. Guidelines for initiation of warfarin. **A,** In the presence of active thrombosis, patients should first receive heparin therapy. Therapeutic levels of heparin should be documented with at least one activated partial thromboplastin time (aPTT) greater than 1.5 times the upper limit of normal before warfarin is initiated. This strategy prevents exacerbation of occult protein C or S deficiency and consequent paradoxic worsening of the thrombotic state. Furthermore, the approach of "loading" patients with warfarin has fallen into disfavor, because high initial doses of warfarin are also likely to precipitate a deficiency of protein C or S. Although no clinical trials have been done to determine the optimum warfarin dosing regimen and duration for pulmonary embolism patients, my preference is intensive anticoagulation therapy with a target International Normalized Ratio of 3.0 to 4.0

with at least 1 year of therapy. I do not proscribe such foods as green, leafy vegetables but instead adjust the dose of warfarin to the patient's diet and other medications.

B, The effect of initiating warfarin therapy on the vitamin K–dependent clotting factors. The prothrombin time measures the vitamin K-dependent activated clotting factors II, VII, IX, and X. The half-life of factor VII is about 6 hours, whereas the half-life of factor II (also known as thrombin) is about 5 days. Therefore, a patient with an elevated prothrombin time within the first few days of receiving warfarin may not be therapeutically anticoagulated. The long half-life of the vitamin K–dependent clotting factors supports the rationale that heparin should be used for at least 5 days, even if the prothrombin time reaches therapeutic levels more quickly.

ADVERSE EFFECTS OF ANTICOAGULATION

DRUG	ADVERSE EFFECT	COMMENTS
Heparin	Bleeding	Search for underlying pathologic lesion (eg, colon cancer if gastrointestinal bleeding) if aPTT <3 times upper limit of normal
	Thrombocytopenia	Occurs commonly but usually without paradoxic thrombosis and usually not clinically relevant because platelet counts usually remain >50,000/mm^3
	↑Transaminase	Occurs commonly but is usually asymptomatic
	Reduced bone density	Evaluated after pregnancy in women requiring >1 m of heparin; diagnosed by bone densitometry; usually asymptomatic
	Hypersensitivity reactions	Rash, hives—may respond to diphenhydramine or topical steroids; rarely characterized by anaphylaxis in the setting of heparin-induced thrombocytopenia
	Skin necrosis	Extremely rare; may be associated with protein C or S deficiency
Warfarin	Bleeding	Investigation for underlying lesion is particularly worthwhile for gastrointestinal bleeding or hematuria, especially if the International Normalized Ratio is <3.0
	Alopecia	Occurs in at least 5% of patients in my practice whom I follow on long-term warfarin
	Skin necrosis	Extremely rare; may be associated with protein C or S deficiency
	Purple toes syndrome	May be from cholesterol embolization

FIGURE 3-18. Adverse effects of heparin and warfarin. Although bleeding is the most obvious side effect of anticoagulation, other adverse effects occur frequently. For example, transaminitis is common among heparin-treated patients [14]. Among patients receiving long-term administration of heparin, reduced bone density is a potentially important but usually asymptomatic side effect [15]. Warfarin-treated patients develop alopecia with surprisingly high frequency. It is reversible when the warfarin is discontinued. Less common is the "purple toes syndrome", which can occur in warfarin-treated patients and which may result from cholesterol embolization [16].

THROMBOLYSIS

CRITERIA FOR THROMBOLYSIS

PRINCIPAL INCLUSION CRITERIA

Massive pulmonary embolism

Anatomically small or moderate size pulmonary embolism with hemodynamic instability (eg, prior cardiopulmonary disease)

Hemodynamically stable, but right ventricular dysfunction detected on baseline echocardiogram

Normal echocardiogram and moderate size pulmonary embolism associated with massive pelvic or leg vein thrombosis

MAJOR EXCLUSION CRITERIA

Intracranial disease

Recent major trauma or surgery

Active bleeding, known bleeding diathesis, or unexplained anemia

Uncontrolled hypertension

FIGURE 3-19. Inclusion and exclusion criteria for thrombolysis. The greatest challenge of thrombolysis for pulmonary embolism is gaining a thorough familiarity of when it should be utilized and, conversely, when it should be withheld.

PROBLEMS WITH UTILIZATION OF THROMBOLYTIC THERAPY

Lack of familiarity with its use, including indications and contraindications

Inadequate response to bleeding complications

Short-term costs that exceed anticoagulation alone due to unnecessary ordering of ancillary tests

Not understanding the limitations of coagulation laboratory tests obtained in the setting of thrombolytic therapy

Forgetting that thrombolysis is an adjunctive therapy that does not prevent recurrent thrombosis

FIGURE 3-20. Problems with thrombolytic therapy. A massive educational campaign has helped train physicians in dealing with potential problems related to thrombolysis among patients evolving acute myocardial infarction. No such program exists for physicians who are contemplating the use of thrombolysis in patients with pulmonary embolism. Listed below are the problems that I have commonly encountered.

HOW TO TREAT BLEEDING COMPLICATIONS OR ALLERGY THAT RESULT FROM ANTICOAGULATION OR THROMBOLYSIS

A

MAJOR BLEEDING	SUGGESTED ACTION
Suspected intracranial bleeding	Discontinue anticoagulation and thrombolysis; obtain head CT scan; consult neurosurgeon
Gastrointestinal bleeding or gross hematuria	Discontinue anticoagulation and thrombolysis
If major bleeding continues despite discontinuation of therapy...	Order 10 U cryoprecipitate; thaw 2 U fresh-frozen plasma; reverse heparin with protamine; transfuse platelets if bleeding time is prolonged; type and cross-match packed red blood cells; obtain endoscopic/surgical consultation
If major bleeding still continues...	Administer epsilon aminocaproic acid as a loading dose of 5 g or 0.1 g/kg intravenously over 30 min, give a continuous infusion of 0.5–1.0 g/h until bleeding is controlled
Expanding groin hematoma	Discontinue anticoagulation and thrombolysis; apply manual pressure to the groin followed by a pressure dressing

B

MINOR BLEEDING	SUGGESTED ACTION
Superficial skin oozing	Apply manual pressure; determine if source is vascular puncture site
Gingival oozing	Pack gingiva with gauze; dental consult if oozing persists
ALLERGY	
Fever	Acetaminophen 1000–1500 mg; hydrocortisone 100 mg IV
Nausea	Diphenhydramine 25–50 mg IV; lorazepam 1–2 mg IV
Chills/rigors	Meperidine 50–100 mg IV; acetaminophen 1000–1500 mg

FIGURE 3-21. How to treat bleeding complications or allergy resulting resulting from anticoagulation or thrombolysis. **A,** Major bleeding complications require urgent action. At a minimum, heparin anticoagulation and thrombolysis should be discontinued immediately. However, the majority of bleeding complications will occur after completing the administration of a thrombolytic regimen of 2 hours or less duration. **B,** Minor bleeding problems rarely require discontinuation of thrombolysis or anticoagulation. Fortunately, most allergic reactions can be readily treated. High doses of acetaminophen (*eg*, 1500 mg) appear particularly effective.

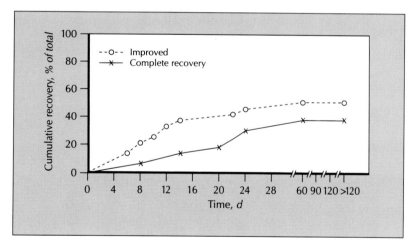

FIGURE 3-22. Efficacy of anticoagulation therapy alone. Patients treated for pulmonary embolism with anticoagulation therapy alone are receiving secondary prevention against recurrent thrombosis but are not receiving primary therapy to lyse the clot that already exists. Residual thrombus may be a nidus for the eventual development of incapacitating pulmonary hypertension. Patients treated with anticoagulation alone also risk persistent thrombosis of the pelvic or deep leg veins, which may make them more susceptible to recurrent pulmonary embolism. With respect to pulmonary perfusion, the illustration portrays results of a classic study among patients who received anticoagulation alone with serial follow-up perfusion lung scans. Only a minority of patients with medium-sized pulmonary embolism had complete recovery evidenced by perfusion lung scans, even after 4 months of follow up. (*Adapted from* Tow and Wagner [17]; with permission.)

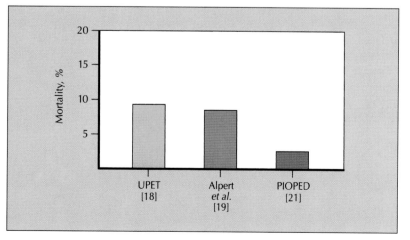

FIGURE 3-23. In-hospital mortality associated with anticoagulation therapy alone. Most studies have indicated high in-hospital mortality among patients treated with anticoagulation therapy alone. This is probably because heparin alone does not reverse right ventricular failure, which is usually the immediate cause of death in patients with acute pulmonary embolism (PE). In the Urokinase Pulmonary Embolism Trial (UPET) [18], the death rate was 9% among patients treated with anticoagulation therapy alone. In a review of 144 consecutive PE patients treated at Peter Bent Brigham Hospital, 12 (8%) died of PE, and only two of the 12 received thrombolytic therapy [19]. In the Minneapolis–St. Paul region (data not shown), the fatality rate for pulmonary embolism in 1984 was 11% for men and 12% for women [20]. In an observational study by Prospective Investigation of Pulmonary Embolism Diagnosis investigators [21], the in-hospital death rate from pulmonary embolism was only 2.5%.

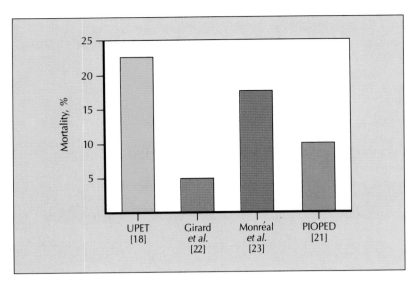

FIGURE 3-24. In-hospital recurrence rate of pulmonary embolism associated with anticoagulation therapy alone. Rates of recurrent pulmonary embolism during initial hospitalization vary widely from study to study. In the Urokinase Pulmonary Embolism Trial (UPET) [18], the rate of recurrence of pulmonary embolism in patients receiving anticoagulation therapy alone was 23%. In a French study of 50 patients, however, the recurrence rate was only 4% with anticoagulation alone [22]. A Spanish study of 38 patients found that 18% had recurrences [23]. In the Prospective Investigation of Pulmonary Embolism Diagnosis observational study [21], the rate of recurrent pulmonary embolism was 8%.

CLASSIC VS CONTEMPORARY PE THROMBOLYSIS

VARIABLE	BEFORE 1990	AFTER 1990
Indications	Hypotension; hemodynamic instability	Hypotension or normotension with accompaning right ventricular hypokinesis
Agents	SK or UK	rt-PA (or SK or UK)
Dosing regimens	250,000 U SK bolus, 100,000 U/h × 24 h; 4400 U/kg UK bolus, 4400 U/kg/h × 12–24 h	100 mg/2 h rt-PA (FDA-approved) or 3,000,000 U/2 h UK (not FDA-approved) or 1,500,000 U/h SK (not FDA-approved)
Coagulation tests	"DIC screens" every 4–6 h during infusion	aPTT at conclusion of thrombolysis
Time window	≤5 d	≤14d
Diagnosis	Mandatory angiography	Angiography or high-probability scan or suggestive echcardiogram (if hypotensive)
Route of drug administration	Locally infused via pulmonary artery catheter	Systemically infused via peripheral vein
Location of patient	ICU	Step-down unit if normotensive; ICU if hypotensive

FIGURE 3-25. Classic (before 1990) versus contemporary (after 1990) pulmonary embolism (PE) thrombolysis. Four PE thrombolysis trials have found that patients treated within 6 to 14 days of new symptoms or signs of PE have as good a response to thrombolytic therapy as patients treated within the first 5 days [1,24,25,31]. A European study showed that locally administered PE thrombolytic agents conferred no advantage over administration of thrombolytic agents through a peripheral vein with respect to efficacy, bleeding complications, or coagulation laboratory parameters [26]. aPTT—activated partial thromboplastin time; ICU—intensive care unit; rt-PA—recombinant tissue-type plasminogen activator; SK—streptokinase; UK—urokinase.

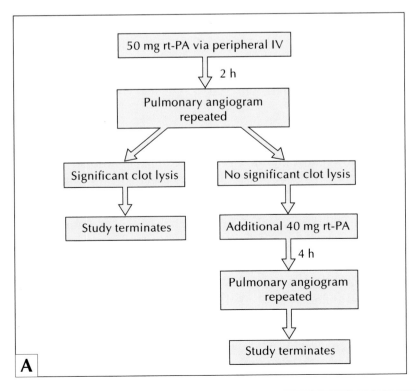

A

FIGURE 3-26. Initial experience with recombinant tissue-type plasminogen activator (rt-PA) for pulmonary embolism (PE). PE Trial #1 [27–29] was an open-label study of 47 patients with angiographically documented PE. This study demonstrated that 50 to 90 mg of rt-PA administered over 2 to 6 hours caused clot lysis in 94% of cases. **A,** All patients received 50 mg of rt-PA over 2 hours, followed immediately by a research angiogram. If clot lysis had not occurred, as judged by the investigator at the time of the angiogram, an additional 40 mg of rt-PA was administered during the next 4 hours and was followed immediately by a third angiogram. Two thirds of the patients had rt-PA administered for longer than 2 hours. During the 3rd and 4th hours of rt-PA therapy, however, an increased frequency of bleeding, particularly at the femoral vein puncture site used for pulmonary angiography, caused us to shorten the duration and raise the dose of rt-PA in subsequent trials. (*continued*)

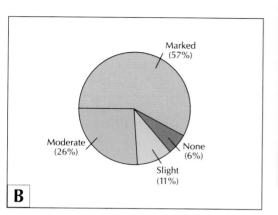

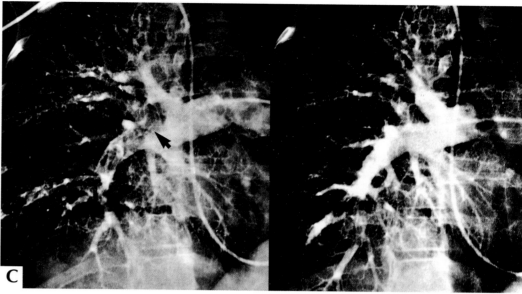

FIGURE 3-26. (*continued*) **B,** Clot lysis within 6 hours was graded as moderate or marked in 83% of the patients and slight in 11%. Among patients with pulmonary hypertension, pulmonary artery pressure decreased during the acute treatment period from 43/17 [27] to 31/13 [19] mm Hg, without any change in systemic artery pressure. **C,** Large filling defect of angiographic contrast agent indicates a subtotally obstructing embolus in the right main pulmonary artery (*arrow* in *left panel*). After a 2-hour infusion of rt-PA through a peripheral vein (*right panel*), there is pronounced resolution, with some residual thrombus in segmental branches. (*Adapted from* Goldhaber and coworkers [27]; with permission.)

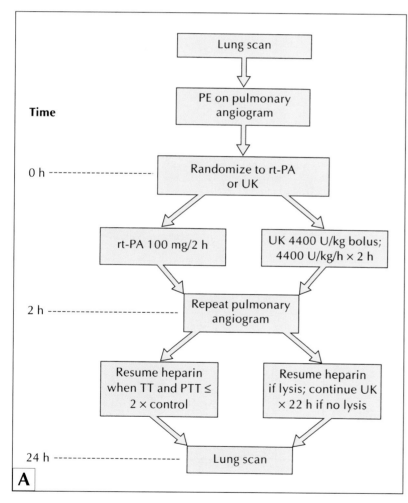

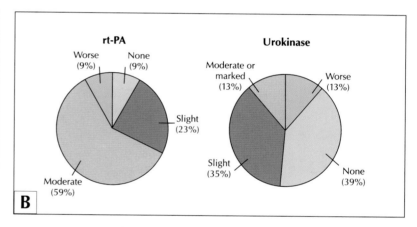

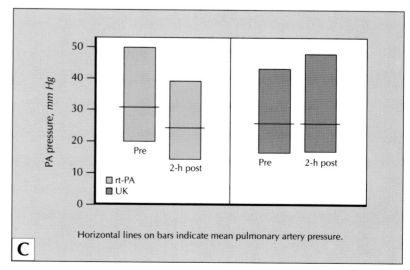

Horizontal lines on bars indicate mean pulmonary artery pressure.

FIGURE 3-27. Recombinant tissue-type plasminogen activator (rt-PA) versus urokinase (UK). Pulmonary embolism (PE) Trial #2 [24] was a randomized trial comparing administration of 100 mg of rt-PA for 2 hours versus 4400 U/kg of UK as a bolus followed by 4400 U/kg/h for up to 24 hours. **A,** The principal end points were improvement on the 2-hour angiogram and 24-hour lung scan compared with the baseline studies. All 45 patients received the full dose of rt-PA, but UK infusions were terminated prema-turely in nine of 23 patients because of allergy in one patient and uncontrollable bleeding in eight others. **B,** After 2 hours, 82% of rt-PA–treated patients showed clot lysis, compared with 48% of UK-treated patients (*P*=0.0008). **C,** Thrombolysis demonstrated by angiography in the rt-PA treated patients was associated with a return of elevated pulmonary artery (PA) pressures toward normal. We concluded that, in the dosing regimens used, rt-PA was more rapid and more safe than UK. (*continued*)

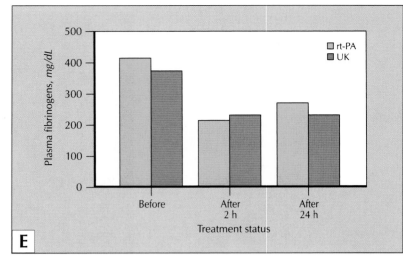

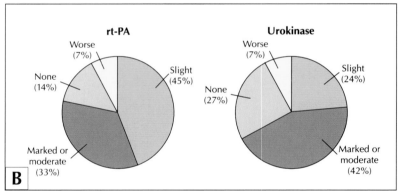

FIGURE 3-27. (*continued*) **D,** After 24 hours, however, there was no difference in scintigraphic improvement between rt-PA and UK patients. **E,** At baseline, 2, and 24 hours after initiation of thrombolysis, the fibrinogen levels were similar in both treatment groups. Despite the increased

rate of bleeding complications among UK-treated patients, there was no difference in fibrinogenolysis between the two treatment groups.

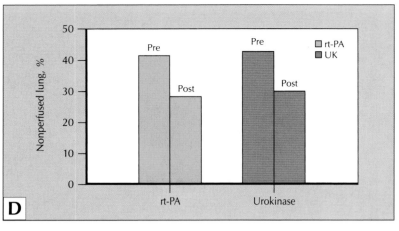

FIGURE 3-28. Moderate clot lysis can result in marked hemodynamic improvement. Pulmonary angiograms (right posterior oblique position) of a 58-year-old man with a 5-day history of dyspnea. *Left panel* shows intraluminal clot in the arteries of the right upper and lower lobe (*arrows*) before treatment. *Right panel* shows evidence of moderate clot lysis (*arrows*) occurring immediately after continuous peripheral intravenous infusion. PRE TX—pretreatment. (*Adapted from* Goldhaber and coworkers [24]; with permission.)

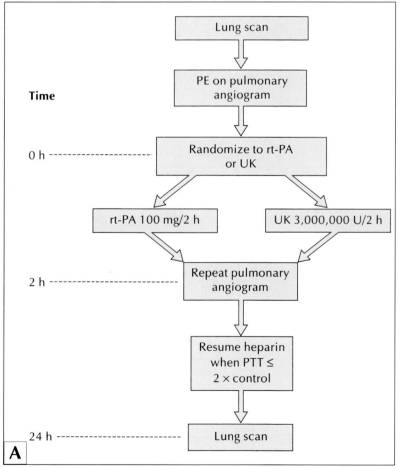

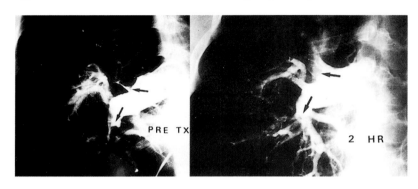

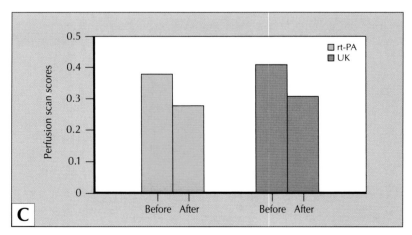

FIGURE 3-29. A short 2-hour thrombolytic infusion is more rapidly effective and safer than a 24-hour infusion. Pulmonary embolism (PE) Trial #3 [25] compressed the 24-hour dose of urokinase (UK) to make it comparable to the high-concentration and short-infusion period that was used for recombinant tissue-type plasminogen activator (rt-PA).

The novel UK dose was 3 million units given over a period of 2 hours with the first million units given as a bolus over 10 minutes (**A**). This trial enrolled 90 patients. Repeat pulmonary angiograms were performed at 2 hours, and repeat lung scans were obtained at 24 hours. These studies were then graded by blinded panels. The results indicated that a 2-hour regimen of rt-PA and the new concentrated 2-hour dosing regimen of urokinase exhibit similar efficacy on follow-up angiograms (**B**) and scans (**C**) as well as similar safety profiles. (*continued*)

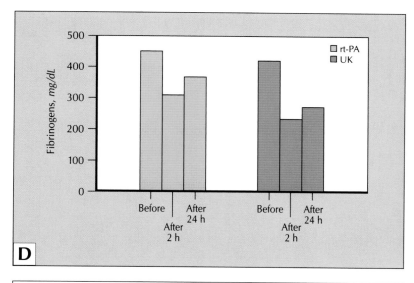

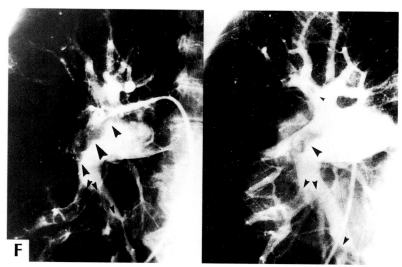

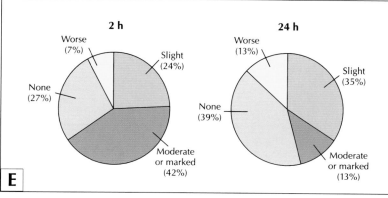

FIGURE 3-29. (continued) Fibrinogenolysis did not differ significantly between the two treatment groups (D). When angiographic clot lysis is compared between this 2-hour UK regimen and the previously used 24-hour UK regimen, the 2-hour regimen is more effective (E). In F, a 71-year-old female subject has a large right interlobar pulmonary artery thrombus with multiple emboli to the basilar segmental arteries (arrowheads) at baseline pulmonary angiography (left panel). The patient was randomized to receive UK and immediately after the end of the 2-hour infusion, the angiogram was repeated (right panel). It revealed moderate clot lysis with reperfusion to the central vessels of the upper and lower lobe, although some peripheral clot persisted (arrowheads).

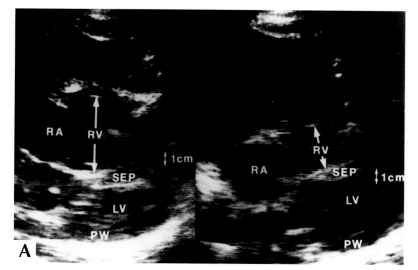

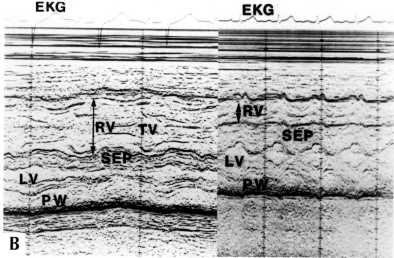

FIGURE 3-30. Thrombolysis improves right ventricular function. In our initial experience with recombinant tissue-type plasminogen activator (rt-PA) for pulmonary embolism (PE), Come et al. [30] performed Doppler echocardiography on seven patients with PE before and after treatment. Within one day of treatment, the right ventricular end-diastolic diameter decreased from an average of 3.9 to 2.0 cm. Right ventricular wall motion, initially graded as mildly, moderately, or severely hypokinetic in one, two, and four patients, respectively, normalized in five patients and improved to mild hypokinesis in two others. Tricuspid regurgitation was present before lytic therapy in six patients but was detected after the completion of lytic therapy in only two patients. There was no tricuspid regurgitation 5 days later in one of the two patients. Early reversal of the hallmarks of right heart failure—right ventricular dysfunction, right ventricular dilatation, and tricuspid regurgitation—suggests that thrombolytic agents might reduce mortality from acute PE.

A, Subcostal two-dimensional images at end-diastole in a PE patient from PE Trial #1 (see Fig. 3-26) who presented with heart failure.

Before rt-PA (left panel), the right ventricle (RV) is markedly enlarged and the diameter of the left ventricle (LV) is reduced. After rt-PA (right panel), a remarkable decrease in RV size and a corresponding increase in LV size are apparent.

B, M-mode echocardiographic recordings of the right ventricle (RV) and left ventricle (LV) from a subcostal transducer position in the same patient as in A before (left panel) and after (right panel) thrombolytic therapy for PE. Before rt-PA treatment, the patient had a markedly enlarged right ventricle, reduced left ventricular chamber size, and paradoxic movement of the interventricular septum. The right ventricle also appeared markedly hypokinetic. After dissolution of pulmonary artery thrombi, documented by pulmonary angiography, the right ventricle became much smaller, and the left ventricle became larger. Paradoxic systolic septal movement was no longer present, and right ventricular wall movement normalized. PW—posterior wall; RA—right atrium; SEP—septum; TV—tricuspid valve. (Adapted from Come and coworkers [30]; with permission.)

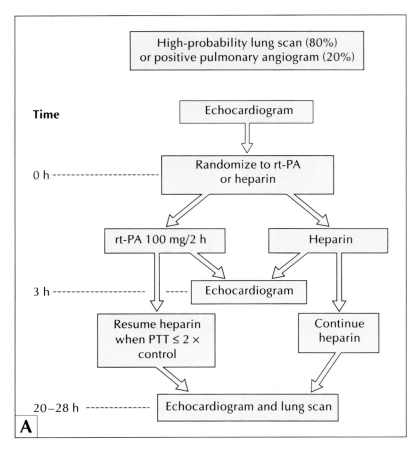

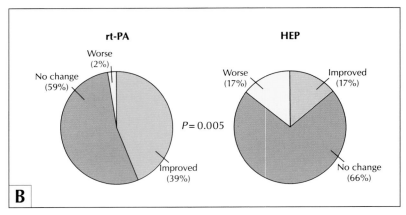

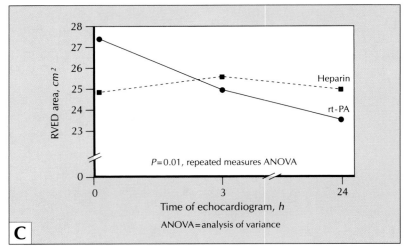

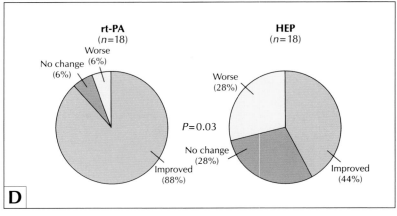

FIGURE 3-31. Recombinant tissue-type plasminogen activator (rt-PA) versus heparin alone: effects on right ventricular function and pulmonary perfusion. The previously observed improvement in right ventricular function with rt-PA (*see* Fig. 3-30) could have been due to heparin and the passage of time rather than to rt-PA. Therefore, PE Trial #4 [1] tested the hypothesis that rt-PA followed by anticoagulants improves right ventricular function and pulmonary perfusion more rapidly than anticoagulation therapy alone (**A**).

Overall, 101 patients were randomized—46 to rt-PA 100 mg/2 h followed by heparin and 55 to heparin alone. This study was the largest thrombolytic agent versus heparin trial that had been undertaken since phase I of Urokinase Pulmonary Embolism Trial [18]. At entry, all patients were hemodynamically stable; no patient presented with an initial systolic artery pressure of less than 90 mm Hg. At baseline, about half of the patients in each treatment group had normal right ventricular function.

Right ventricular wall motion was assessed qualitatively, and right ventricular end-diastolic (RVED) area from the apical four-chamber view was planimetered on serial echocardiograms at baseline, after 3 hours, and after 24 hours. (An abnormally large right ventricular end-diastolic area indicates right ventricular dilatation). Pulmonary perfusion scans were obtained at baseline and after 24 hours. The results indicated that rt-PA (100 mg/2 h) followed by heparin provided striking improvement in right ventricular function and pulmonary perfusion compared with heparin anticoagulation therapy alone.

B, Qualitative assessment of right ventricular wall motion at 24 hours versus baseline demonstrated that 39% of the rt-PA patients improved and 2% worsened; there was 17% improvement and 17% worsening among patients who received heparin alone ($P=0.005$).

C, Quantitative assessment showed that rt-PA patients had a significant decrease in right ventricular end-diastolic area during the first 24 hours after randomization; no improvement was demonstrated among the patients randomized to heparin alone ($P=0.01$). (*Adapted from* Goldhaber and coworkers [1]; with permission.)

D, Among the subset of patients who presented with right ventricular hypokinesis, 88% of the rt-PA patients improved and 6% worsened; 44% of the group receiving only heparin demonstrated improvement and 28% worsened. All adverse clinical events in this trial occurred among the patients who received heparin alone in the setting of baseline right ventricular hypokinesis and who subsequently experienced increased right ventricular dysfunction during the first 24 hours. Most important, no clinical episodes of recurrent PE occurred among rt-PA patients, but five (two fatal and three nonfatal) clinically suspected recurrent PEs occurred in patients randomized to heparin alone ($P=0.06$) within 14 days. All five patients entered the trial with normotension accompanied by right ventricular hypokinesis on echocardiogram, suggesting that patients with this initial echocardiographic finding constitute a high-risk group. Patients receiving rt-PA also had an absolute improvement in pulmonary perfusion of 15% after 24 hours, compared with 2% improvement among patients receiving heparin alone ($P<0.0001$). *See* Fig. 3-15. aPTT—partial thromboplastin time.

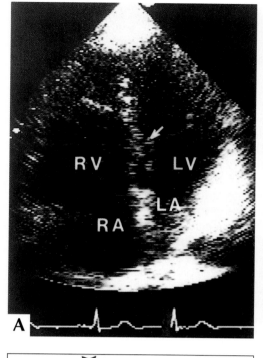

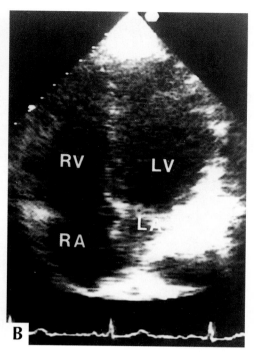

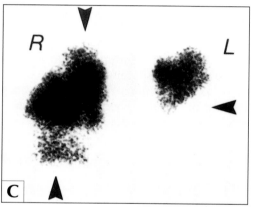

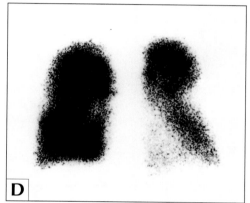

FIGURE 3-32. A hemodynamically stable patient treated with recombinant tissue-type plasminogen activator (rt-PA). **A,** and **B,** Echocardiograms (four-chamber view) in a 53-year-old previously healthy man with a high-probability lung scan for pulmonary embolism. The patient participated in PE Trial #4. Before treatment, the right ventricle was enlarged, and hypokinesis of the right ventricle was moderately severe (*A*). Right ventricular end-diastolic area was 42.9 cm², and the interventricular septum (*arrow*) was displaced toward the left ventricle. Three hours after initiation of rt-PA therapy, the size of the right ventricle became normal (with an end-diastolic area of 25.7 cm²), and the interventricular septum resumed a normal configuration (*B*), right ventricular hypokinesis was reversed, and normal right ventricular function was restored.

Perfusion lung scans before (**C**) and 24 hours after (**D**) initiation of rt-PA therapy for the same patient. On the scan taken before therapy, there is diminished perfusion in the right middle lobe (*lower arrowhead*) and the apical segment of the right upper lobe (*upper arrowhead*) and virtually no perfusion in the left lower lobe. Perfusion is markedly improved on the scan taken after therapy. Less improvement is noted in the left lung, but the irregular perfusion in the apicoposterior segment of the left upper lobe before thrombolytic therapy (*horizontal arrowhead*) is homogeneous after therapy.

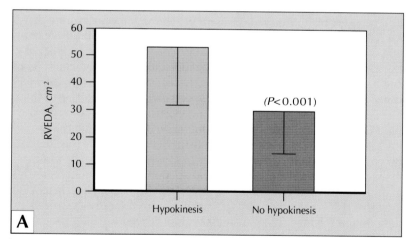

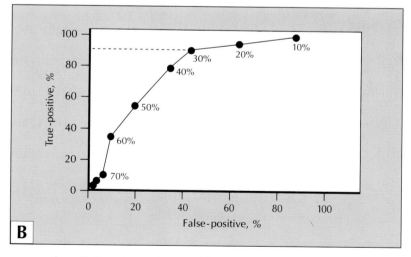

FIGURE 3-33. Relationship between baseline perfusion lung scan and right ventricular function. Although normotensive patients with pulmonary embolism (PE) may have right ventricular (RV) hypokinesis that is obvious on echocardiogram, the disorder may be overlooked on clinical examination because the classic physical findings of right ventricular failure are often not apparent. Such an oversight might result in withholding thrombolytic therapy from a subset of patients that, if treated with heparin alone, are at high risk of recurrent PE. Our research group studied the relationship between right ventricular hypokinesis on baseline echocardiography and the extent of the perfusion deficits on the initial perfusion lung scan [2]. **A,** The magnitude of nonperfused lung was greater in patients with baseline right ventricular hypokinesis (54%±16% of the lung

nonperfused) than in patients with normal right ventricular wall motion at baseline (30%±18% nonperfused lung; *P*<0.001). **B,** Receiver-operating characteristic (ROC) curve analysis revealed that when 30% or more of the lung is not perfused, sensitivity for detecting right ventricular hypokinesis is 92%. This correlation is important because we found that among hemodynamically stable patients who present with PE, all who developed recurrent symptomatic PE (fatal or nonfatal) had right ventricular hypokinesis (13% versus 0% for those with normal RV wall motion; *P*=0.01). Therefore, a strategy of performing echocardiography in those patients with a perfusion scan deficit score of 30% or greater appears to identify most patients at increased risk for recurrent PE.

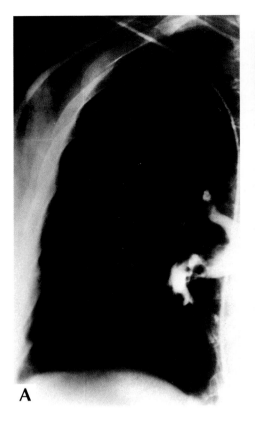

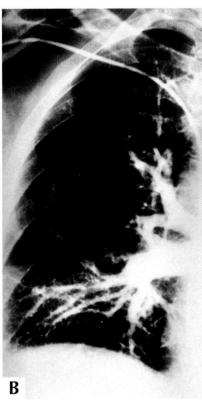

A   **B**

FIGURE 3-34. A reduced dose bolus of recombinant tissue-type plasminogen activator (rt-PA) of 0.6 mg/kg (maximum 50 mg) has generated interest as a method of achieving thrombolysis more rapidly and less expensively than with the Food and Drug Administration (FDA)–approved regimen of 100 mg of rt-PA administered for a period of 2 hours. **A,** Angiogram demonstrating a large embolism of the right main pulmonary artery. The patient was a 64-year-old man who was hemodynamically stable. He received a bolus of 41 mg of rt-PA over a period of 15 minutes. **B,** Two hours later, the angiogram was repeated and showed marked improvement. The patient's baseline fibrinogen level was 670 mg/dL; the fibrinogen nadir was 513 mg/dL, which is much less of a decrement than would be expected with the standard dose of rt-PA. PE Trial #5 [31] tested the hypothesis that a reduced dose of bolus rt-PA (0.6 mg/kg/15 minutes, maximum of 50 mg) would result in fewer bleeding complications than standard 100 mg of rt-PA administered as a continuous infusion over 2 hours among hemodynamically stable patients. Twenty-eight hospitals in the United States, Italy, and Canada participated in this double-blind, double dummy randomized controlled trial. No significant differences were detected between the bolus rt-PA and 2-hour rt-PA with respect to bleeding complications of efficacy. There was, however, less fibrinogenolysis with the bolus dosing regimen.

MECHANICAL INTERVENTIONS

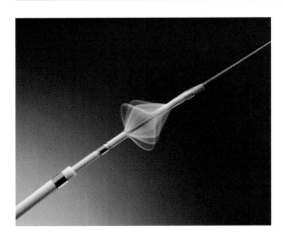

FIGURE 3-35. Mechanical therapy for pulmonary embolism. When thrombolysis alone does not successfully treat massive pulmonary embolism or when patients have major contraindications to thrombolysis, mechanical intervention should be considered. Interventional management can often be undertaken in the cardiac catheterization laboratory. For example, a device called "The Thrombolizer" is undergoing clinical testing. It consists of a 5 F teflon catheter whose distal tip is divided into four 15-mm bends. The high speed mechanical rotation of the catheter (about 100,000 revolutions per minute) causes centrifugal force to open the distal bends and form a soft flexible helical spiral that can pulverize thrombus into microscopic particles within a few seconds [32]. Other catheter-based alternatives include mechanical fragmentation of thrombus with a pulmonary artery catheter [33], simultaneous mechanical clot fragmentation and pharmacologic thrombolysis [34], and suction catheter embolectomy [35, 36]. If these strategies fail, acute surgical pulmonary embolectomy can be undertaken [37]. A nonrandomized comparison of rt-PA thrombolysis with surgical embolectomy showed that both approaches can be lifesaving in the majority of patients with massive PE [38].

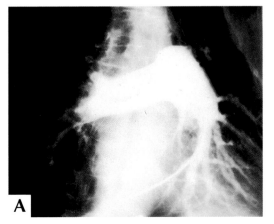

A

FIGURE 3-36. Case presentation of massive pulmonary embolism with hemodynamic instability: combined approach of suction catheter embolectomy and thrombolysis. A 78-year-old woman was admitted to a suburban hospital with severe shortness of breath and persistent hypotension. Blood pressure on admission was 78/51 mm Hg. The patient was given heparin and a Greenfield filter was placed, but the patient was persistently hypoxemic despite nasotracheal intubation for ventilatory support. Pulmonary angiogram demonstrated a massive embolism of the right pulmonary artery (**A**). Melena resulted from the heparin administration, and the patient was transferred to Brigham and Women's Hospital. The medical history revealed heavy cigarette smoking and a remote left thoracoplasty (note the small left lung volume in *A*). The cardiac surgeons declined to perform pulmonary embolectomy because most of the left lung had been removed during the thoracoplasty. Systemic thrombolytic therapy was considered but was believed to be of extraordinarily high risk because of the melena. (*continued*)

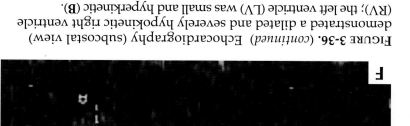

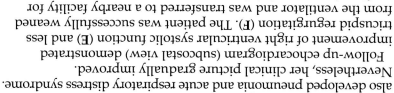

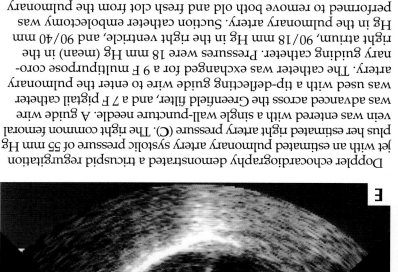

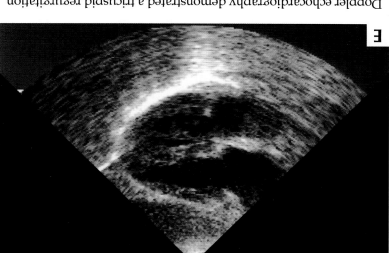

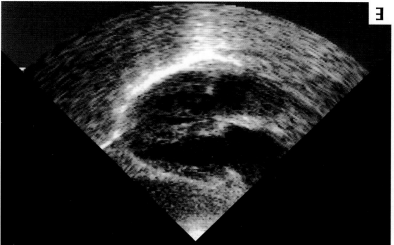

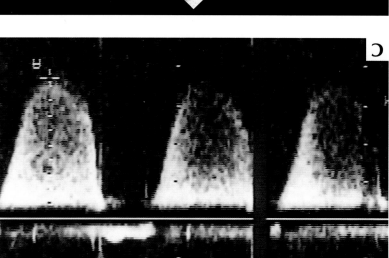

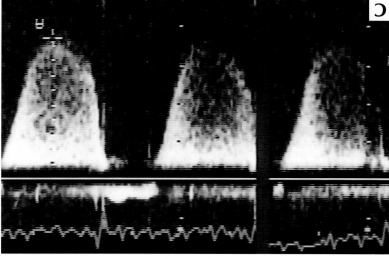

FIGURE 3-36. (*continued*) Echocardiography (subcostal view) demonstrated a dilated and severely hypokinetic right ventricle (RV); the left ventricle (LV) was small and hyperkinetic (**B**).

Doppler echocardiography demonstrated a tricuspid regurgitation jet with an estimated pulmonary artery systolic pressure of 55 mm Hg plus her estimated right atrial pressure (C). The right common femoral vein was entered with a single wall-puncture needle. A guide wire was advanced across the Greenfield filter, and a 7 F pigtail catheter was used with a tip-deflecting guide wire to enter the pulmonary artery. The catheter was exchanged for a 9 F multipurpose coronary guiding catheter. Pressures were 18 mm Hg (mean) in the right atrium, 90/18 mm Hg in the right ventricle, and 90/40 mm Hg in the pulmonary artery. Suction catheter embolectomy was performed to remove both old and fresh clot from the pulmonary artery branches of the upper and lower right lobes. Nevertheless, hypotension persisted. Therefore, an infusion of 50 mg of recombinant tissue-type plasminogen activator (rt-PA) was administered over a period of 15 minutes through the pulmonary artery catheter. D, Pulmonary angiography then demonstrated an approximate 30% reduction in overall clot burden. The patient experienced a retroperitoneal hematoma that required a 12-unit transfusion for correction. She also developed pneumonia and acute respiratory distress syndrome. Nevertheless, her clinical picture gradually improved. Follow-up echocardiogram (subcostal view) demonstrated improvement of right ventricular systolic function (E) and less tricuspid regurgitation (F). The patient was successfully weaned from the ventilator and was transferred to a nearby facility for cardiopulmonary rehabilitation.

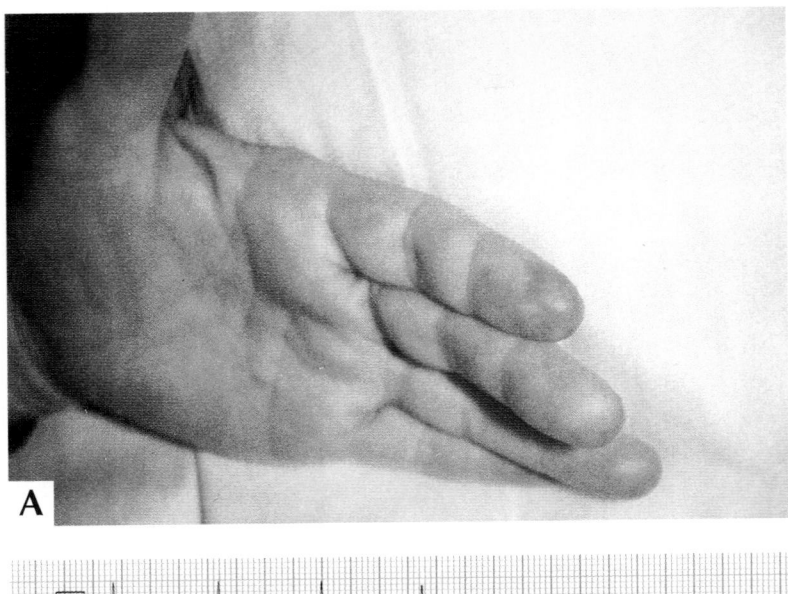

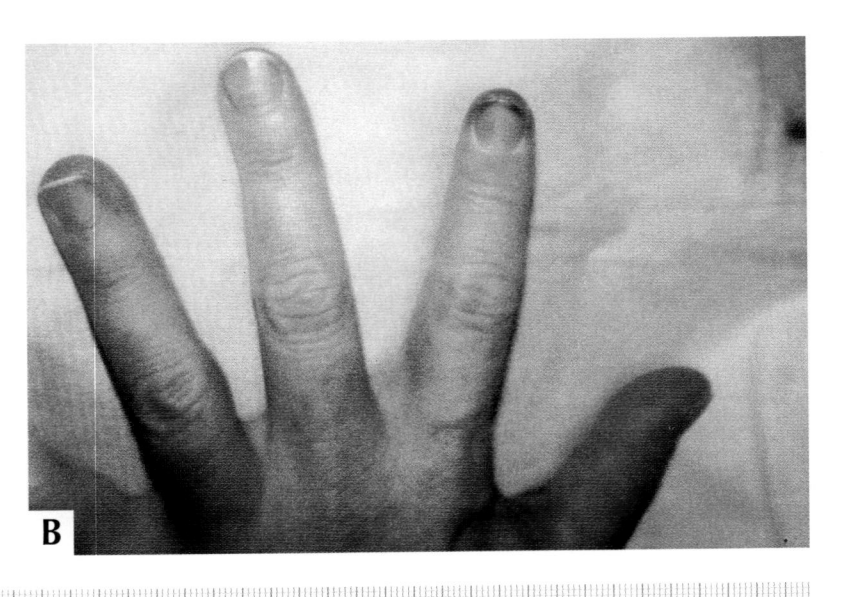

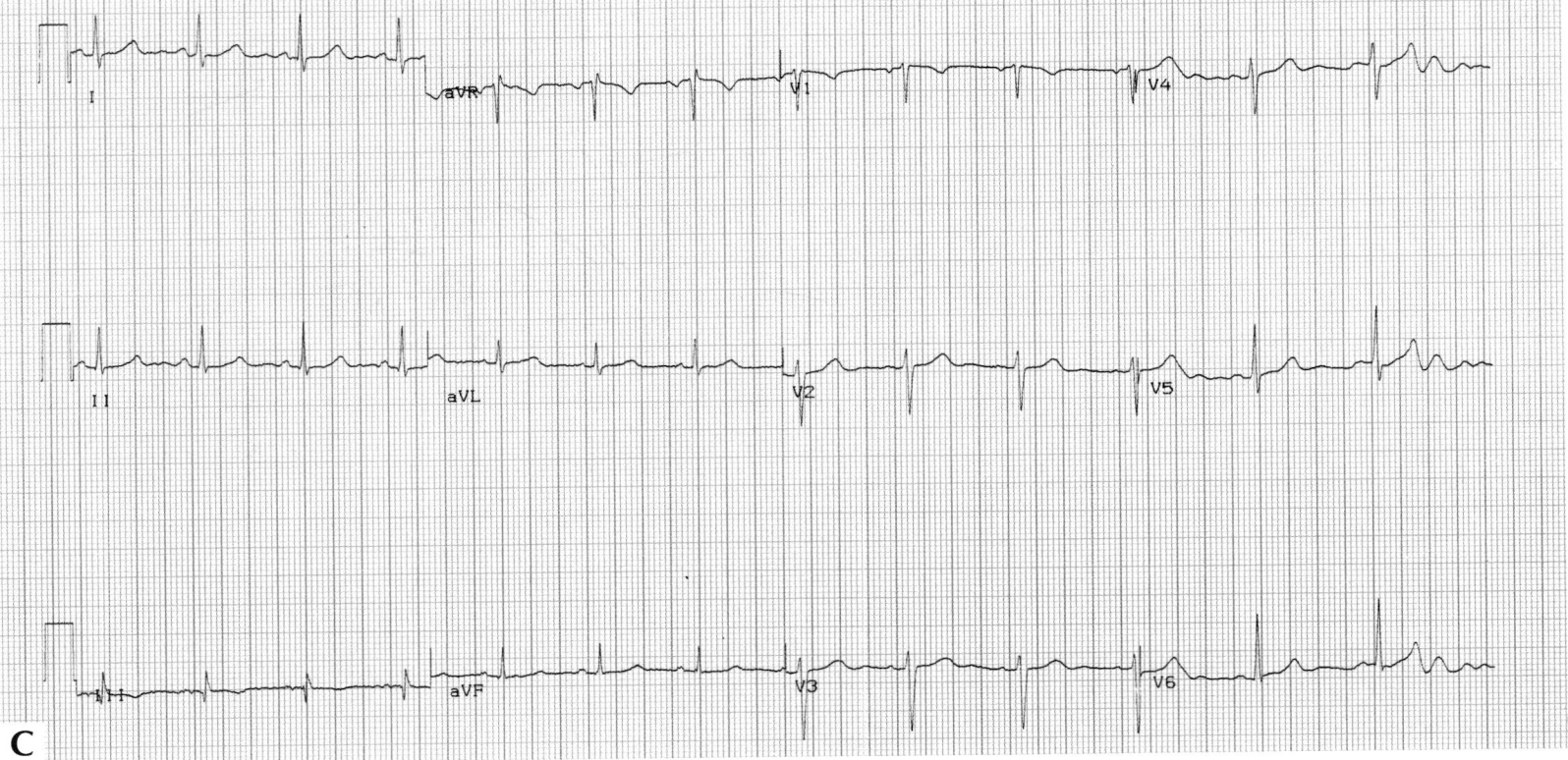

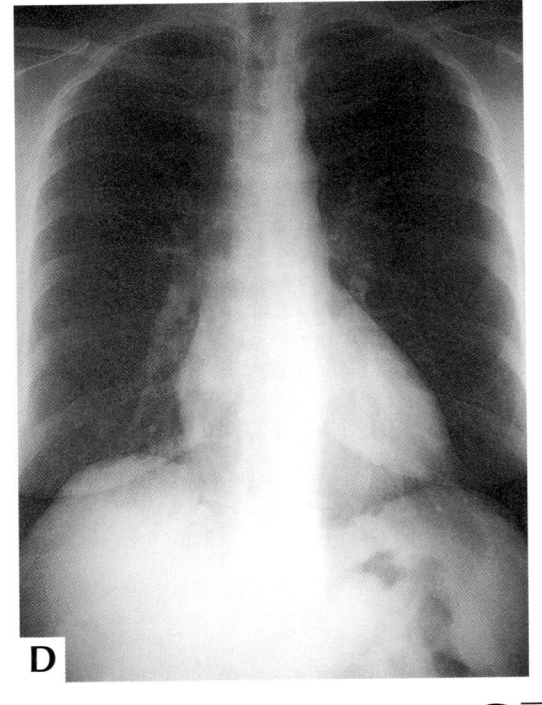

FIGURE 3-37. Case presentation: paradoxical embolism in the setting of moderate-sized pulmonary embolism. A 45-year-old woman presented with a primary complaint of pain in the left index finger and numbness for 2 weeks. During the 3 to 4 days before admission, she suffered sharp, intermittent right-sided pleuritic chest pain. She also complained of a cough with white sputum, sore throat, and mild shortness of breath during the week before admission. Two months previously, the patient had begun taking a low-estrogen oral contraceptive. On examination, she was in no acute distress. Temperature was 99.6°, heart rate was 92 beats per minutes, respiratory rate was 16 per minute, blood pressure was 142/88 mm Hg, and room air saturation was 96%. Chest examination revealed dullness and rales at the posterior zone of the right lower lung. Cardiac examination was unremarkable.

The patient had abnormally purplish second, third and fourth left fingertips (**A**). The tip of the left index finger was cool, cyanotic, and had delayed capillary refill time as well as numbness (**B**). Laboratory examination showed a hematocrit of 31% and idiopathic anemia. Electrocardiogram was normal but suggested an S1Q3T3 pattern, indicative of right heart strain and, at times, associated with pulmonary embolism (**C**). The posteroanterior chest radiograph appeared normal (**D**), but the lateral chest radiograph (**E**) revealed a pleural-based opacity (*arrow*) at the base of the right lung. (*continued*)

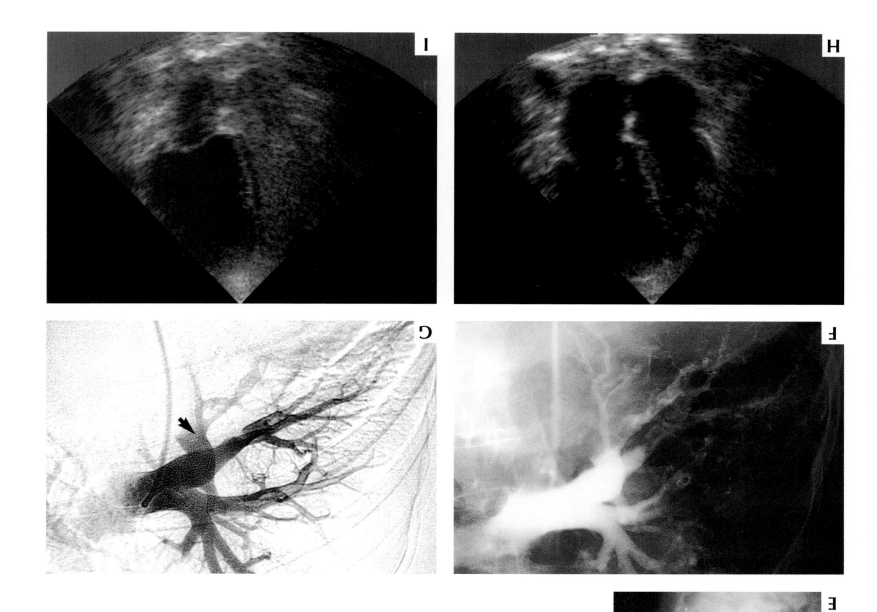

FIGURE 3-37. (continued) Ventilation-perfusion lung scan indicated a low probability for pulmonary embolism. Because of high clinical suspicion for pulmonary embolism, however, the patient underwent diagnostic pulmonary angiography. Right atrial pressure was 13 mm Hg, and pulmonary artery pressure was 45/20 mm Hg.

There were extensive intraluminal filling deficits (arrow) in the anterior segment of the pulmonary artery of the right upper lobe as well as in the vessels of the middle and lower right lobes (F). Subtraction imaging showed a partial cutoff of the pulmonary artery to the right lower lobe (arrow) (G). Echocardiogram showed normal cardiac chambers and normal right and left ventricular function (H); however, a bubble study in which agitated saline was injected into a peripheral vein demonstrated transit of bubbles from the right atrium to the left atrium (arrow) consistent with a diagnosis of patent foramen ovale (I).

Thus, the patient suffered a paradoxic embolism through a patent foramen ovale (which accounted for her cool, cyanotic fingers) as well as extensive pulmonary embolism. Because of the normal right ventricular function and idiopathic anemia, the patient was treated with anticoagulation therapy alone rather than with thrombolytic therapy followed by anticoagulants. She was discharged uneventfully and continues to do well clinically.

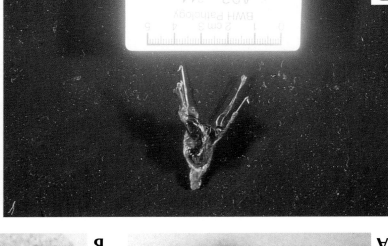

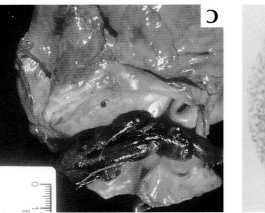

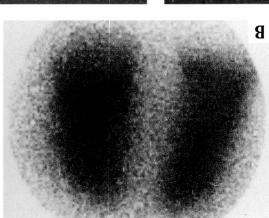

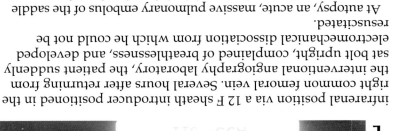

FIGURE 3-38. Failure of a titanium Greenfield filter to prevent fatal pulmonary embolism. A 56-year-old man presented with hypotension (blood pressure 75/60 mm Hg) and shortness of breath 7 weeks after a subarachnoid hemorrhage was treated by clipping of an anterior communicating artery aneurysm and placement of a ventriculostomy tube. Scattered perfusion deficits in the left lower lobe and right upper lobe as well as defects along the fissures in both lobes are demonstrated in this posterior view perfusion lung scan (**A**). The ventilation scan with Xe-133 was normal (**B**). Thus, because of the marked ventilation-perfusion mismatches, the scan was interpreted as revealing a high probability of pulmonary embolism. The patient was not a candidate for anticoagulation because of his recent stroke. Therefore, a titanium Greenfield filter was placed in the inferior vena cava in an infrarenal position via a 12 F sheath introducer positioned in the right common femoral vein. Several hours after returning from the interventional angiography laboratory, the patient suddenly sat bolt upright, complained of breathlessness, and developed electromechanical dissociation from which he could not be resuscitated.

At autopsy, an acute, massive pulmonary embolus of the saddle type with complete occlusion of the left and right pulmonary arteries was found (**C**). The inferior vena cava filter was positioned 2 cm below the left renal vein. Fresh thrombus had adhered to the filter (**D**); however, two of the six filter legs were not extended appropriately. Therefore, the filter legs were deployed every 90° instead of every 60° and did not provide adequate protection against recurrent pulmonary embolism (**E**).

AIR EMBOLISM

Clinical spectrum	
Mild	Nausea, dizziness, dyspnea, confusion
Moderate	Chest pain, tachycardia, tachypnea, localized neurologic deficit
Severe	Coma or cardiopulmonary arrest
Treatment	
	Oxygenation
	Volume expansion to increase right ventricular filling and decrease the space occupied by the air embolus
	Trendelenburg and left lateral decubitus positions
	Aspiration of air through a right heart catheter
	Hyperbaric oxygen

FIGURE 3-39. Embolization of air through a track of a patent central venous catheter generally occurs within the first hour after catheter removal. Therefore, catheter removal should be undertaken with the patient in the Trendelenburg position. The puncture site of the catheter should be covered with antibiotic ointment and an occlusive dressing [39]. Definitive diagnosis can be made by echocardiographic visualization of large "bubbles" of air in the right cardiac chambers [40].

FAT EMBOLISM SYNDROME

Clinical characteristics	Fever
	Increased alveolar-arterial oxygen gradient
	Diffuse chest x-ray infiltrates
	Changes in sensorium
	Irritability, restlessness, confusion, coma
Treatment	Petechiae
	Early immobilization of bone fragments
	Supplemental oxygen
	±Assisted ventilation with PEEP
	±Corticosteroids

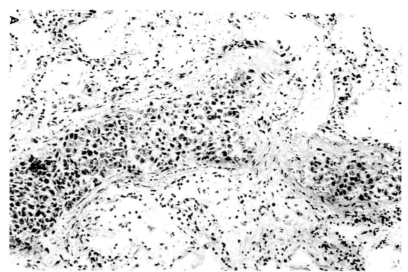

FIGURE 3-40. Fat embolism syndrome tends to occur within 2 days of fracture of the femur, tibia, or fibula. In its most severe form, fat embolism syndrome is characterized by three features: petechial rash, respiratory distress, and central nervous system dysfunction. A mechanical theory to explain the pathogenesis of the syndrome is that intramedullary vein trauma resulting from fracture (or orthopedic surgery) leads to extravasation of marrow fat into the circulation and subsequent embolization to the lungs. Involvement of the skin capillaries and of the brain is thought to occur, in some cases, because of paradoxical embolization through a patent foramen ovale. With aggressive therapy, most patients survive this disorder [41,42].

FIGURE 3-41. Tumor pulmonary embolism. Cancer patients, especially those with metastatic adenocarcinoma, are prone to both thrombotic and tumor pulmonary embolism. In a series of 73 patients with solid malignant tumors and pulmonary embolism, 56 had major thrombotic pulmonary embolism and 17 had major tumor embolism to the lungs. Most presenting symptoms, signs, and associated conditions were similar in the two groups [43], although patients with tumor embolism tend to have more peripheral and more diffuse perfusion deficits on lung scan. Microscopic appearance of tumor emboli in the lumen of a pulmonary artery filled with tumor cells is shown [44]. The primary neoplasm was an infiltrating ductal carcinoma (*Adapted from* Godleski [44]; with permission.)

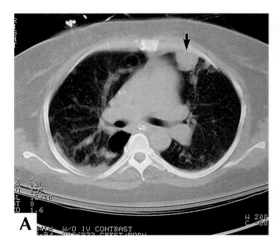
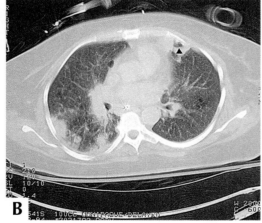
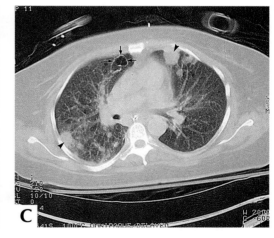

FIGURE 3-42. Case of woman aged 45 years with pyelonephritis. She developed renal vein thrombosis and bacteremia. When she became hypoxic, a spiral computed scan of the chest was obtained. Anteriorly, in the left upper lobe (**A**), is a subpleural density (*arrow*), which subsequently (**B**) gets smaller and contains a cavity (*arrowhead*). In the right lung anteriorly (**C**), a thin-walled cavity is noted (*arrows*). Several other subpleural densities are present (*arrowheads*). These findings are highly suggestive of septic pulmonary emboli.

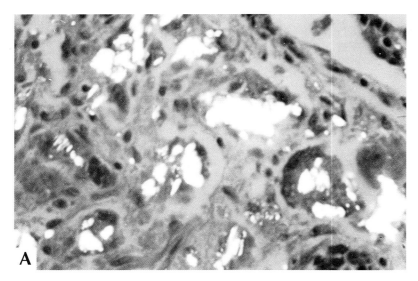

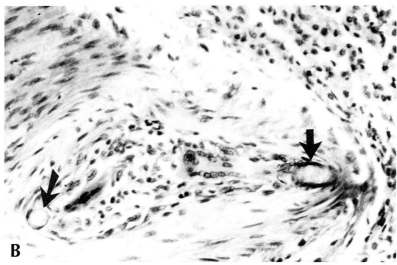

FIGURE 3-43. Pulmonary embolism resulting from self-injection of foreign matter. Foreign matter in the pulmonary vasculature that was injected into a peripheral vein is shown [44]. **A,** Extensive deposition of talc and other crystalline debris in the pulmonary vessels of a heroin addict. This micrograph was taken with polarized light to highlight the foreign matter.

B, A woman was hospitalized for investigation of fever of unknown origin. Eventually, the medical staff discovered that the patient had been injecting herself with foreign matter, including hair and feces. In this micrograph, a hair is seen in a pulmonary vessel. In the vessel lumen a giant cell reaction to foreign bodies (*arrows*) is present. (*Adapted from* Godleski [44]; with permission.)

EMOTIONAL SUPPORT

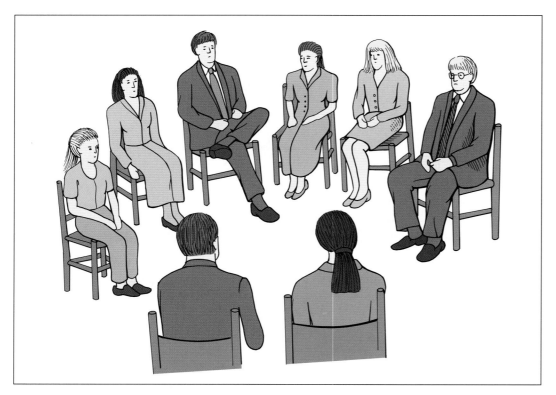

FIGURE 3-44. Pulmonary embolism support group. During hospitalization and outpatient follow-up, patients with pulmonary embolism must deal with a variety of emotional issues superimposed upon their medical problems. In the setting of a noisy hospital or a busy outpatient practice, a patient's psychologic problems that require additional exploration and discussion may not be addressed properly. Therefore, we started a pulmonary embolism support group co-led by a nurse-physician team. Our group meets on a week-night evening once every 3 weeks. The sessions have a component of education regarding the underlying pathophysiology of pulmonary embolism; however, discussion of

common anxieties and living difficulties that occur in the aftermath of pulmonary embolism is emphasized.

Although pulmonary embolism can be as emotionally devastating as myocardial infarction, the general public usually lacks a thorough understanding of this illness, particularly regarding the possibility of long-term disability and incomplete recovery. Young patients with pulmonary embolism repeatedly voice several common themes. Although they usually appear healthy after recovery, such patients have experienced a life-threatening disorder; their outward healthy appearance may make it difficult for them to express their fears about the illness to family and friends. Virtually all patients with pulmonary embolism wonder why they became ill and whether they have an underlying coagulopathy or "bad genes," even if no specific hypercoagulable state can be identified. When anticoagulation is discontinued after an adequate course of therapy, patients become fearful of recurrent embolism and may resist attempts to be weaned from warfarin. They often feel disabled from chronic leg discomfort due to concomitant venous thrombosis of the legs. We can usually ease the emotional burden of pulmonary embolism by setting aside time to discuss the implications of pulmonary embolism with the patient both in individual and group settings.

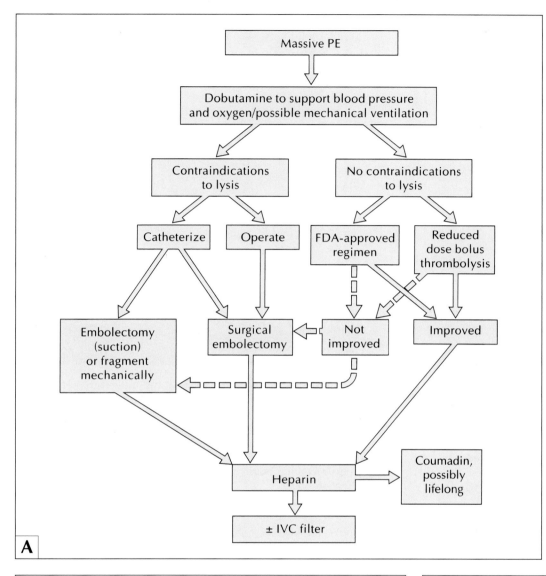

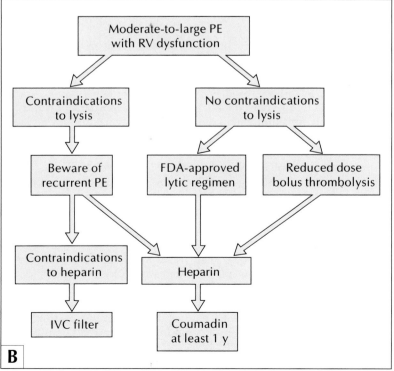

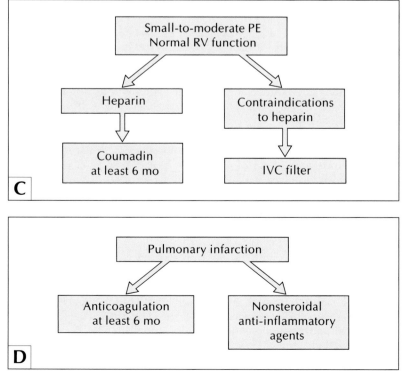

FIGURE 3-45. Protocols for treating different types of pulmonary embolism (PE). The optimal duration of Coumadin has not been studied in patients with pulmonary embolism. **A,** The patient who is hemodynamically compromised can receive an array of pharmacologic or mechanical interventions designed to lyse, remove, and dissipate the embolism while maintaining adequate right ventricular function. Consideration should be given to placement of a filter in the inferior vena cava (IVC) to prevent recurrent embolism that may be fatal in a patient with persistently compromised cardio-pulmonary status.

B, Moderate to large pulmonary embolism with associated right ventricular dysfunction. Although they are normotensive, these patients may benefit from thrombolytic therapy or suction catheter embolectomy not only to reverse right ventricular dysfunction rapidly and hasten pulmonary reperfusion but also to reduce the frequency of such adverse clinical events as recurrent embolism [1].

C, Small to moderate pulmonary embolism with normal right ventricular function. The prognosis of these patients is usually good with anticoagulation therapy alone. **D,** Pulmonary infarction. These patients usually have small pulmonary emboli that lodge in the periphery of the lung, usually near the base. Such patients can usually be managed successfully with anticoagulation and nonsteroidal anti-inflammatory agents. (*continued*)

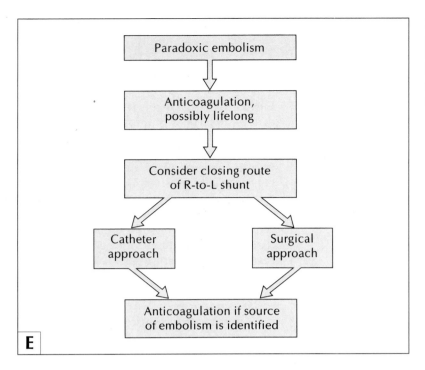

FIGURE 3-45. (*continued*) **E,** Paradoxic embolism. Emboli causing paradoxic embolism are usually too small to be trapped by a filter inserted in the inferior vena cava. Therefore, if the patient is at high risk of paradoxic embolism, transcatheter or surgical closure of a patent foramen ovale (or other causes of right-to-left shunt) should be considered.

REFERENCES

1. Goldhaber SZ, Haire WD, Felstein ML, *et al.*: Alteplase versus heparin in acute pulmonary embolism: randomized trial assessing right ventricular function and pulmonary perfusion. *Lancet* 1993, 341:507–511.

2. Wolfe MW, Lee RT, Feldstein ML, *et al.*: Prognostic significance of right ventricular hypokinesis and perfusion lung scan defects in pulmonary embolism. *Am Heart J* 1994, 127:1371–1375.

3. Stöllberger C, Slany J, Schuster I, *et al.*: The prevalence of deep venous thrombosis in patients with suspected paradoxical embolism. *Ann Intern Med* 1993, 119:461–465.

4. Adler DS: Nonthrombotic pulmonary embolism. *Pulmonary Embolism and Deep Venous Thrombosis.* Edited by Goldhaber SZ. Philadelphia: WB Saunders Co., 1985:209–241.

5. Elliott CG: Pulmonary physiology during pulmonary embolism. *Chest* 1992, 101:163S–171S.

6. Wolfe MW, Skibo LK, Goldhaber SZ: Pulmonary embolic disease: diagnosis, pathophysiologic aspects, and treatment with thrombolytic therapy. *Curr Probl in Cardiol* 1993; 18:585–636.

7. Visner MS, Arentzen CE, O'Connor MJ, *et al.*: Alterations in left ventricular three-dimensional dynamic geometry during acute right ventricular hypertension in the conscious dog. *Circulation* 1983, 67:353–365.

8. Stead RB: Regulation of hemostasis. In *Pulmonary Embolism and Deep Venous Thrombosis.* Edited by Goldhaber SZ. Philadelphia: WB Saunders Co., 1985:27–40.

9. Barritt DW, Jordan SC: Anticoagulant drugs in the treatment of pulmonary embolism: a controlled trial. *Lancet* 1960, 1:1309–1312.

10. Wheeler AP, Jaquiss RDB, Newman JH: Physician practices in the treatment of pulmonary embolism and deep venous thrombosis. *Arch Intern Med* 1988, 148:1321–1325.

11. Basu D, Gallus A, Hirsh J, *et al.*: A prospective study of the value of monitoring heparin treatment with the activated partial thromboplastin time. *N Engl J Med* 1972, 287:324–327.

12. Pineo G, Hull R, Brant R, *et al.*:Introduction of high heparin (H) requirements ("H resistance" as measured by aPTT levels as a predictor of recurrent venous thromboembolism (RVTE) [Abstract]. *Int Angiol* 1994; 13:86.

13. Théry C, Simonneau G, Meyer G, *et al.*: Randomized trial of subcutaneous low-molecular-weight heparin CY 216 (Fraxiparine) compared with intravenous unfractionated heparin in the curative treatment of submassive pulmonary embolism: a dose-ranging study. *Circulation* 1992, 85:1380–1389.

14. Dukes GE Jr, Sanders SW, Russo J, *et al.*: Transaminase elevations in patients receiving bovine or porcine heparin. *Ann Intern Med* 1984, 100:646–650.

15. Ginsberg JS, Kowalchuk G, Hirsh J, *et al.*: Heparin effect on bone density. *Thromb Haemost* 1990, 64:286–289.

16. Hyman BT, Landas SK, Ashman RF, *et al.*: Warfarin-related purple toes syndrome and cholesterol microembolization. *Am J Med* 1987, 82:1233–1237.

17. Tow DE, Wagner NH Jr.: Recovery of pulmonary arterial blood flow in patients with pulmonary embolism. *N Engl J Med* 1967, 276:1053–1059.

18. Urokinase Pulmonary Embolism Trial: a national cooperative study. *Circulation* 1973, 47II:1–108.

19. Alpert JS, Smith R, Carlson J, *et al.*: Mortality in patients treated for pulmonary embolism. *JAMA* 1976, 236:1477–1480.

20. Lilienfeld DE, Godbold JH, Burke GL, *et al.*: Hospitalization and case fatality for pulmonary embolism in the twin cities: 1979-1984. *Am Heart J* 1990, 120:392–395.

21. Carson JL, Kelley MA, Duff A, *et al.*: The clinical course of pulmonary embolism. *N Engl J Med* 1992, 326:1240–1245.

22. Girard P, Mathieu M, Simonneau G, *et al.*: Recurrence of pulmonary embolism during anticoagulant treatment: a prospective study. *Thorax* 1987, 42:481–486.

23. Monréal M, Ruiz J, Salvador R, *et al.*: Recurrent pulmonary embolism: a prospective study. *Chest* 1989, 95:976–979.

24. Goldhaber SZ, Kessler CM, Heit J, *et al.*: Randomized controlled trial of recombinant tissue plasminogen activator versus urokinase in the treatment of acute pulmonary embolism. *Lancet* 1988, 2:293–298.

25. Goldhaber SZ, Kessler CM, Heit JA, *et al.*: Recombinant tissue-type plasminogen activator versus a novel dosing regimen of urokinase in acute pulmonary embolism: a randomized controlled multicenter trial. *J Am Coll Cardiol* 1992, 20:24–30.

26. Verstraete M, Miller GAH, Bounameaux H, *et al.*: Intravenous and intrapulmonary recombinant tissue-type plasminogen activator in the treatment of acute massive pulmonary embolism. *Circulation* 1988, 77:353–360.

27. Goldhaber SZ, Vaughan DE, Markis JE, *et al.*: Acute pulmonary embolism treated with tissue plasminogen activator. *Lancet* 1986, 2:886–889.

28. Goldhaber SZ, Markis JE, Kessler CM, *et al.*: Perspectives on treatment of acute pulmonary embolism with tissue plasminogen activator. *Semin Thromb Hemost* 1987, 13:221–227.

29. Goldhaber SZ, Meyerovitz MF, Markis JE, *et al.* on behalf of the Participating Investigators: Thrombolytic therapy of acute pulmonary embolism: current status and future potential. *J Am Coll Cardiol* 1987, 10:96B–104B.

30. Come PC, Kim D, Parker JA, *et al.* and Participating Investigators: Early reversal of right ventricular dysfunction in patients with acute pulmonary embolism after treatment of intravenous tissue plasminogen activator. *J Am Coll Cardiol* 1987, 10:971–978.

31. Goldhaber SZ, Agnelli G, Levine MN on behalf of the Bolus Alteplase Pulmonary Embolism Group: Reduced dose bolus alteplase vs conventional alteplase infusion for pulmonary embolism thrombolysis. An international multicenter randomized trial. *Chest* 1994, 106:718–724.

32. Dievart F, Fourrier JL, Lefebrvre JM, *et al.*: Treatment of severe pulmonary embolism by means of a high speed rotational catheter (Angiocor thrombolizer): first experience of mechanical thrombolysis in human beings [Abstract]. *J Am Coll Cardiol* 1994, 474A.

33. Brady AJB, Crake T, Oakley CM: Percutaneous catheter fragmentation and distal dispersion of proximal pulmonary embolus. *Lancet* 1991, 338:1186–1189.

34. Essop MR, Middlemost S, Skoularigis J, Sareli P: Simultaneous mechanical clot fragmentation and pharmacologic thrombolysis in acute massive pulmonary embolism. *Am J Cardiol* 1992, 69:427–430.

35. Timsit J-F, Reynaud P, Meyer G, *et al.*: Pulmonary embolectomy by catheter device in massive pulmonary embolism. *Chest* 1991, 100:655–658.

36. Greenfield LJ, Proctor MC, Williams DM, Wakefield TW: Long-term experience with transvenous catheter pulmonary embolectomy. *J Vasc Surg* 1993, 18:450–458.

37. Meyer G, Tamisier D, Sors H, *et al.*: Pulmonary embolectomy: 20-year experience at one center. *Ann Thorac Surg* 1991, 51:232–236.

38. Gulba DC, Schmid C, Borst H-G, *et al.*: Medical compared with surgical treatment for massive pulonary embolism. *Lancet* 1994, 343:565–577.

39. Phifer TJ, Bridges McI, Conrad SA: The residual central venous catheter track–an occult source of lethal air embolism: case report. *J Trauma* 1991, 31:1558–1560.

40. Marcus RH, Weinert L, Neumann A, *et al.*: Venous air embolism: diagnosis of spontaneous right-sided contrast echocardiography. *Chest* 1991, 99:784–785.

41. Guenter CA, Braun TE: Fat embolism syndrome: changing prognosis. *Chest* 1981, 79:143–145.

42. Fabian TC: Unraveling the fat embolism syndrome. *N Engl J Med* 1993, 329:961–963.

43. Goldhaber SZ, Dricker E, Buring JE, *et al.*: Clinical suspicion of autopsy-proven thrombotic and tumor pulmonary embolism in cancer patients. *Am Heart J* 1987, 114:1432–1435.

44. Godleski JJ: Pathology of deep venous thrombosis and pulmonary embolism. In *Pulmonary Embolism and Deep Venous Thrombosis*. Edited by Goldhaber SZ. Philadelphia: WB Saunders Co.; 1985:11–25.

PRIMARY PULMONARY HYPERTENSION

4

CHAPTER

Richard N. Channick

Primary pulmonary hypertension (PPH) is a disorder characterized by chronic elevation in pulmonary vascular resistance because of derangements in either small pulmonary arteries or veins, in the absence of another underlying cardiac or pulmonary disease. Histopathologically, several lesions have been described in PPH: medial hypertrophy of small pulmonary arteries, intimal fibrosis, plexiform lesions, thrombotic lesions, and veno-occlusive lesions. These lesions are not specific to PPH; however, they are recognized in several secondary forms of pulmonary hypertension.

Primary pulmonary hypertension is an uncommon disease, although the exact incidence is unknown. The disease often presents during the third or fourth decade of life. A preponderance in women (1.7:1) has been consistently noted. The precise etiology of PPH is unknown, although associations with exogenous agents [1–3], collagen vascular diseases [4], portal hypertension [5], other autoimmune disorders, and infection with the human immunodeficiency virus [6] have all been recognized. It is likely that PPH is the common end result of a variety of insults to the pulmonary vasculature.

Arriving at the correct diagnosis of PPH requires a high index of suspicion and an orderly diagnostic approach. Dyspnea is the most common presenting symptom, reported in virtually all patients with PPH. Chest pain, easy fatiguability, syncope, hemoptysis, and cough are also common symptoms. Physical examination reveals signs of pulmonary hypertension and, often, overt right heart failure, including elevated jugular venous pressure with prominent V waves, accentuation of the pulmonic component of the second heart sound with fixed splitting, a right-sided precordial lift, S_3, a murmur of tricuspid regurgitation, hepatomegaly, ascites, and peripheral edema.

The diagnostic evaluation of patients with suspected PPH is aimed at excluding secondary causes of pulmonary hypertension. The recommended algorithm includes pulmonary function tests, arterial blood gases, echocardiography, ventilation/perfusion lung scanning, pulmonary angiography, and cardiac catheterization. With these studies, one can eliminate restrictive or obstructive parenchymal lung diseases, hypoventilation syndromes, thromboembolic disease, and congenital heart disease as diagnostic considerations, and arrive at PPH as the diagnosis.

The natural history of PPH is generally unfavorable, with median survival less than 3 years from the time of diagnosis. Outcome is strongly influenced by the magnitude of right heart failure. Treatment includes both supportive (O_2, diuretics, digoxin, warfarin) and more definitive (vasodilators, transplantation) interventions. Approximately 30% of patients with PPH will demonstrate a significant reduction in pulmonary hypertension in response to vasodilators. Patients who respond acutely to these agents appear to have a substantially improved survival compared with nonresponders. The most commonly used vasodilators are oral calcium channel blocking agents; intravenous prostacyclin and inhaled nitric oxide also appear to have promise as chronic vasodilators. Finally, lung transplantation offers a viable option for patients with PPH who do not respond to vasodilators. Single lung transplantation appears to be adequate for restoring right heart function and improving functional status, although the effect of lung transplantation on long-term survival in PPH is not yet known.

BACKGROUND AND EPIDEMIOLOGY

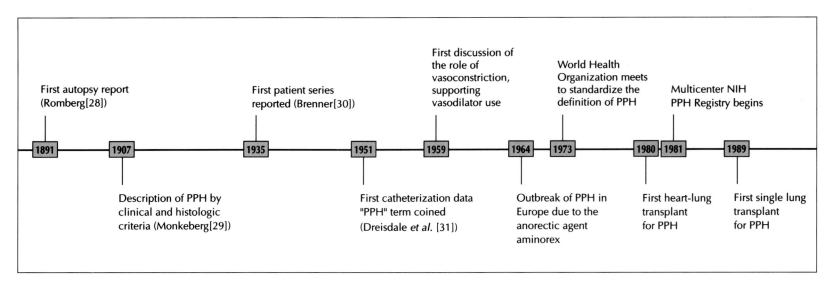

FIGURE 4-1. Major developments in the history of PPH. The advent of catheterization of the right side of the heart led to the evolution of thought about the disease from that of autopsy curiosity to pathophysiologic entity. NIH—National Institutes of Health.

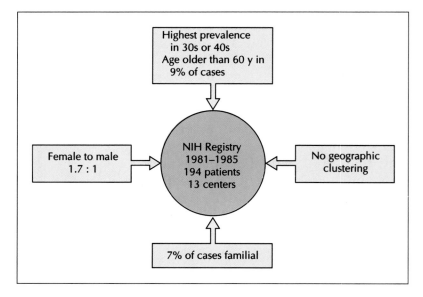

FIGURE 4-2. Epidemiologic characteristics of PPH. These data were obtained through a multicenter National Institutes of Health (NIH) Registry that collected information on 194 patients with PPH between 1981 and 1985 [7]. A female preponderance was seen, although less than previously cited. Twelve percent of patients were black; in that group, the female to male ratio was 4:1. No geographic clusters were found within the United States, but a familial tendency was noted: 7% of the cases were familial. An autosomal-dominant transmission mode with variable penetrance has been hypothesized in familial cases [8].

HISTOPATHOLOGY

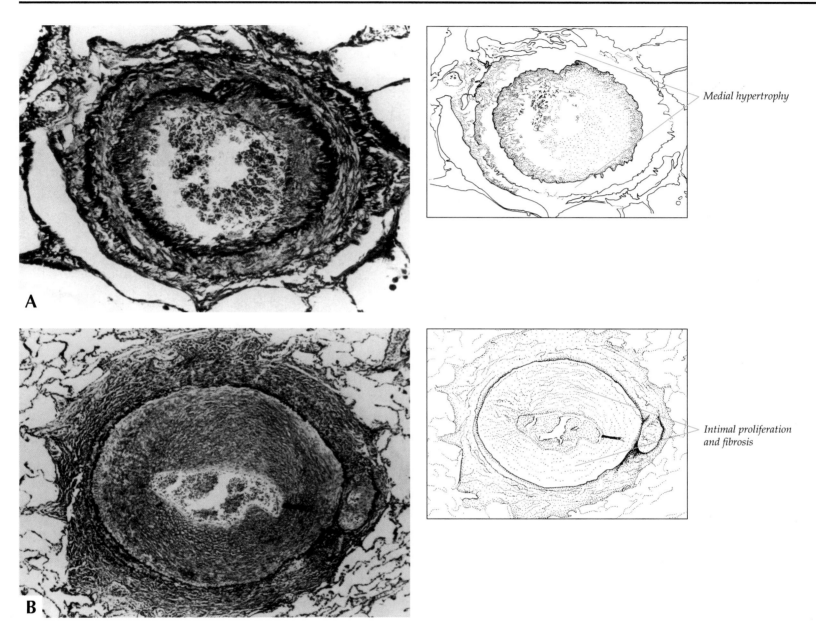

Medial hypertrophy

Intimal proliferation
and fibrosis

FIGURE 4-3. Histopathologic features of PPH. Several lesions have been identified in patients with PPH. **A,** Hypertrophy of the medial layer of muscular arteries is seen to some degree in virtually all cases of PPH. Medial hypertrophy is present in all forms of pulmonary hypertension and probably correlates with the degree of pulmonary arterial pressure elevation. Medial hypertrophy is generally considered a reversible lesion. **B,** Cellular proliferation and concentric fibrosis in the intima. Intimal proliferation may be a primary process or secondary to endothelial cell damage and release of growth factors. Intimal fibrosis may lead to complete obliteration of the vessel lumen. (*continued*)

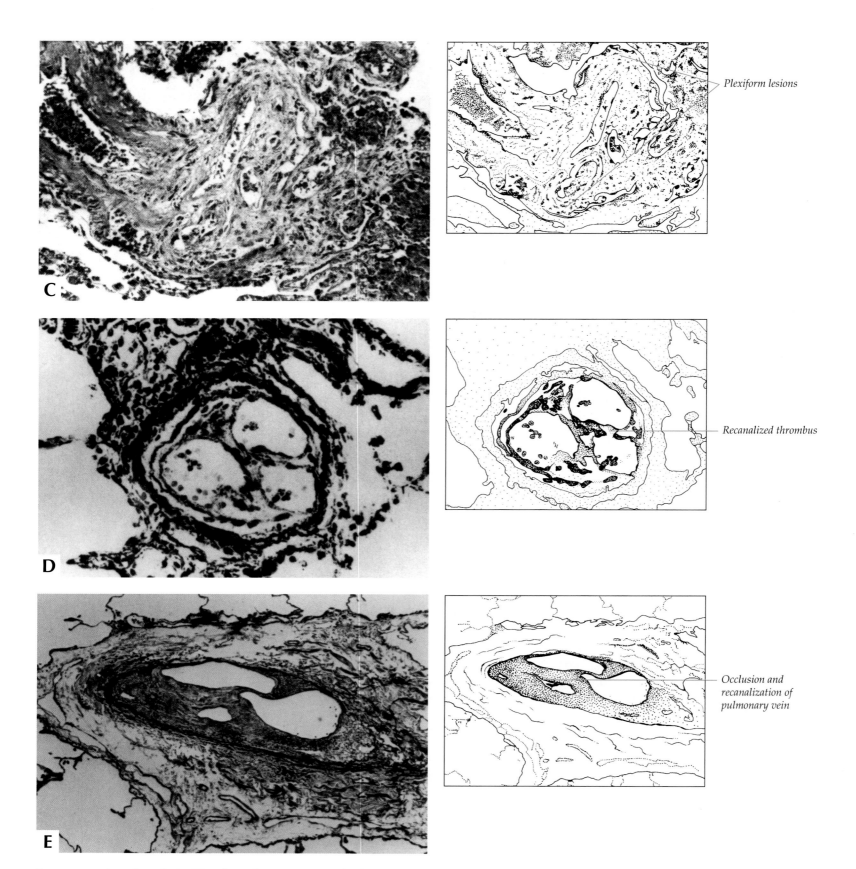

FIGURE 4-3. (*continued*) **C,** Plexiform lesions are multichanneled outpouchings from muscular arterial walls, typically occurring in association with concentric intimal fibrosis. The mechanisms leading to plexiform lesions are not known; they may represent part of the proliferative repair process [9]. Plexiform lesions are not specific to PPH; they have been observed in other forms of precapillary pulmonary hypertension, including chronic thromboembolic disease [10]. **D,** Thrombotic lesions. Organized micro-thrombi with eccentric intimal fibrosis probably represent thrombi in situ due to local hypercoagulability and endothelial damage. These lesions must be distinguished from thromboembolic lesions occurring in large pulmonary arteries. **E,** Pulmonary veno-occlusive disease (PVOD). Arterialization, intimal fibrosis, and occlusion of a pulmonary vein are present. Medial hypertrophy and intimal changes on the arterial side are also seen in PVOD.

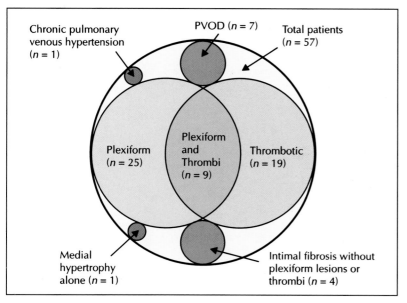

FIGURE 4-4. Frequency of histopathologic lesions in PPH seen in 57 patients in the National Institutes of Health Registry [11]; samples were obtained either by biopsy or at autopsy. The "plexiform" group was characterized by concentric and eccentric intimal fibrosis, and plexiform lesions. The "thrombotic" group was characterized by eccentric intimal fibrosis with recanalized thrombi and no plexiform lesions. Significant overlap between the two groups was found: nine of 25 patients with plexiform lesions also had recanalized thrombi present. Patients with either plexiform lesions or pulmonary veno-occlusive disease (PVOD) had worse survival rates than the thrombotic group. However, no significant hemodynamic differences existed between the groups at the time of presentation. It is likely that the various lesions seen in PPH represent both different stages of the disease and variable responses (*eg*, cellular fibrosis, thrombosis, proliferation) to the same pathogenetic insult.

PATHOGENESIS

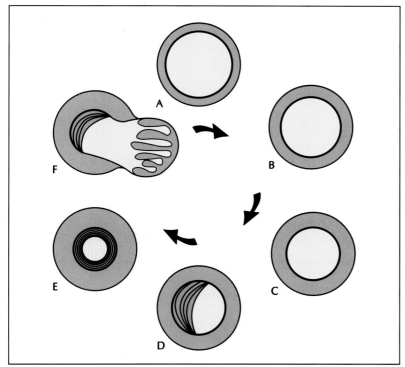

FIGURE 4-5. One potential explanation for the pathogenesis of intimal fibrosis and plexiform lesions is vasoconstriction. Vasoconstriction leads to progressive medial hypertrophy (A, B, C) and elevated pulmonary artery pressure. Elevated pulmonary artery pressure results in endothelial damage and intimal proliferation (D) with concentric fibrosis (E). Plexiform lesions then develop from intimal scarring as part of the repair process (F). A significant role for vasoconstriction in the pathogenesis of PPH is likely in some patients; this group typically responds to vasodilators. The absence of vasoreactivity in the majority of patients with PPH, however, suggests that either 1) PPH can develop as a primary proliferative and fibrotic process without a vasoconstrictive phase or 2) the disease progresses from one of predominantly vasoconstriction and medial hypertrophy to structural lesions that are irreversible. Which of these explanations is most accurate is not known. (*Adapted from* Rich [12]; with permission.)

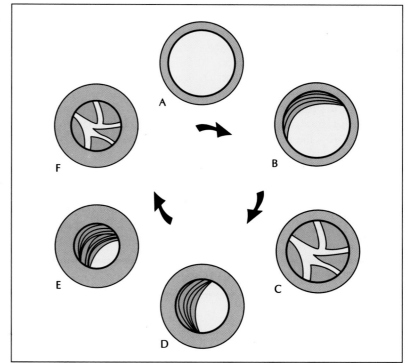

FIGURE 4-6. Development of "thrombotic" lesions (A through F). An initial endothelial defect leads to eccentric intimal fibrosis (B) and thrombosis in situ with recanalization (C). Progressive narrowing of the vessel lumen occurs with resultant elevation in pulmonary artery pressure and secondary medial hypertrophy. The term "thrombotic" may be misleading; this histopathologic entity must be distinguished from the clinical syndrome of proximal thromboembolic disease; the pathogenesis, clinical course, and treatment are entirely different. It should be noted that microscopic evidence for recanalized thrombus may also be seen in proximal thromboembolic pulmonary hypertension. (*Adapted from* Rich [12]; with permission.)

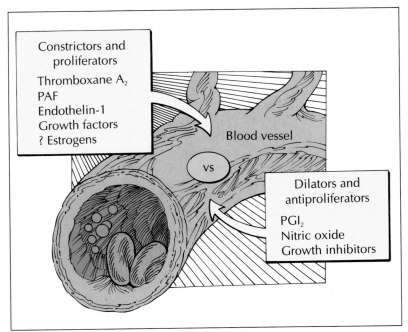

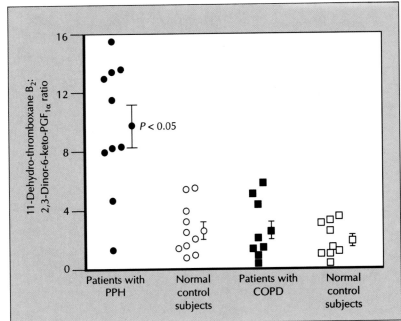

FIGURE 4-7. Potential mediators involved in the pathogenesis and maintenance of PPH. In the normal, high-flow, low-resistance pulmonary vascular bed, a favorable balance exists between endogenous vasodilators (*eg*, PGI_2 [13], nitric oxide [14]) and vasoconstrictors (*eg*, endothelin [15], thromboxane A_2, platelet activating factor [PAF] [16]), and antiproliferators (*eg*, heparin-like substances, nitric oxide) and proliferators (*eg*, platelet-derived growth factor). In response to some insult such as endothelial damage, the balance may change to favor vasoconstriction and cell proliferation. This results in further endothelial damage, thrombosis, and self-perpetuation of the proliferative, constrictive, fibrotic, and thrombotic process and, thus, the clinical syndrome of PPH. Individual susceptibility also likely plays some role in the development of PPH.

FIGURE 4-8. Demonstration of an increase in the ratio of urinary thromboxane A_2 metabolites to PGI_2 metabolites in patients with PPH. An increase in this ratio would favor vasoconstriction, platelet aggregation, and cell proliferation. As with other mediators, the alterations in thromboxane A_2 and PGI_2 may represent an important pathogenetic derangement, or it may merely be a marker of the disease. *T-bars* represent SEM. COPD—chronic obstructive pulmonary disease. (*Adapted from* Christman and coworkers [13]; with permission.)

CLINICAL FEATURES AND DIAGNOSIS

CLINICAL MANIFESTATIONS

SYMPTOMS IN PRIMARY PULMONARY HYPERTENSION

Dyspnea	Palpitations
Chest pain	Syncope
Easy fatiguability	Leg swelling
Cough	Hemoptysis

FIGURE 4-9. Common symptoms in PPH. Dyspnea is the presenting symptom in over 60% of cases and is present, at some stage in the disease, in virtually all patients [17]. The mechanisms of dyspnea in PPH are not clear; activation of pulmonary artery stretch receptors, parasympathetic activation, and impaired cardiac function have all been suggested as possible causes of dyspnea in these patients. Chest pain may be nonspecific or due to right ventricular ischemia. A persistent dry cough can be debilitating to some patients. Syncope is more common in the latter stage of the disease; mechanisms of syncope in these individuals include arrhythmias and sudden decreases in right ventricular preload such as those produced by coughing or the Valsalva maneuver.

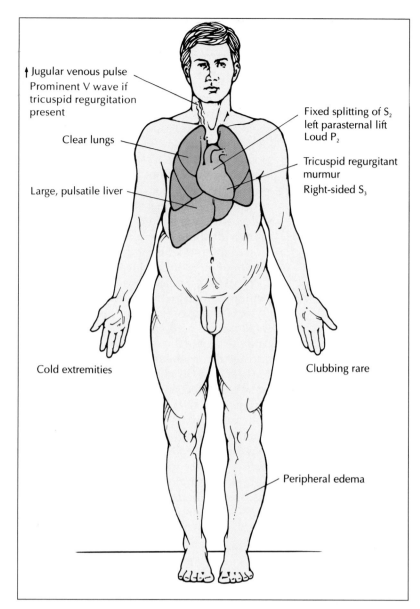

Figure 4-10 labels:
- ↑ Jugular venous pulse Prominent V wave if tricuspid regurgitation present
- Clear lungs
- Large, pulsatile liver
- Cold extremities
- Fixed splitting of S₂ left parasternal lift Loud P₂
- Tricuspid regurgitant murmur Right-sided S₃
- Clubbing rare
- Peripheral edema

FIGURE 4-10. Common signs in PPH. These findings are nonspecific signs present in patients with pulmonary hypertension from any cause. Of note, physical examination can help to exclude secondary pulmonary hypertension (*eg,* the absence of clubbing makes congenital heart disease with Eisenmenger's physiology less likely; an unremarkable lung examination argues against parenchymal lung disease.)

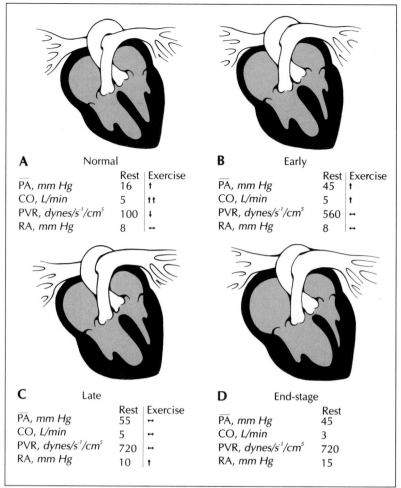

A Normal

	Rest	Exercise
$\overline{PA}$, *mm Hg*	16	↑
CO, *L/min*	5	↑↑
PVR, *dynes/s⁻¹/cm⁵*	100	↓
RA, *mm Hg*	8	↔

B Early

	Rest	Exercise
$\overline{PA}$, *mm Hg*	45	↑
CO, *L/min*	5	↑
PVR, *dynes/s⁻¹/cm⁵*	560	↔
RA, *mm Hg*	8	↔

C Late

	Rest	Exercise
$\overline{PA}$, *mm Hg*	55	↔
CO, *L/min*	5	↔
PVR, *dynes/s⁻¹/cm⁵*	720	↔
RA, *mm Hg*	10	↑

D End-stage

	Rest
$\overline{PA}$, *mm Hg*	45
CO, *L/min*	3
PVR, *dynes/s⁻¹/cm⁵*	720
RA, *mm Hg*	15

FIGURE 4-11. The pathophysiology of PPH. **A,** In the normal pulmonary vascular bed, pulmonary vascular resistance (PVR) is low at rest. With exercise, cardiac output (CO) rises substantially. However, because the normal pulmonary vascular bed is quite distensible and closed vascular beds can be recruited, pulmonary artery pressure ($\overline{PA}$) rises only modestly. Calculated PVR, therefore, decreases with exercise. **B,** In early PPH, $\overline{PA}$ and PVR rise. There is some loss of vascular recruitment and distensibility; thus, PVR does not decrease normally with exercise. Cardiac reserve, however, is still adequate and the heart responds to exercise. These patients are generally only minimally symptomatic. **C,** With more advanced disease, cardiac reserve becomes impaired. CO remains normal at rest, but does not increase appropriately with exercise. These patients have significant exertional symptoms, but not overt right-sided heart failure. **D,** In end-stage PPH, resting CO is reduced, and signs of right ventricular failure are present. With the reduction in CO, $\overline{PA}$ may actually decrease at this stage, although this obviously does not represent improvement in the disease. RA—right atrial pressure.

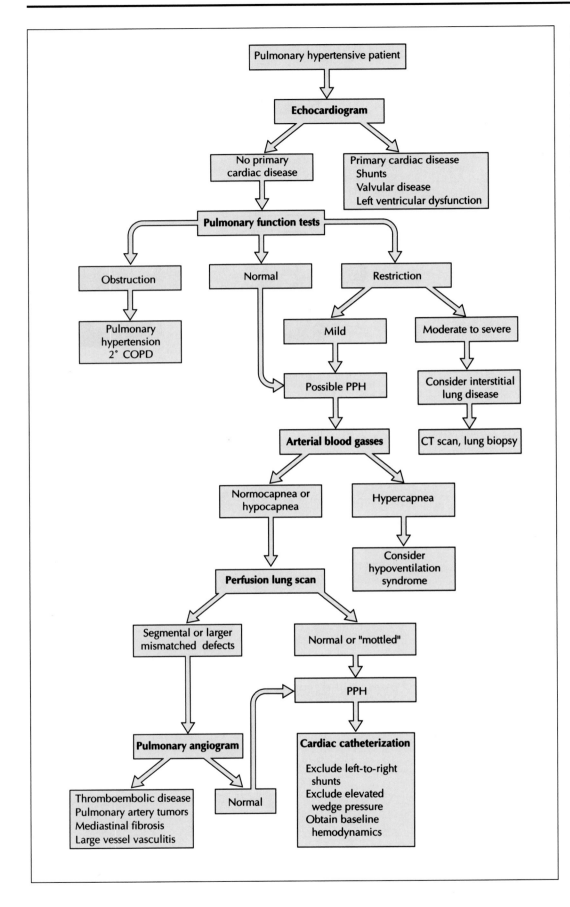

FIGURE 4-12. Diagnostic approach. An orderly approach with the stepwise elimination of possible secondary causes can yield the diagnosis of PPH with a high degree of accuracy. Important diagnostic points include the following. 1) Interstitial lung disease does not lead to significant pulmonary hypertension unless quite severe (lung volumes < 50%); therefore, mild restriction should not lead the clinician to attribute the pulmonary hypertension to interstitial lung disease. In the National Institutes of Health Registry of PPH, in fact, a mild restrictive defect was common, with an average total lung capacity of 80% of predicted in these individuals. 2) Although perfusion lung scans may underestimate the degree of obstruction in chronic thromboembolic pulmonary hypertension [18], the absence of *any* segmental or larger defects is highly accurate in distinguishing PPH from chronic thromboembolic pulmonary hypertension [19]. 3) In a small number of cases, uncertainty will remain, even following pulmonary angiography. In these instances, we have found pulmonary angioscopy to be useful in assessing the proximal vascular bed. COPD—chronic obstructive pulmonary disease; CT—computed tomography.

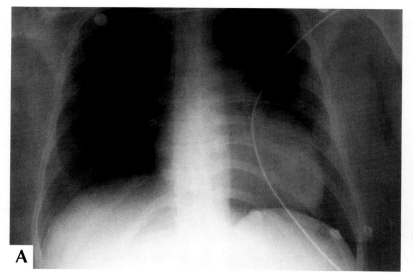

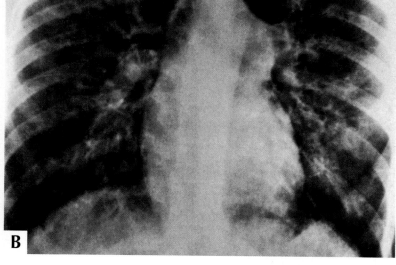

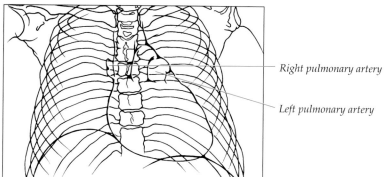

Right pulmonary artery

Left pulmonary artery

FIGURE 4-13. Chest radiographs. **A**, Classic PPH. Right-sided cardiomegaly is clearly present. Bilateral enlargement of the proximal pulmonary arteries, with rapid "pruning" of vessels, is noted. Peripheral lung fields appear hypolucent. **B**, Pulmonary veno-occlusive disease. Cardiomegaly and pulmonary artery enlargement are also noted. In addition, diffuse interstitial edema is present. The constellation of right ventricular and pulmonary artery enlargement, interstitial edema, and the absence of mitral stenosis or left atrial problems is highly suggestive of pulmonary veno-occlusive disease.

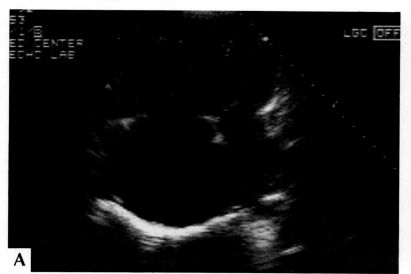

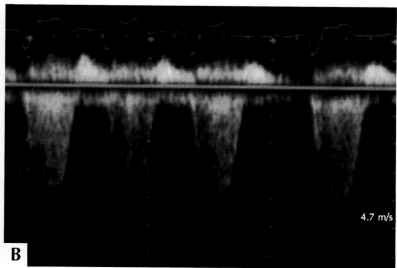

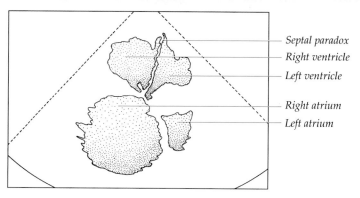

Septal paradox
Right ventricle
Left ventricle
Right atrium
Left atrium

FIGURE 4-14. A, Echocardiogram of a patient with PPH. The typical echocardiogram of a patient with PPH demonstrates enlargement of the right atrium (RA) and right ventricle, and a normal or reduced left ventricular chamber size. Reversal of the normal septal curvature, indicating right ventricular pressure overload, is also seen. An inverse relationship between pulmonary vascular resistance and left ventricular internal dimension has been found [7]. **B**, Doppler ultrasound of the tricuspid regurgitant jet in a patient with PPH. The peak flow velocity (v) correlates with a pulmonary artery systolic pressure of $4v^2$ + RA pressure; in the illustrated case: pulmonary artery systolic = $4(4.7)^2$ + RA or 88 mm Hg + RA.

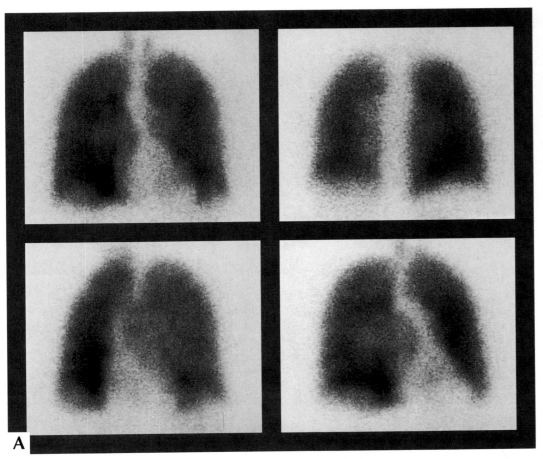

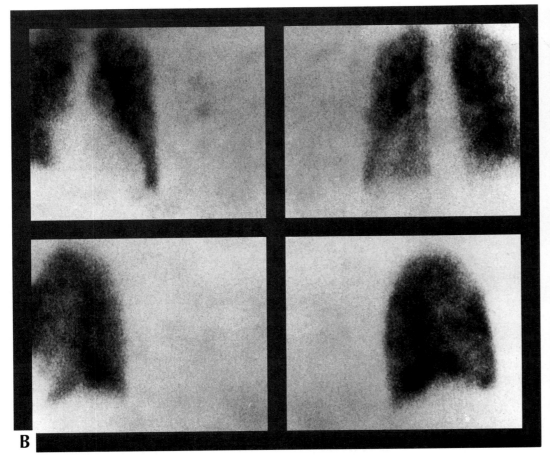

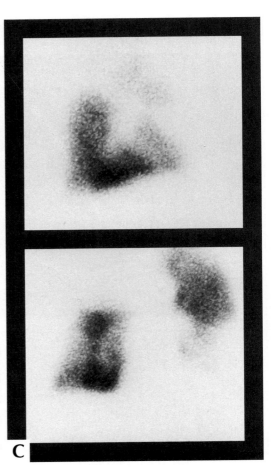

FIGURE 4-15. Perfusion lung scan patterns in PPH. The perfusion scan can be normal (*panel A*) or can demonstrate a "mottled" appearance, with multiple, diffuse, small defects (*panel B*). This scan is in clear contrast to the patient with chronic thromboembolic pulmonary hypertension (*panel C*), in whom segmental or larger, usually multiple, mismatched perfusion defects are seen. Perfusion scanning is entirely safe in patients with even very severe pulmonary hypertension and is a mandatory step in the evaluation of these patients.

A

B

C

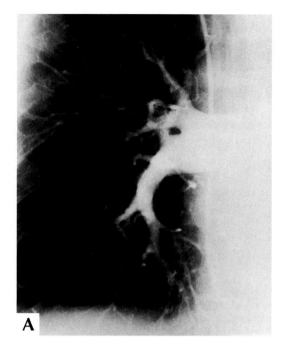

A

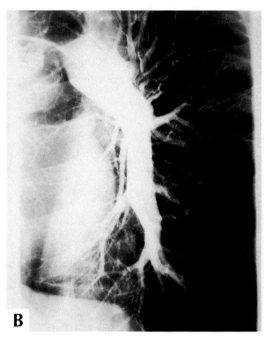

B

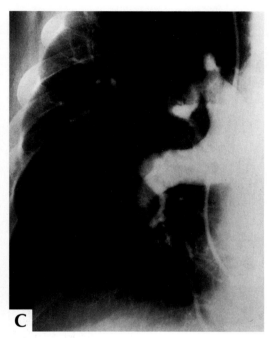

C

FIGURE 4-16. Pulmonary angiograms. **A**, The normal angiogram demonstrates a diffuse branching pattern with smoothly tapering vessels and branches leading to the periphery of the lung. **B**, In PPH, pulmonary angiography demonstrates marked "pruning" of small vessels with absent peripheral flow. No segmental or larger vascular abnormalities are noted. **C**, In contrast, the angiogram in a patient with chronic thromboembolic pulmonary hypertension characteristically demonstrates proximal pulmonary artery irregularity, abnormal narrowing of the proximal vessel, and large areas with absent flow. PA—pulmonary artery.

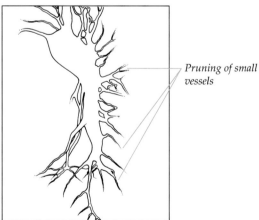

Pruning of small vessels

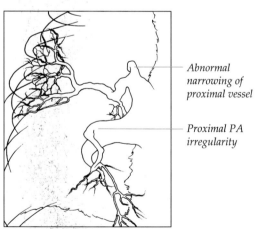

Abnormal narrowing of proximal vessel

Proximal PA irregularity

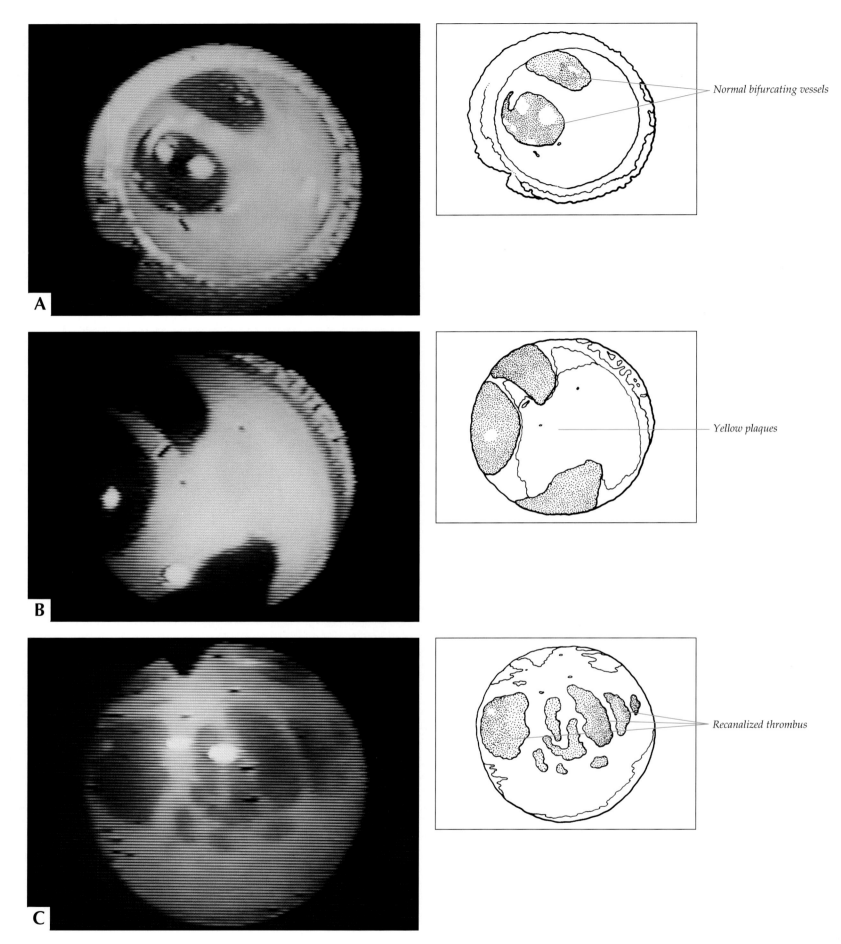

FIGURE 4-17. Pulmonary angioscopy. The segmental and lobar vessels are visualized through the wall of a clear balloon attached to a fiberoptic scope. **A**, The vessel wall is normally smooth and glistening; normal bifurcating vessels are seen. **B**, In PPH, yellow plaques on the vessel wall may be visualized; this finding is a nonspecific manifestation of elevated pulmonary artery pressure. **C**, In chronic thromboembolic pulmonary hypertension, marked irregularity of the vessel wall with evidence of recanalized thrombus is noted in a lobar vessel.

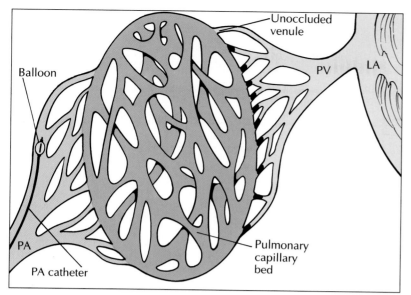

FIGURE 4-18. Pathophysiology of pulmonary veno-occlusive disease. Thrombotic or fibrotic obstruction of small pulmonary veins and venules results in interstitial pulmonary edema and secondary pulmonary arterial (PA) changes. On catheterization of the right side of the heart, wedge pressure will be elevated if the catheter is in an obstructed segment. However, if the pulmonary artery catheter is placed into a vascular segment containing an unobstructed vein, the wedge pressure will accurately reflect left atrial (LA) pressure. Therefore, multiple wedge pressure measurements in several sites are useful when considering a diagnosis of pulmonary veno-occlusive disease. PV—pulmonary vein.

NATURAL HISTORY AND PROGNOSIS

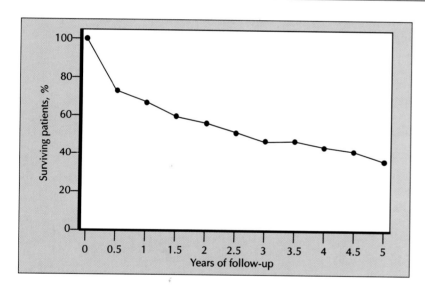

FIGURE 4-19. The natural history of PPH, from the National Institutes of Health Registry. Median survival was 2.9 years, with 5-year survival less than 40% [20]. Right ventricular failure accounted for 63% of deaths, and sudden death, 7%. Despite the generally poor clinical course, a subgroup of patients manifest survival of 10 years or more; and there are isolated reports of patients surviving more than 20 years with documented PPH.

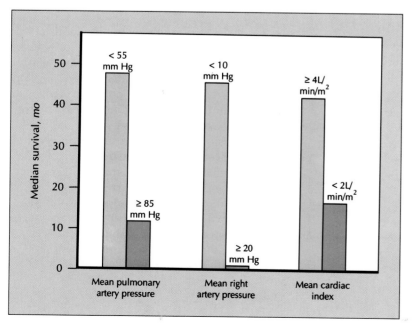

FIGURE 4-20. Variables most strongly correlating with survival are right atrial pressure, mean pulmonary arterial pressure, and cardiac index. Right atrial pressure is consistently the strongest single predictor of survival. In addition, functional classification, mixed venous oxygen saturation, and response to vasodilators are predictors of outcome. An equation has been derived to predict survival in the individual patient:

$$P(t) = [H(t)]^{A(x,y,z)}$$
$$H(t) = [0.88 - 0.14t + 0.01t^2]$$
$$A(x,y,z) = e^{(0.007325x + 0.0526y - 0.3275z)}$$

where $P(t)$ represents a patient's chance of survival at t years; x is mean pulmonary arterial pressure; y is mean atrial pressure; and z is cardiac index. This equation has been validated in prospective studies, and is useful in informing a patient of his or her outlook and in assessing the effectiveness of various interventions on survival. (*Adapted from* D'Alonzo and coworkers [20]; with permission.)

TREATMENT

OVERVIEW

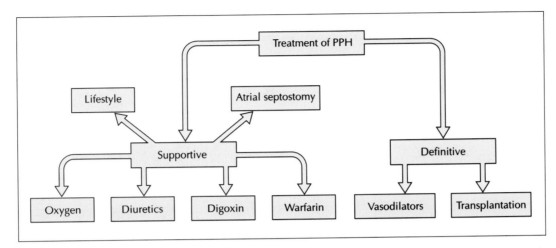

FIGURE 4-21. Treatment options in PPH. Therapeutic interventions may be supportive if aimed at symptomatic relief, or "definitive" if significant survival prolongation is possible; no treatment in PPH is truly curative. Limitation of activity is strongly recommended; even low levels of exertion can result in inadequate cardiac output and worsening of pulmonary hypertension. Also, pregnancy is contraindicated; numerous reports have described decompensation in PPH patients who become pregnant. Oxygen therapy is not generally useful, as most patients are not hypoxemic. However, some patients will demonstrate significant oxygen desaturation upon exercising, due to impaired cardiac reserve. In this group, supplemental oxygen is indicated. Diuretics are useful in relieving symptoms of right-sided heart failure, such as hepatic congestion, ascites, and peripheral edema. These agents, however, must be used with extreme caution, as the right ventricle is quite preload-dependent in these patients and precipitous reductions in intravascular volume can be hazardous. The efficacy of digoxin in right ventricular failure is unproven; some authors, however, recommend its use, especially in patients receiving vasodilators with negative inotropic properties [21]. (*See following* for discussion of warfarin, atrial septostomy, vasodilators, and transplantation).

VASODILATORS

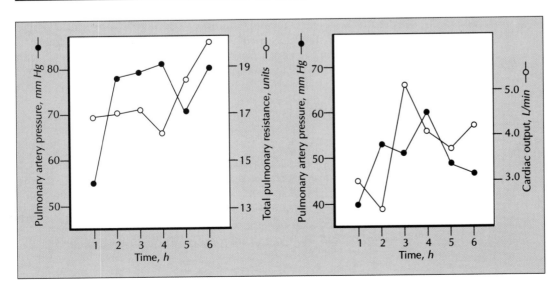

FIGURE 4-22. Significant spontaneous fluctuations in pulmonary artery pressure, cardiac output, and pulmonary vascular resistance are demonstrated in two patients with PPH. This phenomenon is important to consider when evaluating the response to vasodilators in PPH. Based on the substantial spontaneous variability that is observed in these measurements, it has been demonstrated that at least a 22% decrease in pulmonary artery pressure and a 36% decrease in pulmonary vascular resistance must occur to attribute an effect to a vasodilator drug and not to chance alone. (*Adapted from* Rich and coworkers [22]; with permission.)

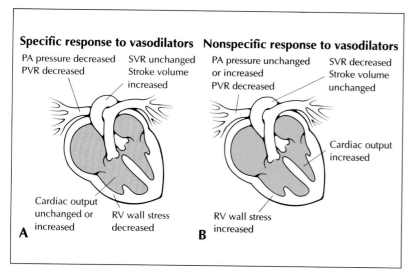

Specific response to vasodilators

PA pressure decreased
PVR decreased

SVR unchanged
Stroke volume increased

Cardiac output unchanged or increased

RV wall stress decreased

A

Nonspecific response to vasodilators

PA pressure unchanged or increased
PVR decreased

SVR decreased
Stroke volume unchanged

Cardiac output increased

RV wall stress increased

B

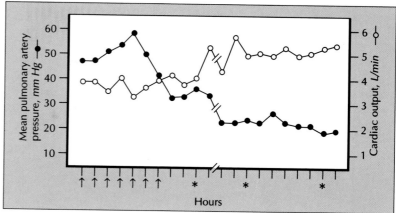

FIGURE 4-24. The response to nifedipine in one patient with PPH. Twenty milligrams of nifedipine was given every hour (*arrows*) until a fall in pulmonary artery pressure occurred. This graph demonstrates that extremely high doses of oral calcium channel blockers are often required to elicit a favorable hemodynamic response. Patients who respond to high doses of calcium channel blockers generally tolerate these doses surprisingly well, with minimal side effects. Intravenous prostacyclin, PGE_1, hydralazine, and adenosine have also been used acutely to test for vasoresponsiveness in PPH. It is mandatory that patients being tested initially for vasodilator responsiveness be studied in a monitored setting with a pulmonary artery catheter in place. *Asterisks* represent repeated doses of nifedipine (120 mg). (*Adapted from* Rich [12]; with permission.)

FIGURE 4-23. Two hemodynamic responses that can occur with vasodilator therapy. **A**, Vasodilator treatment results in dilation of the pulmonary arterial bed. This results in decreased pulmonary artery (PA) pressure and pulmonary vascular resistance (PVR), decreased right ventricular (RV) afterload, decreased septal compression of the left ventricle, and improved cardiac performance. This is a favorable response to vasodilators, and occurs in approximately 25% of patients with PPH. **B**, A more common response to systemic vasodilators, seen in at least 50% of patients. In these patients, vasodilators also lead to reduction in calculated PVR. However, this decrement in PVR is due to a rise in cardiac output secondary to systemic vasodilatation. In this case, PA pressure remains the same or even increases. Thus, RV afterload remains high and RV preload increases; this response will lead to increased RV wall stress, worsening left ventricular compression, systemic hypotension, and, often, worsened symptoms. A fall in PA pressure *in addition to* a fall in PVR should, therefore, be observed to classify a patient as having a favorable response to systemic vasodilators. SVR—systemic vascular resistance.

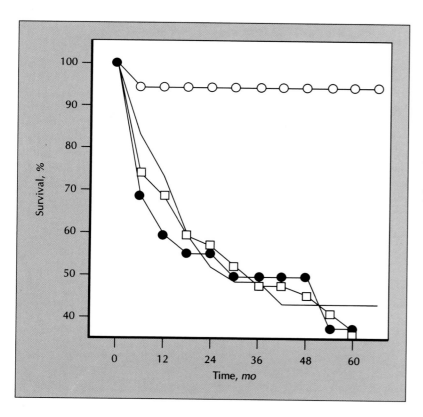

FIGURE 4-25. Survival curves in patients who responded acutely to calcium channel blockers (nifedipine or diltiazem) and were continued on treatment with one of these agents (*open circles*), compared with patients in the same study who did not respond favorably to calcium channel blockers (*solid line*), patients from the NIH Registry treated at the study institution (*solid circles*), and patients in the NIH Registry Cohort (*open squares*). This is the first evidence of improved survival with long-term pharmacologic therapy for PPH. The group that responded to calcium channel blockers also had a sustained reduction in pulmonary arterial pressure, pulmonary vascular resistance, and right ventricular chamber size diameter; symptoms were significantly alleviated. (*Adapted from* Rich and coworkers [23]; with permission.)

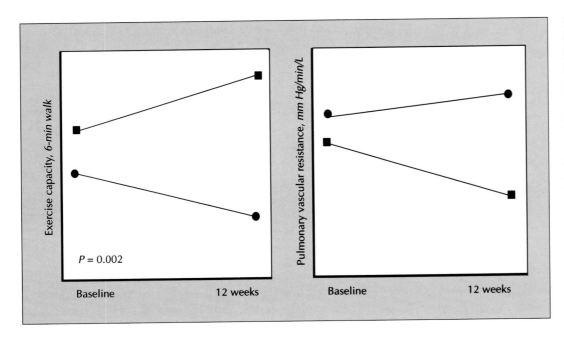

FIGURE 4-26. Hemodynamic and clinical effects of chronic prostacyclin infusions [24]. Patients from several centers were randomly assigned to receive either conventional therapy plus prostacyclin (*closed squares*) or conventional therapy alone (*closed circles*). Prostacyclin was delivered via an infusion pump through an indwelling Hickman catheter. At 12 weeks, exercise capacity, pulmonary arterial pressure, pulmonary vascular resistance, and cardiac output were improved in the prostacyclin group. Survival was also greater in patients receiving prostacyclin. Of interest, the improvements seen in the prostacyclin group were not predicted by the short-term response to this agent. Several patients who had little hemodynamic response during the acute infusion improved significantly over the 12-week period. The mechanisms underlying this disparity are not clear.

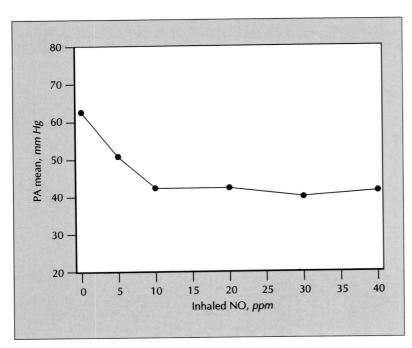

FIGURE 4-27. Dose-response curve for inhaled nitric oxide (NO) in a patient with PPH. A significant reduction in pulmonary (PA) pressure occurred with as little as 5 ppm of NO gas. When delivered by inhalation, NO has been found to be a potent vasodilator that is entirely selective for the pulmonary vascular bed. No adverse symptoms or systemic hemodynamic effects have been seen in 16 patients with PPH studied by the author (Channick, unpublished data). Similar to responses found with other vasodilators, approximately 30% of patients have had favorable responses to inhaled NO; the remainder presumably have "fixed" vascular disease.

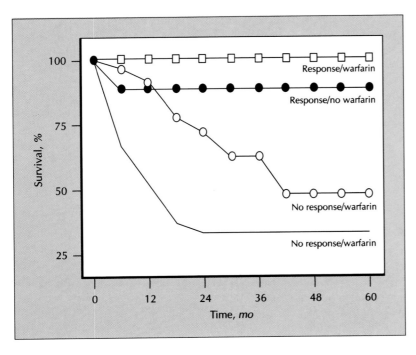

FIGURE 4-28. Survival in patients with PPH treated with warfarin. In the group of patients who did not respond favorably to oral calcium channel blockers, those who were on warfarin had a significantly better survival than the nonresponders who were not maintained on warfarin. This was not a controlled study; definitive conclusions cannot be made. In the responder group, warfarin had no effect on survival, although overall survival was excellent in this group, independent of warfarin therapy. Most authors now recommend anticoagulant therapy in patients with PPH. (*Adapted from* Rich and coworkers [23]; with permission.)

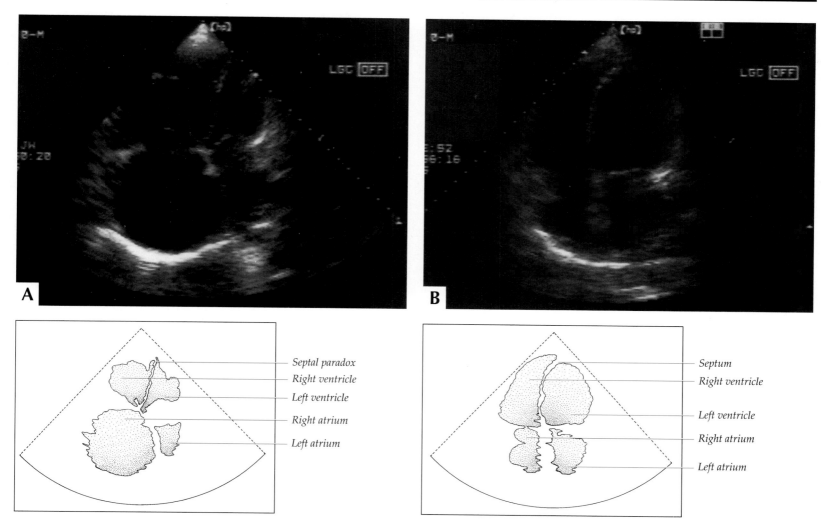

FIGURE 4-29. Echocardiogram before (*panel A*) and after (*panel B*) single lung transplantation in a patient with PPH. Right ventricular (RV) internal dimension decreased markedly with resolution of septal paradox. This underlines the point that single lung transplantation in PPH, even in the setting of severe RV dysfunction, is successful in reversing RV failure; heart-lung transplantation is not necessary.

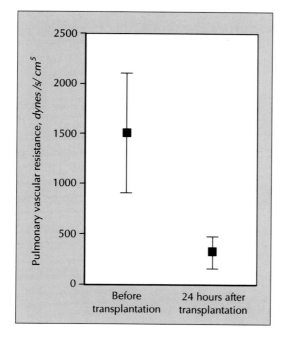

FIGURE 4-30. Pulmonary vascular resistance before and 24 hours after single lung transplantation in seven patients with PPH (UCSD Medical Center experience, unpublished data). Single lung transplantation generally leads to immediate, significant reductions in pulmonary arterial pressure and pulmonary vascular resistance. Most patients have returned to class I or II New York Heart Association functional status. Complications following single lung transplantation include infection, acute rejection, stenosis at the bronchial anastomotic site, and bronchiolitis obliterans. Recurrence of PPH in the transplanted lung has not occurred. Survival at 1 year (all US centers combined) is approximately 60% [25]; longer survival data are not yet available. Which patients with PPH should be referred for lung transplantation is still not entirely clear. It is generally felt that patients with significant functional impairment who do not respond to vasodilators but who have not yet developed severe right ventricular failure (hepatic dysfunction, refractory ascites) are appropriate potential candidates for single lung transplantation.

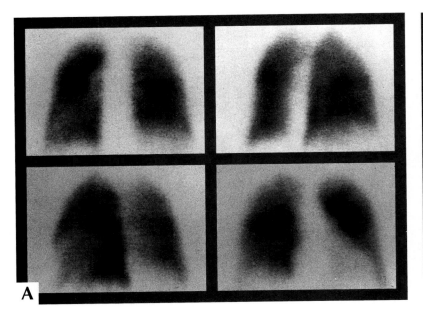
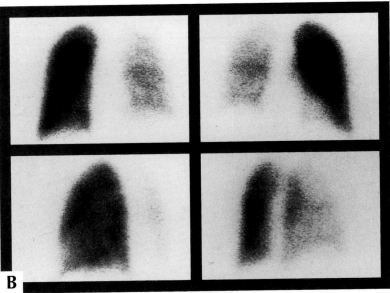

FIGURE 4-31. Perfusion lung scans before (*panel A*) and 1 month after (*panel B*) single lung transplantation in one PPH patient. Following transplantation, perfusion shifts almost entirely to the transplanted lung (low vascular resistance bed). This blood flow imbalance results in an increase in alveolar dead space (the native lung is ventilated but not perfused) and, thus, minute ventilation requirements increase. This derangement in the ventilation-perfusion ratio might be expected to lead to increased perceived dyspnea. However, the improvement in cardiac function that occurs after single lung transplantation more than outweighs the increase in dead space and, therefore, dyspnea is markedly improved.

ATRIAL SEPTOSTOMY

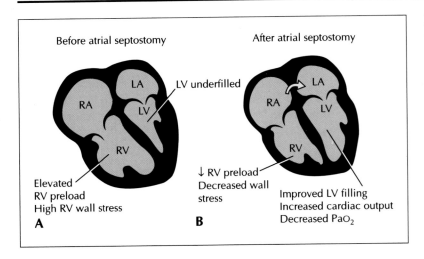

FIGURE 4-32. Physiologic effects of balloon atrial septostomy. In end-stage PPH, the right ventricle (RV) is massively dilated and under great wall stress; the left ventricle (LV) is severely underfilled. Cardiac output is often reduced to the point of prerenal azotemia, cerebral hypoperfusion, and metabolic acidosis. By creating a small atrial septal defect, blood will be shunted to the left side of the heart. This will result in decreased RV preload and wall stress, increased left ventricular filling, and improved cardiac output. Of course, right-to-left shunting will also occur, leading to a decrease in arterial oxygen content. However, if the improvement in cardiac output is significant enough, oxygen delivery will increase. The size of the septostomy created is critical; too small a defect will have no significant effect; too large a defect will lead to refractory hypoxemia. A septostomy of approximately 8 to 10 mm is generally recommended. LA—left atrium; PaO_2—partial pressure of oxygen, arterial; RA—right atrium.

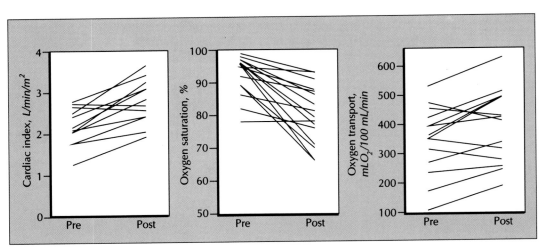

FIGURE 4-33. Hemodynamic and gas exchange effects of balloon atrial septostomy in 12 patients [26]. In several of these patients, balloon septostomy resulted in a significant improvement in cardiac output, marked diuresis, and improved oxygen delivery. This and other recent studies [27] provide evidence that balloon septostomy may be a useful palliative therapy, possibly serving as a bridge to lung transplantation in patients for whom more conventional therapy is failing. (*Adapted from* Nihill and coworkers [26]; with permission.)

FUTURE

FUTURE QUESTIONS

Can a cohesive schema explain the pathogenesis and course of PPH?

Can long-term pharmacologic therapy (eg, PGI_2, NO) remodel the pulmonary vasculature toward normal?

Who and when to transplant?

FIGURE 4-34. Important unanswered questions. Although great progress has been made in understanding the pathogenesis of PPH, in recognition of the clinical disease and its natural history, and in treatment, several important questions remain. 1) How do the many, apparently important, pathogenetic mechanisms fit together? Is there a single cohesive scheme that can explain the development and clinical course of PPH, or are there many individual schemata? 2) Can long-term pharmacologic therapy, possibly aimed at specific mediator defects, actually reverse the process and lead to remodeling of the pulmonary vascular bed toward normal? 3) What is the optimal timing for lung transplantation? Which patients should be referred for lung transplantation? Does lung transplantation prolong survival in appropriately selected patients?

REFERENCES

1. Gurtner HP: Aminorex and pulmonary hypertension. *Cor Vasa* 1985, 27:160–171.

2. Gomez-Sanchez MA, Saine de la Calzada C, Gomez-Pajuelo C, *et al.*: Clinical and pathologic manifestations of pulmonary vascular disease in the toxic oil syndrome. *J Am Coll Cardiol* 1991, 18:1539–1545.

3. Tazelaar HD, Myers JL, Drage CW, *et al.*: Pulmonary disease associated with L-tryptophan–induced eosinophilic myalgia syndrome: clinical and pathology features. *Chest* 1990, 97:1032–1036.

4. Salerni R, Rodnan GP, Leon DF: Pulmonary hypertension in the CREST syndrome variant of progressive systemic sclerosis (scleroderma). *Arch Intern Med* 1977, 86:394–399.

5. Hadengue A, Behayoun MK, Lebrec D, *et al.*: Pulmonary hypertension complicating portal hypertension: prevalence and relation to splanchnic hemodynamics. *Gastroenterology* 1991, 100:520–528.

6. Speich R, Jenni R, Opravil M, *et al.*: Primary pulmonary hypertension in HIV infection. *Chest* 1991, 100:1268–1271.

7. Rich S, Dantzker DR, Ayres SM, *et al.*: Primary pulmonary hypertension: a national prospective study. *Ann Intern Med* 1987, 107:216–223.

8. Loyd JE, Primm RK, Newman JH: Familial primary pulmonary hypertension: clinical patterns. *Am Rev Respir Dis* 1984, 129:194–197.

9. Smith P, Heath D, Yacoub M, *et al.*: The ultrastructure of plexogenic pulmonary arteriopathy. *J Pathol* 1990, 160:111–121.

10. Moser KM, Bloor CM: Pulmonary vascular lesions occurring in patients with chronic major vessel thromboembolic pulmonary hypertension. *Chest* 1993, 103:685–692.

11. Pietra GG, Edwards WD, Kay JM, *et al.*: Histopathology of primary pulmonary hypertension: a qualitative and quantitative study of pulmonary blood vessels from 58 patients in the National Heart, Lung, and Blood Institute primary pulmonary hypertension registry. *Circulation* 1989, 80:1198–1206.

12. Rich S: Primary pulmonary hypertension. *Prog Cardiovasc Dis* 1989, 31:205–238.

13. Christman BW, McPherson CD, Newman JH, *et al.*: An imbalance between the excretion of thromboxane and prostacyclin metabolites in pulmonary hypertension. *N Engl J Med* 1992, 327:70–75.

14. Dinh Xuan AT, Higenbottam TW, Clelland CA: Impairment of endothelium-dependent pulmonary artery relaxation in chronic obstructive lung disease. *N Engl J Med* 1991, 324:1539–1547.

15. Stewart DJ, Levy RD, Cernacek P, *et al.*: Increased plasma endothelin-1 in pulmonary hypertension: marker or mediator of disease. *Ann Intern Med* 1991, 114:464–496.

16. Ohar JA, Waller KS, Dahms TE: Platelet-activating factor induces selective pulmonary arterial hyperreactivity in isolated perfused rabbit lungs. *Am Rev Respir Dis* 1993, 148:158–163.

17. Hughes JD, Rubin LJ: Primary pulmonary hypertension: an analysis of 28 cases and a review of the literature. *Medicine* 1986, 65:56–72.

18. Ryan KL, Fedullo PF, Davis GB, *et al.*: Perfusion scan findings understate the severity of angiographic and hemodynamic compromise in chronic thromboembolic pulmonary hypertension. *Chest* 1988, 98:1180–1185.

19. Fedullo PF, Fishmann AJ, Moser KM: Pulmonary perfusion scans in primary pulmonary hypertension. *Chest* 1983, 127:82–86.

20. D'Alonzo GG, Barst RJ, Ayres SM, *et al.*: Survival in patients with primary pulmonary hypertension: results from a national prospective registry. *Ann Intern Med* 1991, 115:343–349.

21. Rich S, Brundage BH: High-dose calcium channel blocking therapy for primary pulmonary hypertension: evidence for long-term reduction in pulmonary arterial pressure and regression of right ventricular hypertrophy. *Circulation* 1987, 76:135–141.

22. Rich S, D'Alonzo GE, Dantzker DR, *et al.*: Magnitude and implications of spontaneous hemodynamic variability in primary pulmonary hypertension. *Am J Cardiol* 1985, 55:159–163.

23. Rich S, Kaufman E, Levy PS: The effect of high doses of calcium-channel blockers on survival in primary pulmonary hypertension. *N Engl J Med* 1992, 327:76–81.

24. Long W, Rubin LJ, Barst RJ, *et al.*: Influence of treatment with continuous infusion prostacyclin on survival in PPH. *Ann Intern Med* 1994, in press.

25. The Registry of the International Society for Heart and Lung Transplantation: ninth official report-1992. *J Heart Lung Transplant* 1992, 11:599–606.

26. Nihill MR, O'Laughlin MP, Mullins CE: Effects of atrial septostomy in patients with terminal cor pulmonale due to pulmonary vascular disease. *Cathet Cardiovasc Diagn* 1991, 24:166–172.

27. Kerstein D, Garofano RP, Hsu DT, *et al.*: Efficacy of blade balloon atrial septostomy in advanced pulmonary vascular disease [abstract]. *Am Rev Respir Dis* 1992, 145:A717.

28. Romberg E: Urer sklerose der lungenarterien. *Dtsch Arch Klin Med* 1891, 48:197.

29. Monkeberg JG: Ube die genuine arterioskerose den lungenarterie. *Dtsch Med Wochenschr* 1907, 33:1243.

30. Brenner O: Pathology of the vessels of the pulmonary circulation. *Arch Intern Med* 1935, 56:211–219.

31. Dreisdale DT, Schultz M, Michtom RJ: Primary pulmonary hypertension: 1. Clinical and hemodynamic study. *Am J Med* 1951, 11:686–705.

HIGH ALTITUDE PULMONARY EDEMA

Robert B. Schoene

In the past, pulmonary edema has been classified into two types: 1) edema caused by an increase in intravascular hydrostatic forces, as occurs in congestive heart failure, and 2) edema caused by inflammation, which results in a leak of plasma and/or protein-rich fluid from the intra- to extravascular space in the lung. The former is characterized by low protein concentrations in the alveolar fluid, while the latter is not. The characterization of pulmonary edema fluid is useful in providing insight into the mechanism of the leakage.

High altitude pulmonary edema (HAPE) is a form of edema that occurs in healthy individuals who ascend to a high altitude without adequate time for acclimatization [1,2]. Such edema is characterized by normal left ventricular function [3,4], high pulmonary artery pressure [3–7], very high protein concentrations in the alveolar fluid [8,9], lack of sepsis or trauma, and rapid resolution in most cases. The pathophysiologic mechanism remains elusive, but some intriguing clues provide important insight into the cause of the leak; such mechanisms may also be important in other forms of clinical pulmonary edema. The purpose of this chapter is to review the clinical presentation of HAPE, and to discuss its pathophysiology, including the roles of high pressure and inflammation in the mechanism of HAPE.

CHAPTER

5

PHYSIOLOGIC ADAPTATIONS

OVERVIEW FOR HIGH ALTITUDE ACCLIMATIZATION

A

SYSTEM	RESPONSE	EFFECT	TIME COURSE
Pulmonary	Increase in alveolar ventilation	Raises alveolar and arterial oxygen content	Immediate and progressive
Cardiovascular	Increase in cardiac output	Increases oxygen delivery	Transient, usually returns to sea level values
Cardiopulmonary	Increase in pulmonary vascular tone	Optimizes ventilation-perfusion match in lungs	Immediate and ongoing

B

SYSTEM	RESPONSE	EFFECT	TIME COURSE
Hematologic	Erythropoiesis	Increases O_2-carrying capacity	1–2 wk
	Left-shift in O_2-hemoglobin dissociation curve 2° to respiratory alkalosis	Improves O_2-loading at the alveolar-capillary interface (especially at extreme altitude)	Immediate and progressive
Tissues	Increase in capillary and mitochondrial density	Optimize oxygen availability to mitochondria	Weeks
	Stimulation of oxidative enzyme activity	Improve oxidative capabilities	

FIGURE 5-1. Overview of high altitude acclimatization. This table outlines the body's adaptation to high-altitude hypoxia (**A** and **B**). In a low oxygen environment, this process optimizes oxygen delivery from the air to the blood to the tissues. Each of these changes follows a different time course, which involves an immediate increase in ventilation and an improvement in ventilation and perfusion match, an increase in red blood cells, and tissue adaptations, which occur over several weeks.

CLINICAL EPIDEMIOLOGY

CLINICAL SETTING

Rapid ascent (1–2 d) to 3000 m (can be seen as low as 2500 m)

Symptoms of acute mountain sickness in first 12–48 h followed by HAPE

Preceding or concomitant viral illness, (eg, upper respiratory illness)

Susceptible individual (one or more previous episodes of HAPE)

Re-entry HAPE (usually children living at moderate altitude, 2700–4000 m, who travel to low altitude and return to home)

FIGURE 5-2. High altitude pulmonary edema (HAPE) is usually associated with one or more settings that may provide insight into pathophysiologic mechanisms. These associations are not consistent, however [6,10]. HAPE usually occurs when there has not been enough time for the body to adapt (*see* Fig. 5-1), *eg*, rapid ascent, especially if symptoms of acute mountain sickness (a milder form of altitude illness) precede HAPE. Individuals with a concomitant or prior viral illness, as well as those who have had previous bouts of HAPE, may also be more susceptible.

FIGURE 5-3. Characteristics that may be present in patients with HAPE. Inherent characteristics, such as blunted, as opposed to brisk, ventilatory responses to hypoxia and brisk hypoxic pulmonary vasoconstriction, may result in even more accentuated pulmonary hypertension than is usual [3,4,7,11–14]. This augmented stress on the pulmonary microvasculature is an important factor in the leak of fluid into the interstitial and alveolar spaces.

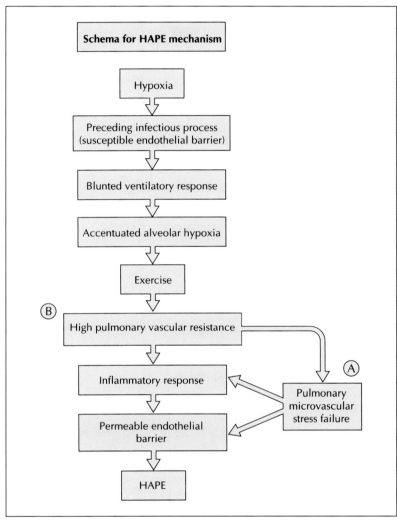

FIGURE 5-4. Possible pathways for HAPE. Two related pathways have been proposed to explain the mechanism of HAPE. During exposure to ambient hypoxia, a blunted ventilatory response leads to accentuated alveolar hypoxia, which is the stimulus for the pulmonary vasoconstrictive response that appears to be inherently greater in HAPE patients. There is also some evidence that in most cases of HAPE there is a preceding or concomitant viral illness that may cause an inflammatory response. As a result, the endothelium is primed and vulnerable to further physical stress or inflammation. Pathway A suggests that physical stress is the primary cause of capillary leakage. However, exposure of the basement membrane may also cause an inflammatory response. Pathway B acknowledges the presence of high intravascular pressure but indicts an initiating and ongoing inflammatory response as the primary cause of endothelial permeability.

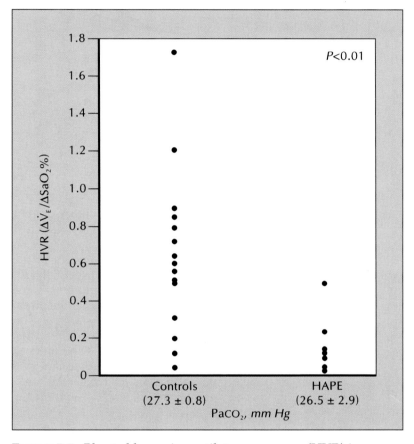

FIGURE 5-5. Blunted hypoxic ventilatory response (HVR) in patients with HAPE, both during and after the clinical course of HAPE, compared with controls. The data suggest that a blunted HVR results in more profound hypoxemia upon ascent and predisposes some individuals to HAPE. In fact, all but one patient had a markedly blunted HVR. Actual depression of ventilation, which was demonstrated by a paradoxic increase in ventilation with administration of oxygen [15], was found in several subjects. (*Adapted from* Hackett and coworkers [15]; with permission.)

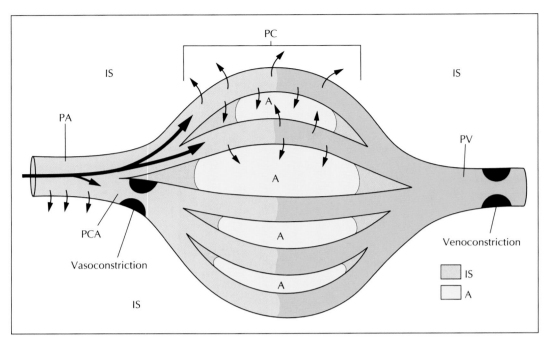

FIGURE 5-6. Sites of possible hypoxic pulmonary vasoconstriction at which high intravascular pressure may lead to extravascular leakage. At high altitudes, hypoxic pulmonary vasoconstriction may occur in a patchy or homogeneous pattern. Accentuated intravascular pressure at sites proximal to the vasoconstriction may lead to stretching of the endothelial layer and leakage of fluid rich in protein and cells into the interstitial and alveolar space (A). The figure represents the pulmonary microvasculature with interstitial (IS) and alveolar space. If vasoconstriction occurs at the precapillary arteriole (PCA), blood flow to the distal alveoli is decreased, and hydrostatic pressure in the proximal PCA and blood flow to the nonconstricted areas are increased. Fluid leakage could occur in the proximal PCA and the pulmonary capillary (PC), which becomes a site of overperfusion and stress on the capillary endothelium. Some hypoxic pulmonary venoconstriction at the pulmonary venules (PV) may occur, which could lead to similar forces in the proximal vasculature. All of these mechanisms are speculative. PA—pulmonary artery.

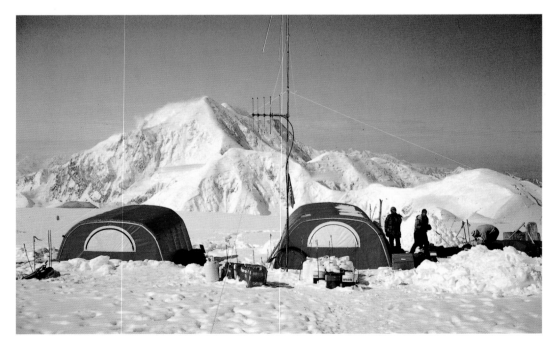

FIGURE 5-7. Site of Denali Medical Research Project where important research on HAPE took place in the 1980s. This camp was located 4400 m above sea level near the West buttress of Mt. McKinley in Alaska. Dr. Peter Hackett directed research teams in a number of studies on the pathophysiology of forms of altitude illness at this location for 7 years. In May and June of each year, climbers ascended the mountain quickly with heavy loads in extreme cold. The climbers provided a large number of subjects, many of whom suffered altitude illness.

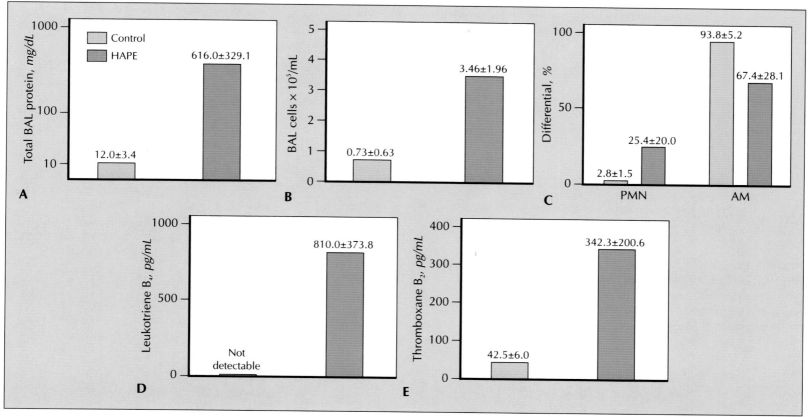

FIGURE 5-8. Evidence for high permeability leakage, cellular response, and inflammatory and vasoconstrictive mediators. Bronchoalveolar lavage (BAL) performed in HAPE patients at 4400 m above sea level on Denali in the Mt. McKinley Park in Alaska provided intriguing information regarding leakage of fluid. **A,** Total protein concentrations in the BAL fluid of controls and HAPE subjects demonstrates protein levels that are 50 times greater in HAPE. **B,** Total cell counts are close to five times higher in HAPE BAL. **C,** The differential counts on the cells in BAL of controls and HAPE subjects shows that there is a preponderance of alveolar macrophages (AM) in HAPE victims but that there is also a modest increase in neutrophils. **D,** There are very high levels of leukotriene B_4, a strong chemotactic mediator, in the HAPE BAL. **E,** Thromboxane B_2, a vasoactive mediator, is also significantly higher in HAPE BAL. The numbers above each bar indicate mean ± SD. PMN—polymorphonuclear leukocytes.

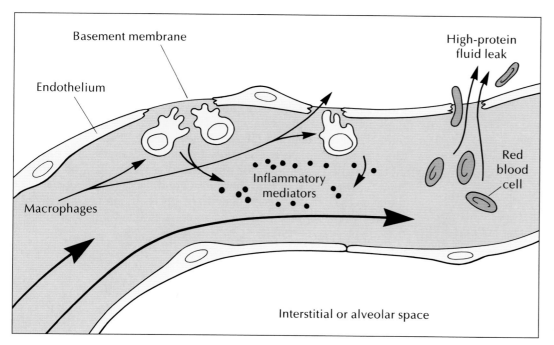

FIGURE 5-9. Possible role of inflammation in the reduced permeability of HAPE. Although the role of inflammation is not clear, the presence of a preceding viral illness in many patients and of inflammatory mediators in the bronchoalveolar lavage fluid suggests an important primary or secondary role for inflammation. A preceding viral illness in some patients may make the pulmonary vessels and endothelium more susceptible to the subsequent stresses of high intravascular pressure. An alternate but not exclusive hypothesis would be that high pressure leads to stretching of the endothelial barrier and exposure of the basement membrane, which in turn incites an inflammatory response. Further study of the clinical course of the disease is necessary to define the true role of inflammation.

SIGNS AND SYMPTOMS

EARLY

Most victims have preceding AMS (headache, loss of appetite, lethargy, nausea and vomiting, trouble sleeping)

Decreased exercise tolerance, dyspnea at rest, dry cough with tachycardia, tachypnea, cyanosis, and low-grade fever

LATE

Severe dyspnea, confusion, cough productive of pink frothy sputum that may proceed to coma and death

FIGURE 5-10. Early recognition of HAPE is critical because early intervention can save the life of the patient. These signs and symptoms provide important information for the sojourner and party members to avoid severe illness or death. AMS—acute mountain sickness.

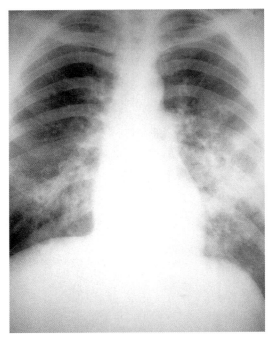

FIGURE 5-11. The chest radiograph of a patient with HAPE shows a normal cardiac silhouette and patchy infiltrates, which usually start in the right middle lobe and spread diffusely. All patterns of infiltrates have been described, however. The pulmonary arteries may be prominent.

PREVENTION OF HAPE

FIRST-TIME SOJOURNERS TO 3000 m

Awareness of signs and symptoms of AMS and HAPE

Slow ascent, monitoring symptoms, optimizing acclimatization

Use of acetazolamide (125 mg BID) if symptoms of AMS occur; may be helpful to prevent progression of AMS to HAPE (no data available)

INDIVIDUALS REQUIRING RAPID ASCENT AS A PART OF A RESCUE OR A MILITARY TEAM

Acetazolamide (125 mg BID) to minimize AMS

Nifedipine-XL (30 mg BID) for first several days

HAPE-SUSCEPTIBLE INDIVIDUALS

Slow, graded ascent with careful monitoring of AMS symptoms; do not ascend farther if symptoms occur and persist

Nifedipine-XL (30 mg BID) for first several days

FIGURE 5-12. Guidelines to provide critical measures for the prevention of HAPE in several scenarios. Medical personnel must be cognizant of each person's high altitude medical history and of the time course of ascent in order to anticipate HAPE and recognize the early signs and symptoms. This way, severe HAPE can be treated easily and successfully. This table lists three types of individuals who ascend to high altitudes who are exposed to the risk of getting HAPE [2,3,5,6,11,12,16,17]. AMS—acute mountain sickness.

TREATMENT OF HAPE

Descent of ≥1000 m if possible should alleviate many of the symptoms and prevent progression of the disease

Use of nifedipine-XL may be helpful (little data are yet available proving efficacy of nifedipine for treatment)

Low-flow oxygen, if available

Use of hyperbaric therapy by portable bags is helpful in improving the condition until descent is possible

Use of continuous positive airway pressure mask in expiratory positive airway pressure mode may be a temporizing measure to improve gas exchange while victim is descending or while he or she can't descend

FIGURE 5-13. Guidelines for the treatment of HAPE provide therapeutic modalities that should prevent serious illness or death once HAPE is recognized in the clinical setting [5,16–18]. The main objective is to anticipate the evolution of HAPE in its early phases. At this point, the patients are ambulatory and can descend before they become too ill to help themselves and become a danger to themselves or to other members of the party. If descent is delayed because of orthopedic trauma or severe weather, other modalities, if available, can be used.

REFERENCES

1. Houston CS: Acute pulmonary edema of high altitude. *N Engl J Med* 1960, 263:478–480.

2. Singh I, Khanna PK, Srivastava MC, *et al.*: Acute mountain sickness. *N Engl J Med* 1969, 280:175–184.

3. Hultgren HN, Lopez CE, Lundberg E, Miller H: Physiologic studies of pulmonary edema at high altitude. *Circulation* 1964, 29:393–408.

4. Hultgren HN, Grover RF, Harley LH: Abnormal circulatory responses to high altitude in subjects with a previous history of high altitude pulmonary edema. *Circulation* 1971, 44:759–770.

5. Bartsch P, Maggiorini M, Ritter M, *et al.*: Prevention of high altitude pulmonary edema by nifedipine. *N Engl J Med* 1991, 325:1284–1289.

6. Hackett PH, Rennie D, Levine HD: The incidence, importance, and prophylaxis of acute mountain sickness. *Lancet* 1976, 2:1149–1154.

7. Yagi H, Yamada H, Kobayashi T, Sekiguchi M: Doppler assessment of pulmonary hypertension induced by hypoxic breathing in subjects susceptible to high altitude pulmonary edema. *Am Rev Respir Dis* 1990, 142:796–801.

8. Schoene RB, Hackett PH, Henderson WR, *et al.*: High altitude pulmonary edema: characteristics of lung lavage fluid. *JAMA* 1986, 256:63–69.

9. Schoene RB, Swensen ER, Pizzo CJ, *et al.*: The lung at high altitude: broncho-alveolar lavage in acute mountain sickness and pulmonary edema. *J Appl Physiol* 1988, 64:2605–2613.

10. Scoggin CH, Hyers TM, Reeves JT, Grover RF: High altitude pulmonary edema in the children and young adults of Leadville, Colorado. *N Engl J Med* 1977, 297:1269–1273.

11. Bartsch P, Haeberli A, Franciolli M, *et al.*: Coagulation and fibrinolysis in acute mountain sickness and beginning pulmonary edema. *J Appl Physiol* 1989, 66:2136–2144.

12. Hackett PH, Creagh CE, Grover RF, *et al.*: High altitude pulmonary edema in persons without the right pulmonary artery. *N Engl J Med* 1980, 302:1070–1073.

13. Hackett PH, Rennie ID, Hofmeister SE, *et al.*: Fluid retention and relative hypoventilation in acute mountain sickness. *Respiration* 1982, 43:321–329.

14. Hyers TM, Scoggin CH, Will DH, *et al.*: Accentuated hypoxia at high altitude in subjects susceptible to high altitude pulmonary edema. *J Appl Physiol* 1979, 46:41–46.

15. Hackett PH, Roach RC, Schoene RB, *et al.*: Abnormal control of ventilation in high altitude pulmonary edema. *J Appl Physiol* 1988, 64:1268–1272.

16. Oelz O, Maggiorini M, Ritter M, *et al.*: Nifedepine for high altitude pulmonary edema. *Lancet* 1989, 2:1241–1244.

17. Reeves JT, Schoene RB: When lungs on mountains leak. *N Engl J Med* 1991, 325:1306–1307.

18. Schoene RB, Roach RC, Hackett PH, *et al.*: High altitude pulmonary edema and exercise at 4,400 meters on Mount McKinley: effect of expiratory positive airway pressure. *Chest* 1985, 87:330–333.

Surgical Interventions

ACUTE PULMONARY EMBOLECTOMY

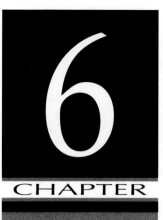

6

CHAPTER

Guy Meyer, Daniel Tamisier, Philippe Reynaud, and Hervé Sors

Open pulmonary embolectomy was first attempted in 1908 by Trendelenburg [1], but none of his patients survived the operation. The first surgical success was reported by Kirschner [2] in 1924. In 1960, Allison *et al.* [3] described a technique of bilateral embolectomy through the main pulmonary artery, which used venous inflow occlusion to produce a temporary circulatory arrest. However, the overall mortality rate for this operation remains 60%. Since 1962, cardiopulmonary bypass has been used for pulmonary embolectomy, thereby allowing a substantial reduction in the operative mortality rate. Cardiopulmonary bypass is considered by most surgeons to be the best operative procedure. Venous inflow occlusion or unilateral embolectomy might be indicated when cardiopulmonary bypass is not available or when the full heparinization required for cardiopulmonary bypass is contraindicated. Recently, transvenous procedures for embolectomy have been undertaken in the catheterization laboratory. The role of these interventional procedures is evolving.

Whatever the procedure, the role of pulmonary embolectomy in the treatment of massive pulmonary embolism remains controversial. Because of its high mortality, embolectomy ideally should be attempted only in those patients who will not survive without surgery. However, as Sautter [4] stated 15 years ago, "The identification of an unequivocal set of circumstances or findings which indicate those patients who will die without embolectomy remains to be made." In our opinion, pulmonary embolectomy should be considered for hemodynamically compromised patients if thrombolytic therapy is contraindicated and for those with a deteriorating hemodynamic condition despite intensive medical treatment, particularly thrombolytic therapy.

PULMONARY EMBOLECTOMY UNDER CARDIOPULMONARY BYPASS

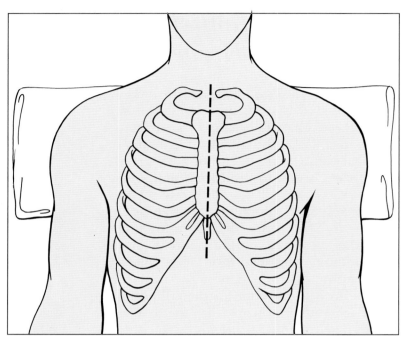

FIGURE 6-1. Surgical approach. As soon as the decision to attempt pulmonary embolectomy is made, the operating room is quickly prepared with an anesthesiologist and surgical teams. Due to the high risk of cardiac arrest, monitoring equipment (electrocardiograph, radial artery cannula, venous catheters, urethral catheter, thermistor probes) is installed prior to anesthesia. The patient is placed on his or her back and a pad is placed behind the chest. A straight vertical midline skin incision is performed, and the sternum is quickly split with an electric saw. The pericardium is then opened lengthwise in the midline, followed by the application of pericardial stay sutures.

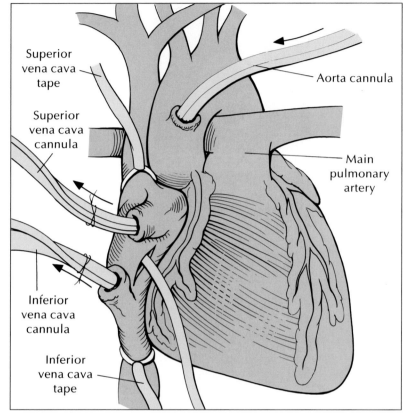

FIGURE 6-2. Preparation for bypass. Most patients are critically ill and severely compromised hemodynamically. Consequently, some surgical teams use preoperative circulatory support with cannulation of the femoral vessels while the patient is under local anesthesia. Nevertheless, performing the sternotomy and installing the bypass through the aorta and venae cava could, depending on the case, be quicker than dividing the femoral vessels. Purse-string sutures for aortic and venous cannulation are installed. The patient is heparinized and the arterial cannula placed in the ascending aorta. The venae cava are cannulated and tapes are placed around them. The cardiopulmonary bypass is quickly started. The venous tapes are closed, the right atrium is opened, and a suction device is installed to drain the coronary sinus outflow. The embolectomy is conducted under normothermia without aortic cross-clamping, and the temperature is maintained to avoid ventricular fibrillation.

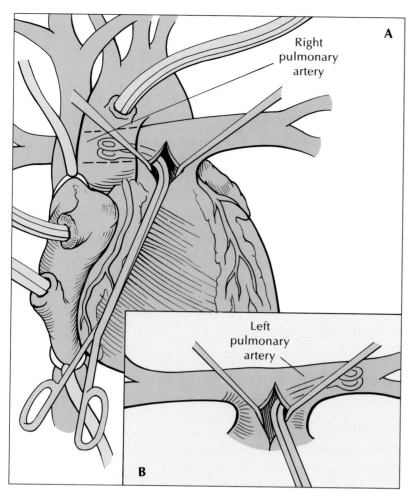

FIGURE 6-3. Right (**A**) and left (**B**) pulmonary artery embolectomy. A lengthwise incision of the main pulmonary artery is performed and the edges of the incision are retracted. Usually, clots can be easily removed. Common bile duct forceps are used to explore the main pulmonary artery and its branches. A standard suction catheter is gently introduced in the pulmonary branches and extracts the distal clots. The pleurae can also be opened for massaging both lungs in order to dislodge peripheral clots. The right atrium and ventricle are explored and the inferior vena cava is flushed for residual clots. The pulmonary trunk and the right atrium are then closed up with continuous sutures. Cardiopulmonary bypass is then discontinued, the cannulae are removed, and protamine is administered. If a caval interruption is performed concomitantly, a caval clip is inserted before the chest is closed.

PULMONARY EMBOLECTOMY WITHOUT CARDIOPULMONARY BYPASS

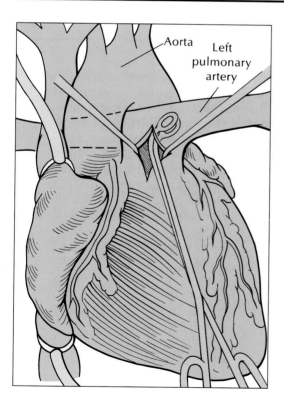

FIGURE 6-4. Venous inflow occlusion. Installation of the patient on the operating table and sternotomy are performed in the same manner. Tapes with tourniquets are placed around the superior and inferior venae cava in order to cross-clamp the vessels and dry out the right cardiac chambers. In less than 2 minutes the surgeon opens the pulmonary trunk and quickly extracts most clots. The pulmonary artery is immediately closed with a lateral clamp and sutured after the caval tapes have been released. This operation is hazardous because important blood loss may occur through the pulmonary arteriotomy and because a brief circulatory arrest is induced by the interruption of the venous return.

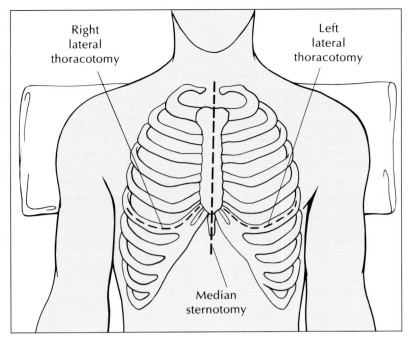

FIGURE 6-5. Surgical approach for unilateral pulmonary embolectomy. When clots are located primarily in one of the main pulmonary branches, embolectomy can be performed without circulatory arrest. The surgical approach of pulmonary branches is possible through a left or right lateral thoracotomy. This approach is not fully satisfactory, however, due to the following factors: the lateral position of the patient could provoke hemodynamic side effects; contralateral migration of clots is possible; the surgical exposure is precarious; and cardiac massage becomes difficult. Therefore, when possible, standard median sternotomy should be performed.

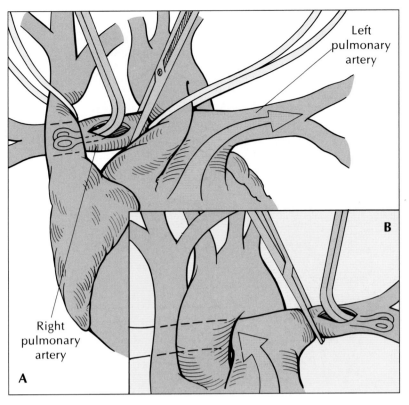

FIGURE 6-6. A, After complete dissection between the ascending aorta and the superior vena cava, the right pulmonary artery is cross-clamped. The cardiac output is derived through the left pulmonary artery. A lengthwise incision of the right pulmonary artery is undertaken and the embolectomy is performed according to the standard technique. B, Because of its anatomic location, dividing the left pulmonary artery is more difficult. The left pulmonary artery is cross-clamped and embolectomy is performed in the same manner.

RESULTS

OPERATIVE MORTALITY FROM PULMONARY EMBOLECTOMY UNDER CARDIOPULMONARY BYPASS

STUDY	PATIENTS, n	DEATHS, n	MORTALITY, %
Cross and Mowlem [5]	115	65	56
Stansel et al. [6]	10	3	30
Gentsch et al. [7]	10	3	30
Berger [8]	17	4	23
Heimbecker et al. [9]	12	1	8
Reul and Beall [10]	17	6	35
Tschirkov et al. [11]	24	7	29
Eisenmann et al. [12]	54	6	11
Bottzauw et al. [13]	23	6	26
Glassford et al. [14]	20	8	40
Soyer et al. [15]	17	4	23
Mattox et al. [16]	40	22	55
Gray et al. [17]	71	21	30
Boulafendis et al. [18]	16	5	31
Meyer et al. [19]	96	36	37
Schmid et al. [20]	27	12	44
Meyns et al. [21]	30	6	20
Total	599	215	36

FIGURE 6-7. Operative mortality from pulmonary embolectomy under cardiopulmonary bypass. These figures refer to deaths that occurred intraoperatively or during the remainder of the hospitalization. Because isolated case reports mainly include successful procedures, reports of less than 10 cases are excluded here. To avoid duplication of data, the initial results of some institutions, which were included in subsequent reports, are also excluded. In the most recent reports, the mortality rates average 20% to 40%.

OPERATIVE MORTALITY FROM PULMONARY EMBOLECTOMY WITHOUT CARDIOPULMONARY BYPASS

STUDY	PATIENTS, n	DEATHS, n	MORTALITY, %
Cross and Mowlem [5]	22	13	59
Eisenmann et al. [12]	51	40	78
Clarke and Abrams [22]	55	22	40
Total	128	75	59

FIGURE 6-8. Operative mortality from pulmonary embolectomy without cardiopulmonary bypass. The data here refer to the classic Trendelenburg operation [1], venous inflow occlusion embolectomy, and unilateral embolectomy. The results of these three operations are published mainly as case reports. Only one survey and two relatively large series are available for analysis. In the survey published by Cross and Mowlem [5], all three procedures were employed. In the other series, most of the patients underwent operations by venous inflow occlusion.

PREDICTIVE FACTORS OF OPERATIVE MORTALITY

VARIABLE	ALL PATIENTS	NONSURVIVORS	SURVIVORS	P VALUE
Male, %	52	64	45	0.07
Associated HLD, %	11	19	7	0.06
Shock %	81	92	75	0.04
Cardiac arrest, %	25	39	17	0.02
No preoperative thrombolysis, %	69	81	62	0.05
Age, y	52±14	55±12	50±15	0.06
Cardiac index, $L/min/m^2$	2.0±0.7	1.8±0.5	2.1±0.8	0.06
TPRI, U/m^2	18.4±8.8	20.6±9.2	17.1±6.5	0.06

FIGURE 6-9. Preoperative factors that might affect hospital mortality were evaluated by univariate and multivariate analysis in 96 consecutive patients operated at one center [19]. Clinical variables, including sex, age, associated heart or lung disease (HLD), shock, cardiac arrest, date of embolectomy, delay between the first episode of pulmonary embolism and operation, preoperative thrombolytic therapy, as well as hemodynamic preoperative measurements, were evaluated by univariate analysis. Multivariate analysis was performed by stepwise logistic regression on the eight variables that were different at the 10% level between survivors and nonsurvivors. Cardiac arrest ($P=0.025$) and previous cardiopulmonary disease ($P=0.045$) were identified as the two variables predictive of operative death that increased the operative mortality by 3.4 and 4.7, respectively. TPRI—total pulmonary resistance index.

POSTOPERATIVE COMPLICATIONS

COMPLICATION	n
Lethal	
Right heart failure	38
Brain damage	20
Sepsis	10
Pulmonary hemorrhage	10
Diagnostic error (no PE)	7
Recurrent embolism	2
Miscellaneous	7
Nonlethal	
ARDS	11
Sepsis	10
Bleeding	9
Brain damage	6
Acute renal failure	5
Heparin-induced thrombocytopenia	5

FIGURE 6-10. Postoperative complications. Right heart failure is the most frequent cause of death during pulmonary embolectomy. Brain damage usually results from prolonged cardiac arrest before operation. Septic postoperative complications are due mainly to mediastinitis. The very high mortality encountered in patients embolectomized with an erroneous diagnosis of pulmonary embolism (PE) highlights the need for an objective diagnostic method when surgery is considered. The risk of subsequent fatal PE during the postoperative course prompted us and others to perform a vena cava interruption either by clipping or by filter insertion immediately after the operation. Postoperative adult respiratory distress syndrome (ARDS) and preoperative hemorrhagic pulmonary edema are also frequent complications of pulmonary embolectomy and are most probably related to ischemia/reperfusion injury. There were 94 deaths resulting from postoperative complications among 273 patients studied [7–9,11,15,16,19–21], and 46 nonlethal complications among 126 patients studied [19,21]. Miscellaneous lethal complications included ARDS, bleeding, and fat emboli.

EMBOLECTOMY USING GREENFIELD'S CATHETER DEVICE

TECHNIQUE AND OPERATIVE PROCEDURE

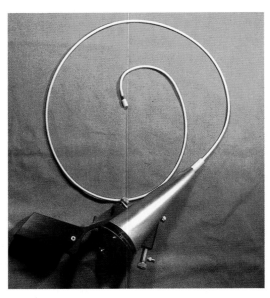

FIGURE 6-11. Transvenous pulmonary embolectomy was first attempted in humans by Greenfield in 1971 [23]. The embolectomy device is a 10 F steerable catheter (Meditech Inc., Watertown, MA) with a suction cup attached at the tip. Due to the cup's large size, a transcutaneous approach is not possible and the catheter is inserted through surgical venotomy. A steerable handle is used to control the progression of the catheter through the right cardiac chambers and the pulmonary arterial branches.

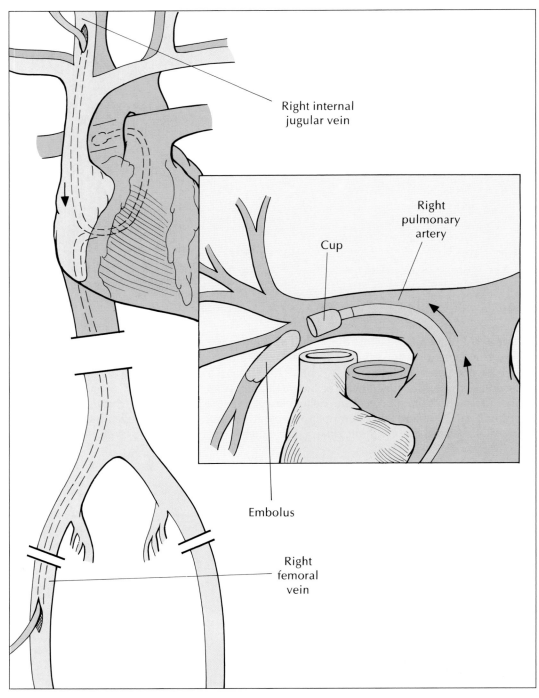

FIGURE 6-12. The catheter is introduced through a right jugular or femoral venotomy after local anesthesia. The catheter is then advanced through the right side of the heart and is positioned in the pulmonary artery under fluoroscopic control. Repeated injections of contrast medium through the catheter allow visualization of the clots and an optimal positioning of the distal cup.

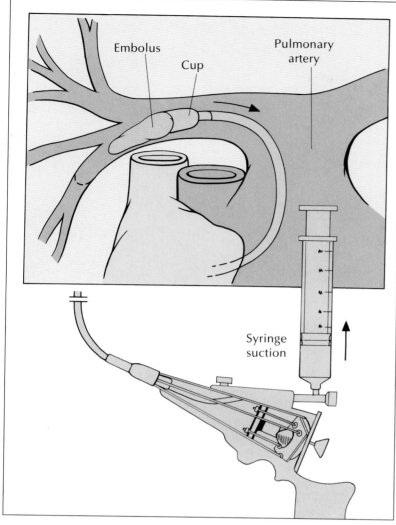

FIGURE 6-13. Under fluoroscopic control, the catheter's cup is advanced close to the clot inside a lobar or segmental pulmonary arterial branch. Syringe suction is then applied at the proximal end of the catheter to aspirate the embolus in the cup. Sustained syringe suction is used to hold the clot in the cup as the catheter is withdrawn. The absence of aspirated blood in the syringe confirms the capture of the embolus within the cup.

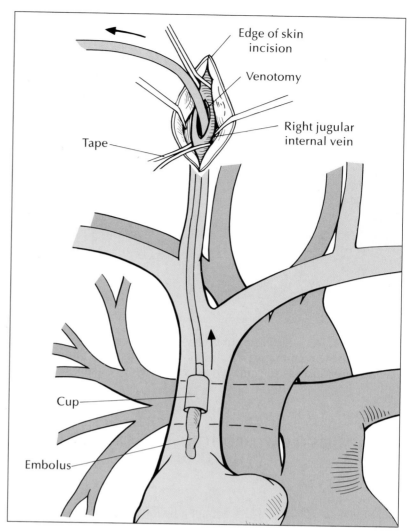

FIGURE 6-14. The catheter is then carefully withdrawn from the pulmonary artery through the right heart and vena cava. During this procedure, syringe suction is maintained to hold the clot in the cup. The procedure may have to be repeated several times in order to obtain a significant angiographic or hemodynamic improvement. At the end of the procedure, a vena cava filter is inserted through the venotomy.

RESULTS

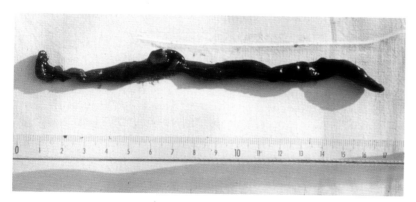

FIGURE 6-15. Thrombi of different sizes can be removed by catheter embolectomy. Most often 3- to 5-cm long clots are obtained after several passages of the catheter. When the clots are fresh and unattached to the pulmonary arterial wall, 17-cm long clots can be removed, thereby producing rapid hemodynamic improvement.

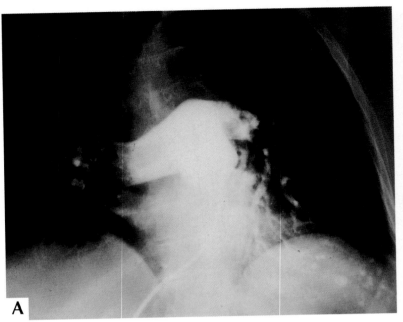

A

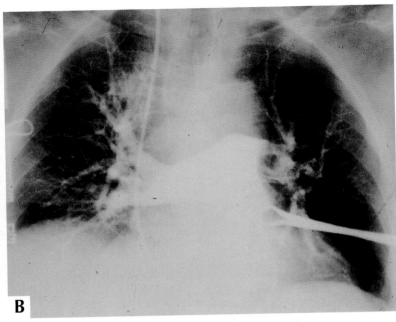

B

FIGURE 6-16. A, Selective pulmonary arteriogram before embolectomy showing a massive pulmonary embolism. **B,** The same patient after successful transvenous embolectomy using Greenfield's catheter device: the angiogram shows a significant improvement in the pulmonary vascular flow.

RESULTS FROM EMBOLECTOMY BY GREENFIELD'S CATHETER DEVICE

STUDY	PATIENTS, n	SUCCESSES, n	POSTOPERATIVE DEATHS, n
Greenfield *et al.* [24]	46	35	14
Timsit *et al.* [25]	18	11	5

FIGURE 6-17. Results from embolectomy by Greenfield's catheter device. *Success* is defined as significant clot extraction during the procedure. Failures are related mainly to the presence of adherent and organized old clots (subacute recurrent pulmonary embolism). Death could be caused by irreversible right heart failure when the procedure has failed, brain damage, or underlying disease. Catheterization of the pulmonary artery with the device requires a skilled physician. However, even with highly professional competence, this procedure is unsuccessful in some patients (18 failures in the 64 patients reported). These limitations may account for the infrequent use of the technique, despite impressive results in the two published series.

OTHER PROCEDURES

OTHER PROCEDURES

Ultrasound-assisted aspiration
Kensey procedure
Fragmentation by angiographic catheters
Laser-assisted embolectomy
Rotating basket catheter

FIGURE 6-18. Various other procedures have been used for pulmonary embolectomy. Ultrasound-assisted aspiration is effective *in vitro*, but *in vivo* experiments are scarce even in animal models. The ultrasound-assisted aspiration catheter is a 1-mm diameter ultrasound probe connected to a 250-W power generator and a piezoceramic transducer with a frequency of 27 kHz. The probe is inserted in a 7 F to 9 F untapered catheter connected to a roller pump for transcatheter suction [26]. The Kensey catheter is an 8 F catheter containing a torsional drivewire that revolves a distal head at a speed of up to 100,000 rpm. During the operation, irrigation fluid is supplied through the catheter and is directed laterally to the rotating tip for cooling purposes. This device was used in 11 dogs with experimental pulmonary embolism produced by injection of allogeneic clots prepared *in vitro*. In six of the dogs the clots were readily fragmented after 5 to 10 seconds of activation of the catheter but in the other five animals, catheterization of the pulmonary artery was not possible [27]. Fragmentation by angiographic catheters, laser-assisted embolectomy, and the rotating basket catheter are described in Figs. 6-19, 6-20, and 6-21, respectively.

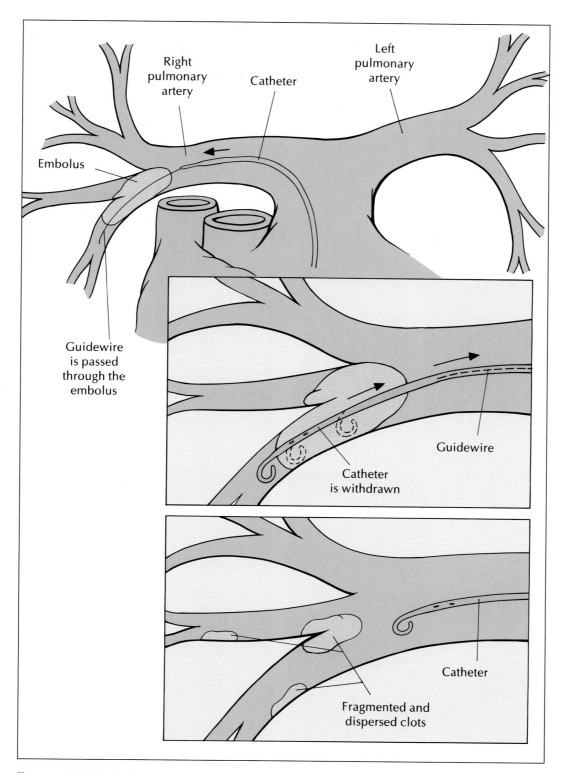

FIGURE 6-19. Embolectomy using angiographic catheters. **A,** A standard angiographic catheter mounted on a J wire is advanced to the pulmonary trunk. Injections of contrast medium are used to visualize the clots. The thrombus is first pushed forward by advancing the catheter. The guidewire is then passed through the embolus and the catheter is advanced over the wire. The wire is withdrawn, thereby allowing the catheter's tip to assume its normal shape. **B,** The catheter is then withdrawn, resulting in a fragmentation of the thrombus. Successful attempts at this simple and attractive method have been reported in only a few patients [28,29].

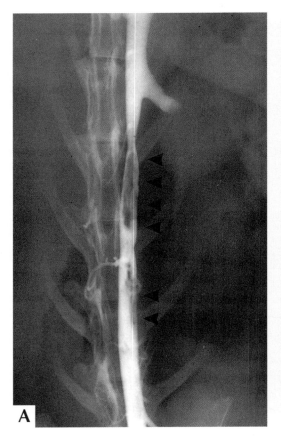 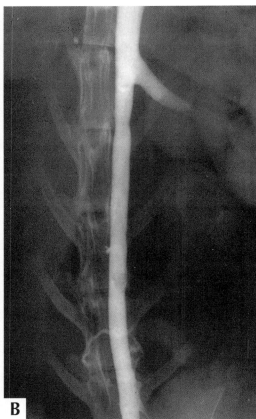

FIGURE 6-20. Laser-assisted thrombectomy. **A,** Subtotal thrombosis (*arrowheads*) of the inferior vena cava created in a New Zealand male rabbit. After surgical dissection, a woolen thread is inserted into the vena cava below the renal veins [30]. Clamps are placed 2 cm apart and left in place for 30 minutes and 5 to 45 IU of thrombin are injected. The laser is a pulsed dye laser connected to a 180-μm optical fiber inserted in a catheter. **B,** Complete recanalization of the inferior vena cava in the same rabbit after laser irradiation. Recanalization was completely achieved in five animals and a partial result was obtained in seven out of a total of 12. Perforation of the vena cava occurred in five rabbits and was related to noncoaxial placement of the fiber [30].

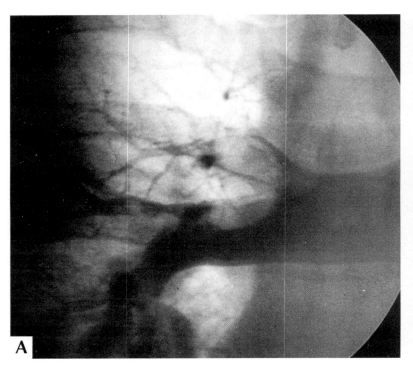 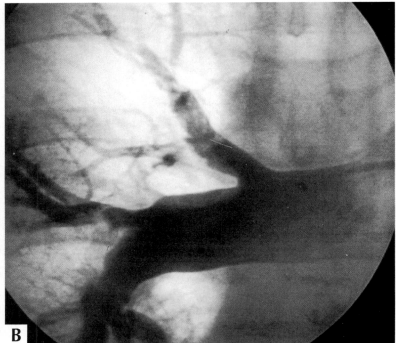

FIGURE 6-21. Angiograms before (**A**) and after (**B**) embolectomy using the rotating basket catheter. The rotating basket catheter is a 7 F hollow metal spiral with a self-expandable basket consisting of four spiral-shaped wires at the tip of the catheter. An impeller mounted at the center of the basket is connected to an external drive system. The catheter is introduced in a sheath and the basket is expanded distally to the clot. The impeller is then rotated at 100,000 rpm for several seconds [31]. (Courtesy of Dr. Lefevre, Lille, France.)

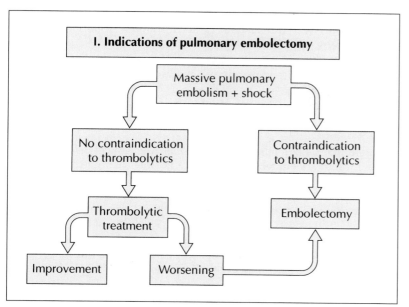

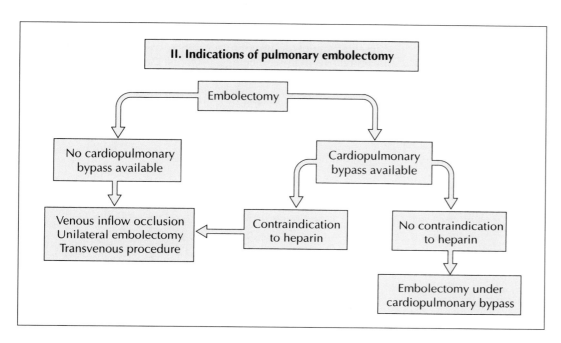

FIGURE 6-22. Almost 90% of the patients in a state of shock who were mistakenly diagnosed as having pulmonary embolism, and subsequently operated on, do not survive. Confirmation of pulmonary embolism by angiography or ventilation-perfusion scan is mandatory before embolectomy is undertaken. In our opinion, pulmonary embolectomy should only be considered for patients with clinical signs of shock despite inotropic support when thrombolytic therapy has failed or is contraindicated. Although clinical criteria have been proposed for the definition of shock in massive pulmonary embolism, they have not been evaluated prospectively. As a result, the decision regarding pulmonary embolectomy depends on the particular evaluation by each individual physician. In our experience [19], thrombolytic therapy is not associated with an increased number of postoperative complications and fatalities. Consequently, thrombolytic therapy does not preclude embolectomy.

FIGURE 6-23. When available, pulmonary embolectomy under cardiopulmonary bypass is the most desirable procedure. When cardiopulmonary bypass is not available, a unilateral embolectomy may be undertaken when the vascular obstruction mainly involves one lung. However, in massive pulmonary embolism, both sides are most often involved and embolectomy must be performed with venous inflow occlusion. Transvenous procedures based in the catheterization laboratory are not available in most centers and their routine clinical use requires additional evaluation.

REFERENCES

1. Trendelenburg F: Ueber die operative behandlung der embolie der lungenarterie. *Arch Klin Chir* 1908, 86:686–700.

2. Kirschner M: Ein durch die Trendelenburgsche operation geheilter fall von embolie der arterie pulmonalis. *Arch Klin Chir* 1924, 133:312–359.

3. Allison PR, Dunhill MS, Marshall R: Pulmonary embolism. *Thorax* 1960, 15:273–283.

4. Sautter RD: Treatment of massive pulmonary embolism. *Chest* 1977, 71:127–128.

5. Cross FS, Mowlem A: A survey of the current status of pulmonary embolectomy for massive pulmonary embolism. *Circulation* 1967, 35(suppl 1):86–91.

6. Stansel HC, Hume M, Glenn WWL: Pulmonary embolectomy: results in ten patients. *N Engl J Med* 1967, 276:717–721.

7. Gentsch TO, Larsen PB, Daughtry DC, *et al.*: Community-wide availability of pulmonary embolectomy with cardiopulmonary bypass. *Ann Thorac Surg* 1969, 7:97–103.

8. Berger RL: Pulmonary embolectomy with preoperative circulatory support. *Ann Thorac Surg* 1973, 16:217–226.

9. Heimbecker RO, Keon WJ, Richards KU: Massive pulmonary embolism. *Arch Surg* 1973, 107:740–746.

10. Reul GJ, Beall AC: Emergency pulmonary embolectomy for massive pulmonary embolism. *Circulation* 1974, 50(suppl II):236–240.

11. Tschirkov A, Krause E, Elert O, *et al.*: Surgical management of massive pulmonary embolism. *J Thorac Cardiovasc Surg* 1978, 75:730–733.

12. Eisenmann B, Kretz JG, Heitz A, *et al.*: Massive pulmonary embolism: a series of 59 successful emergency pulmonary embolectomies. *Prog Respir Res* 1980, 13:151–158.

13. Bottzauw J, Vejlsted HJ, Albrechtsen O: Pulmonary embolectomy using extracorporeal circulation. *Thorac Cardiovasc Surg* 1981, 29:320–322.

14. Glassford DM, Alford WC, Burrus GR, *et al.*: Pulmonary embolectomy. *Ann Thorac Surg* 1981, 32:28–32.

15. Soyer R, Brunet AP, Redonnet M, *et al.*: Follow-up of surgically treated patients with massive pulmonary embolism: with reference to 12 operated patients. *Thorac Cardiovasc Surg* 1982, 30:103–108.

16. Mattox KL, Feldtman RW, Beall AC, *et al.*: Pulmonary embolectomy for acute massive pulmonary embolism. *Ann Surg* 1982, 195:726–731.

17. Gray HH, Morgan JM, Paneth M, *et al.*: Pulmonary embolectomy: indications and results. *Br Heart J* 1987, 57:572.

18. Boulafendis D, Bastounis E, Panayiotopoulos YP, *et al.*: Pulmonary embolectomy (answered and unanswered questions). *Int Angiol* 1991, 10:187–194.

19. Meyer G, Tamisier D, Sors H, *et al.*: Pulmonary embolectomy: a 20-year experience at one center. *Ann Thorac Surg* 1991, 51:232–236.

20. Schmid C, Zietlow S, Wagner TOF, *et al.*: Fulminant pulmonary embolism: symptoms, diagnostics, operative technique, and results. *Ann Thorac Surg* 1991, 52:1102–1107.

21. Meyns B, Sergeant P, Flameng W, *et al.*: Surgery for massive pulmonary embolism. *Acta Cardiol* 1992, 47:487–493.

22. Clarke DB, Abrams LD: Pulmonary embolectomy: a 25-year experience. *J Thorac Cardiovasc Surg* 1986, 92:442–445.

23. Greenfield LJ, Bruce TA, Nichols TB: Transvenous pulmonary embolectomy by catheter device. *Ann Surg* 1971, 174, 881–886.

24. Greenfield LJ, Proctor MC, Williams DM, *et al.*: Long-term experience with transvenous catheter pulmonary embolectomy. *J Vasc Surg* 1993, 18:450–458.

25. Timsit JF, Reynaud P, Meyer G, *et al.*: Pulmonary embolectomy by catheter device in massive pulmonary embolism. *Chest* 1991, 100:655–658.

26. Schmitz-Rode T, Günther RW, Müller-Leisse C: US-assisted aspiration thrombectomy: in vitro investigations. *Radiology* 1991, 178:677–679.

27. Stein PD, Sabbah HN, Basha MA, *et al.*: Mechanical disruption of pulmonary emboli in dogs with a flexible rotating-tip catheter (Kensey catheter). *Chest* 1990, 98:994–998.

28. Brady AJB, Crake T, Oakley CM: Percutaneous catheter fragmentation and distal dispersion of proximal pulmonary embolus. *Lancet* 1991, 338:1186–1189.

29. Essop MR, Middlemost S, Skoularigis J, *et al.*: Simultaneous mechanical clot fragmentation and pharmacologic thrombolysis in acute massive pulmonary embolism. *Am J Cardiol* 1992, 69:427–430.

30. Meyer G, Makowski S, Steg PG, *et al.*: Percutaneous pulsed dye laser recanalization of experimental venous thrombosis. *Am Heart J* 1991, 122:1177–1180.

31. Dievart F, Fourrier JL, Lefebvre JM, *et al.*: Treatment of severe pulmonary embolism by means of a high speed rotational catheter (Angiocor Thrombolizer): first experience of mechanical thrombolysis in human beings. *J Am Coll Cardiol* 1994, 24:474A.

A Multidisciplinary Approach to Chronic Thromboembolic Pulmonary Hypertension

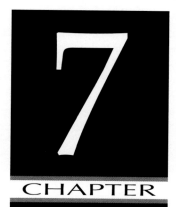

7

CHAPTER

Peter F. Fedullo, William R. Auger, Richard N. Channick, Stuart W. Jamieson, and Kenneth M. Moser

The usual natural history of pulmonary embolism is total embolic resolution, or resolution leaving minimal residua, with restoration of a normal symptomatic and hemodynamic status. However, for reasons yet to be determined, embolic resolution is incomplete in a small subset of patients. Irregular patterns of organization and recanalization occur, leaving fibrotic, endothelialized remnants that obstruct major pulmonary arteries. This failure of resolution may lead to obstruction of sufficient magnitude to decrease significantly the cross-sectional area of the pulmonary vascular bed and increase pulmonary vascular resistance. This, in turn, may result in the syndrome of chronic thromboembolic pulmonary hypertension (CTEPH).

The presenting complaint and physical examination of patients with CTEPH vary depending on the extent of pulmonary vascular obstruction and right ventricular performance. The one symptom that is common to all is dyspnea. Early in the course of the disease, the physical findings may be quite subtle. Later in the course, obvious evidence of right ventricular hypertrophy or overt right ventricular failure may be present. The major goals of the diagnostic evaluation are to establish the presence and degree of pulmonary hypertension, to define its chronic thromboembolic basis, and to confirm surgical accessibility. The procedure that best confirms the diagnosis and establishes surgical feasibility is the pulmonary angiogram. Pulmonary angioscopy may be indicated if pulmonary angiographic findings do not define precisely the extent or proximal extension of the occluding thrombi.

The decision to proceed to thromboendarterectomy is based on a number of objective and subjective factors. The chronic thromboemboli must be surgically accessible. The presence of pulmonary vascular obstruction should be responsible for hemodynamic or ventilatory impairment at rest or with exercise. The presence of concurrent disease must also be considered since this influences operative risk and long-term functional outcome. Finally, the patient must be willing to accept the mortal and morbid risks of the procedure. Sternotomy with cardiopulmonary bypass and periods of hypothermic circulatory arrest is the surgical procedure of choice. Significant surgical experience is necessary since the neointima may often be deceptive and is often not easily recognizable as chronic thrombi. The procedure is not an embolectomy but rather a true endarterectomy, which requires careful dissection of chronic endothelialized material from the native intima to restore pulmonary artery patency. In addition to complications common to other forms of cardiac surgery, patients undergoing thromboendarterectomy have two unique complications: acute reperfusion edema and pulmonary vascular "steal."

Overall operative and perioperative mortality in 471 patients undergoing pulmonary thromboendarterectomy at the UCSD Medical Center has been 9.8%. Between 1990 and 1993, 275 patients underwent thromboendarterectomy with an overall mortality of 6.2%. This improvement in outcome is largely the result of increased experience and close interaction among members of a multidisciplinary team aware of the challenging problems these patients present in the evaluative, surgical, and postoperative phases of their care. The immediate and long-term hemodynamic and symptomatic improvement among survivors has been gratifying. Relief of pulmonary vascular obstruction leads to a decrease in pulmonary artery pressures and an improvement in cardiac output even when the right ventricle is severely compromised prior to surgery. Functional improvement, present at the time of discharge, continues for 12 months as the postoperative anemia, reperfusion edema, and pulmonary artery steal resolve, and as conditioning and nutritional status improve. The majority of patients return to class I New York Heart Association functional status.

PATHOGENESIS AND NATURAL HISTORY

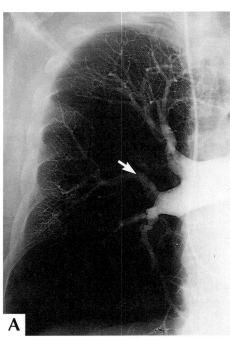
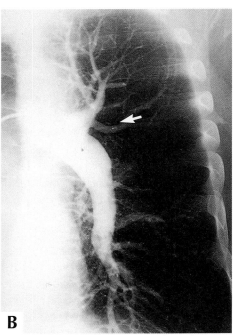

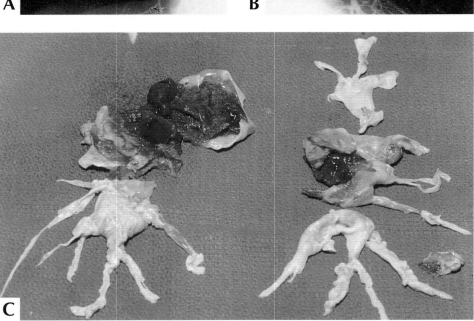

FIGURE 7-1. Although once considered to be a rare autopsy curiosity, chronic thromboembolic pulmonary hypertension (CTEPH) is now recognized with increasing frequency since improved diagnostic approaches were developed and effective therapeutic initiatives became available [1–10]. A distinction must be made between major-vessel CTEPH, which involves the main, lobar, and segmental pulmonary arteries and for which effective surgical intervention is available, and the thromboembolic arteriopathy variant of primary pulmonary hypertension [11–13].

A, Right-sided pulmonary angiogram demonstrating abrupt narrowing of the descending pulmonary artery with the absence of right-middle and lower lobe flow (*arrow*).

B, Left-sided pulmonary angiogram demonstrating the irregularity of the descending left pulmonary artery with diminished flow to the lingula and left lower lobe (*arrow*).

C, Chronic occluding thrombi obtained at the time of pulmonary thromboendarterectomy.

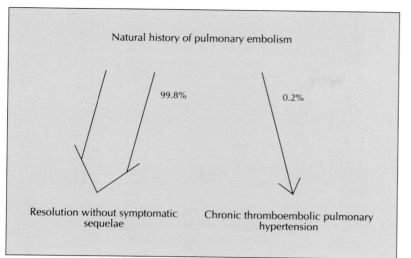

Natural history of pulmonary embolism

99.8%   0.2%

Resolution without symptomatic   Chronic thromboembolic pulmonary
sequelae   hypertension

FIGURE 7-2. The natural history of most pulmonary emboli is total resolution or resolution leaving minimal residua with restoration of normal pulmonary hemodynamics [14–17]. Over the past several decades, however, an alternate natural history has been identified in a small minority of embolic survivors. In these patients, an embolic event, which is commonly not diagnosed or treated during its acute phase, results in organized, recanalized residua that obstruct or significantly narrow major pulmonary arteries. Given obstruction of sufficient magnitude to substantially increase right ventricular afterload, pulmonary hypertension, right ventricular failure, and death may ensue [1–6, 18–20].

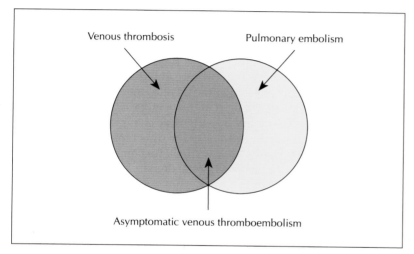

Venous thrombosis   Pulmonary embolism

Asymptomatic venous thromboembolism

POTENTIAL BASIS FOR FAILURE OF NORMAL THROMBOEMBOLIC RESOLUTION

Abnormal endogenous fibrinolytic mechanism

Thrombotic predisposition leading to multiple thromboembolic recurrences

Inadequate initial therapy

Uncommon manifestation of the normal spectrum of embolic disease

FIGURE 7-3. The majority of patients with chronic thromboembolic pulmonary hypertension do not have a history of a documented acute thromboembolic event. This lack of a clear-cut history probably reflects the frequency with which the diagnoses of both venous thrombosis and pulmonary embolism are overlooked in the population at large. In PIOPED (Prospective Investigation of Pulmonary Embolism Diagnosis), for example, only 11% of patients with angiographically confirmed pulmonary emboli had clinical evidence of venous thrombosis. Furthermore, rather than being a dramatic event as commonly perceived, the clinical presentation of acute embolism may often be subtle or silent.

Approximately 50% of patients with proximal vein thrombosis, although asymptomatic from a cardiopulmonary standpoint, will have perfusion scan findings consistent with embolism [21]. It is estimated that most pulmonary emboli are either never diagnosed and adequately treated or result in death before effective therapy can be instituted [22]. Although many patients with chronic thromboembolic disease are unable to provide a history of a documented thromboembolic event, they can often provide a history of unexplained chest pain or dyspnea, one or more episodes of "pleurisy" or atypical pneumonia, or instances of lower extremity "cellulitis" or "muscle strain," which may have represented their acute thromboembolic event.

FIGURE 7-4. One of the most intriguing questions regarding the pathogenesis of chronic thromboembolic pulmonary hypertension is why normal embolic resolution does not occur always. No consistent pattern of low tissue plasminogen activator activity or high plasminogen activator inhibitor-1 activity has been detected [23]. The search for other fibrinolytic defects remains under active investigation. The only identifiable thrombotic predisposition has been the presence of anticardiolipin antibodies in approximately 10% of patients. Less than 1% of patients have had deficiencies of antithrombin III, protein C, or protein S [2]. Although thromboembolic recurrence has occurred in certain patients, it has not proven to be the case in the majority of patients in whom sequential perfusion scans are available for review. It is possible that these patients, the majority of whom did not have the diagnosis of embolism made or treatment instituted at the time of their initial embolic event, represent an uncommon segment of the normal spectrum of pulmonary embolic disease in which endogenous fibrinolytic mechanisms are overcome by the age, extent, or location of the obstructing embolus.

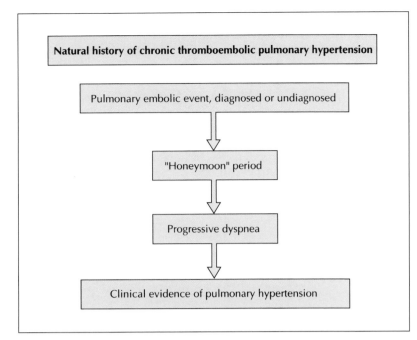

FIGURE 7-5. Because the majority of patients present late in the course of their disease, the exact hemodynamic evolution of their pulmonary hypertension has not been defined precisely. The history of such patients, however, has been well described [1–4]. Even when extensive occlusion follows an acute thromboembolic event, a patient may carry on relatively normal activities. Following an asymptomatic period that may range from months to years, worsening exertional dyspnea, hypoxemia, and right ventricular failure ultimately ensue. Considerable delay often occurs before the diagnosis of CTEPH is considered in a patient with dyspnea of undetermined etiology.

It is essential that pulmonary vascular disease be considered in any patient with dyspnea in whom no compelling cause can be established. Many patients have carried the diagnoses of asthma, chronic obstructive lung disease, interstitial lung disease, coronary artery disease, or psychogenic dyspnea for years before the diagnosis of CTEPH was considered. Increased recognition of this disease entity as a potential cause of dyspnea or pulmonary hypertension has represented a major advance, transforming what was once considered to be an autopsy curiosity or immutable cause of death into a disease entity with effective, well-defined diagnostic and therapeutic goals.

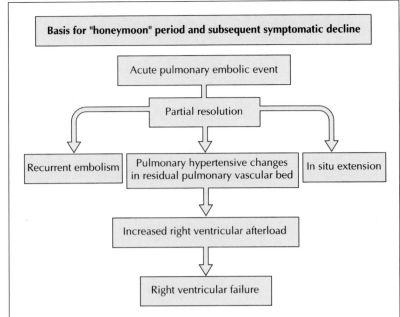

FIGURE 7-6. Retrospective observations suggest that the basis for this asymptomatic "honeymoon period," followed by a period of symptomatic decline, is related to the development of secondary pulmonary hypertensive changes in the open pulmonary vascular bed. Whether these secondary hypertensive changes are the consequence of an unidentified mediator or the direct result of high pulmonary artery pressures or flows, they further increase right ventricular afterload, placing additional demands on the right ventricle.

In a study of 31 patients with CTEPH, Moser and Bloor [24] demonstrated a full range of pulmonary hypertensive lesions, including plexogenic lesions, in the small pulmonary arteries. It is interesting that the pulmonary hypertensive lesions occurred not only in lung regions served by patent proximal vessels but also in lung regions distal to completely and partially obstructed proximal vessels. Alternatively, symptomatic decline may be related to retrograde extension of embolic obstruction proximal to a partially obstructing lesion as a result of turbulent or sluggish flow. Finally, although unusual in our experience, embolic recurrence can further increase pulmonary vascular resistance.

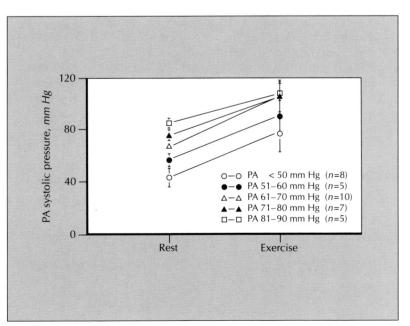

FIGURE 7-7. Rest and exercise hemodynamics in 35 patients with CTEPH and resting pulmonary artery (PA) systolic pressures less than 90 mm Hg [25]. Significant increases in PA pressure occurred with exercise regardless of the resting PA pressure. It is possible that early in the course of CTEPH increases in PA pressures during exercise are partially compensated for by recruitment or distention of normal vessels within the residual pulmonary vascular bed. Over time, the development of secondary pulmonary hypertensive changes in that open pulmonary vascular bed abolishes these compensatory mechanisms, resulting in further increases in right ventricular afterload and eventually in overt right ventricular failure.

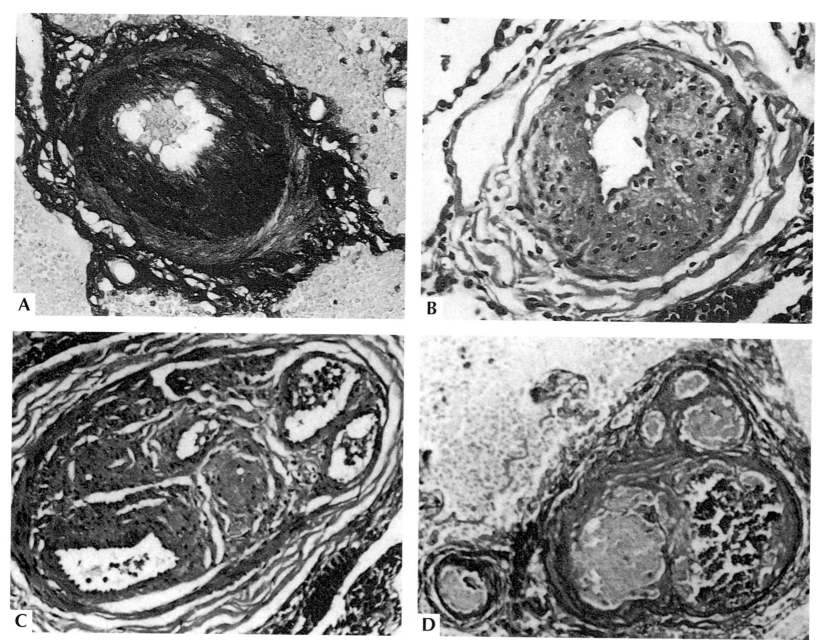

FIGURE 7-8. Secondary pulmonary hypertensive changes in the small muscular arteries and arterioles in CTEPH [24]. These lesions occur not only in vessels served by open proximal vessels but also in lung regions distal to partially and completely obstructed proximal vessels. The lesions identified include medial hypertrophy, concentric and eccentric intimal fibrosis, thrombotic lesions, and plexogenic lesions. The time course over which such lesions develop in CTEPH is unknown. However, the development of such lesions may play a role in the symptomatic and hemodynamic deterioration these patients experience over time. These findings also indicate that the etiologic basis for pulmonary hypertension cannot be established by lung biopsy. **A,** This muscular pulmonary artery shows asymmetric fibroelastosis of the intima. Fibroelastic changes are present in the intima inside of a relatively intact internal elastin.

B, This muscular pulmonary artery shows marked proliferation of longitudinal intimal fibromuscular tissue involving the entire circumference of the vessel.

C, This enlarged muscular pulmonary artery contains an obstructive lesion comprising multiple, thin-walled vascular channels and slits. A small central sclerotic zone is present.

D, This pulmonary artery has two large channels in its main lumen that may represent recanalization of an organized thromboembolus. Also, there is aneurysmal expansion of the vessel wall with several smaller vascular channels present as well.

CLINICAL PRESENTATION AND DIAGNOSIS

Exertional dyspnea
Chest pain
Syncope or near-syncope
Edema
Hemoptysis
Cough

FIGURE 7-9. Symptomatic presentation of CTEPH. Dyspnea, either at rest or with exercise, is the presenting symptom in virtually all patients with CTEPH. As a subjective complaint, dyspnea must be considered in the context of a patient's lifestyle. Early in the course of their disease, patients may remain active but complain of a decrease in exercise tolerance. The key is to consider pulmonary vascular disease in a patient with exertional dyspnea or an unexplained decline in exercise tolerance when no compelling cause can be established.

The mechanisms of dyspnea in CTEPH include an increase in dead space ventilation, resulting in high minute ventilation demands, and an inability of cardiac output to meet metabolic demands. Exertional chest pain may be related to right ventricular ischemia as the hypertrophied right ventricle outstrips its blood supply. Syncope or near-syncope usually does not occur until the later stages of the disease and may be related to sudden decreases in right ventricular preload associated with coughing or the Valsalva maneuver or to an inability of the right ventricle to augment cardiac output with exercise. Lower extremity edema may be a consequence of right ventricular failure or may be a manifestation of a post-phlebitic syndrome.

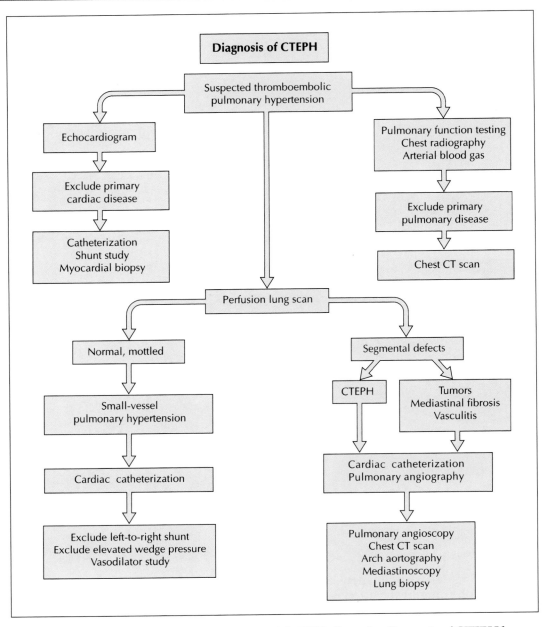

FIGURE 7-10. Diagnostic algorithm in suspected CTEPH. Once the diagnosis of CTEPH has been considered, the diagnostic approach, under most circumstances, is relatively straightforward. Competing cardiac diagnoses (cardiomyopathy, valvular disease shunt) and pulmonary diagnoses (parenchymal lung disease, hypoventilation syndrome) can be excluded by the appropriate application of echocardiography, pulmonary function testing, arterial blood gas evaluation, and, if indicated, high-resolution chest computed tomography (CT). In patients with CTEPH, findings on standard laboratory tests are subtle early in the disease and become obvious only as the disease progresses. Secondary polycythemia may develop as a result of longstanding hypoxemia. Abnormal liver or renal function studies may result from ventricular failure and a reduced cardiac output.

After competing diagnoses have been excluded, ventilation-perfusion scanning provides an excellent, low-risk, noninvasive means of distinguishing between pulmonary hypertension due to potentially operable CTEPH and obliterative, small-vessel pulmonary hypertension. Cardiac catheterization and pulmonary angiography are necessary to establish the degree of pulmonary hypertension, to confirm the diagnosis of chronic thromboembolic disease, to establish surgical accessibility, and to exclude potential competing diagnoses. While the pulmonary angiogram usually completes the diagnostic sequence, other studies may be indicated. CT of the chest to evaluate the mediastinum can be useful in excluding the possibility of fibrosing mediastinitis or mediastinal tumors. Arch aortography may be useful when vasculitis is suspected. Finally, pulmonary angioscopy has proven useful in confirming the presence of chronic thromboembolic obstruction and in determining the location of its proximal extent.

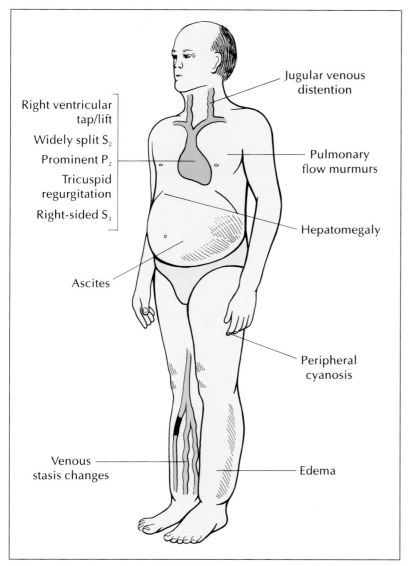

FIGURE 7-11. Findings on physical examination are influenced by the degree of pulmonary hypertension and right ventricular dysfunction present. Although the examination may be deceptively normal early in the course of the disease, obvious findings of right ventricular hypertrophy or failure may be present later. One finding that should be sought diligently is the presence of flow murmurs over the lung fields, a result of turbulent flow through a partially obstructing or recanalized thrombus [26]. These often subtle murmurs, similar to those heard in congenital branch stenosis or with pulmonary arteriovenous fistulas, are high-pitched and blowing in quality, accentuated during inspiration, and frequently heard only during brief periods of breath-holding. This is an important sign because such a murmur has not been reported in patients with primary pulmonary hypertension, which is an often-competing diagnosis.

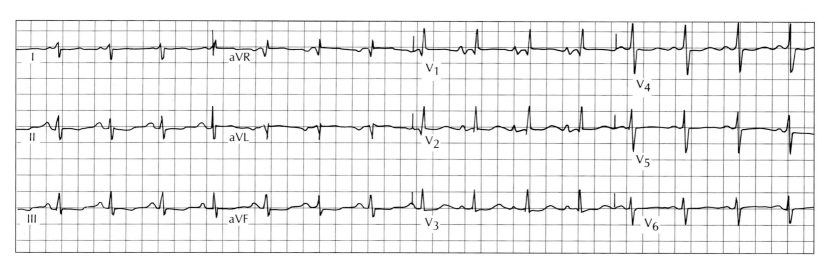

FIGURE 7-12. Electrocardiogram in CTEPH. Typical findings of right axis deviation, right atrial abnormality, and right ventricular hypertrophy are present. Earlier in the course of the disease, before significant right ventricular hypertrophy has developed, the electrocardiogram may be normal.

A. PULMONARY FUNCTION REPORT*

	NORMAL PREDICTED VALUES	BASELINE OBSERVED	% PREDICTED
Lung volumes			
Vital capacity, *L*	4.57	3.08[†]	67
FRC (body box), *L*	2.86	1.76[†]	62
RV (body box), *L*	1.71	0.89[†]	52
TLC (body box), *L*	6.1	3.97[†]	65
RV/TLC (body box), %	27	22	—
Flow rates			
FVC, *L*	4.57	3.08[†]	67
FEV1, *L*	3.58	2.43[†]	68
FEV1/FVC, %	78	79	
FEF25–75, *L/s*	3.96	2.2	56
Peak expiratory flow, *L/s*	8.5	7.3	85
FEF25%, *L/s*	8.3	5.1[†]	62
FEF50%, *L/s*	5.7	2.4[†]	41
FEF75%, *L/s*	2.1	0.8[†]	41
Peak inspiratory flow, *L/s*	5.3	4.6	86
Airway resistance			
Raw, *Inspiratory cm H$_2$O/L/s*	<2.5	2.6	—
Diffusing capacity			
DLCO, *mL CO/min/mm Hg*	32.2	20[†]	62
TLC single breath, *L*	6.1	4.39[†]	72
Maximum respiratory pressures			
MIP at RV, *cm H$_2$O*	>70	155	—
MEP at TLC, *cm H$_2$O*	>100	175	—

*Patient age, 31 years; height, 177 cm; weight, 114 kg; date of study, 2-15-92.
[†]Indicates a value outside the limits of normalcy.

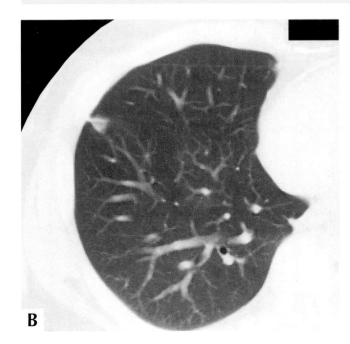

B

FIGURE 7-13. **A,** Pulmonary function report in a patient with chronic thromboembolic disease. Pulmonary function testing is usually within normal limits. Although the majority of patients do have a reduction in the single breath diffusing capacity for carbon monoxide (DLCO), a normal value does not exclude the diagnosis. As illustrated by the reduced TLC, approximately 20% of patients demonstrate a mild to moderate restrictive defect [27]. This defect may be related in part to scarring from areas of prior infarction and result in consideration of an interstitial rather than pulmonary vascular process.

B, Chest computed tomography scan demonstrating a peripheral, wedge-shaped area of infarction in a zone of lung served by an occluded proximal vessel. Pulmonary function studies may also demonstrate a mild obstructive defect as a result of bronchial hyperemia related to the large bronchial arterial collateral circulation these patients develop. FEF—forced expiratory flow rate; FEV$_1$—forced expiratory volume at 1 second; FRC—functional residual capacity; FVC—forced vital capacity; MEP—maximal expiratory pressure; MIP—maximal inspiratory pressure; RV—residual volume; TLC—total lung capacity.

EXERCISE STUDY*

	Rest	0.6	1.0	1.5
Speed, *mph*	Rest	0.6	1.0	1.5
Duration, *min*	15:00	02:00	02:00	04:00
Position	Standing	Standing	Standing	Standing
Room air	20.9	20.9	20.9	20.9
Arterial blood gas				
Pa_{O_2}, *mm Hg*	79	—	—	47
Pa_{CO_2}, *mm Hg*	23	—	—	23
pH	7.47	—	—	7.41
$P(A-a)_{O_2}$, *mm Hg*	44	—	—	79
O_2Hb (co-oximeter), %	94.8	—	—	80
Sa_{O_2} (ear oximeter), %	95.9	91.5	86.7	82.5
Expired gases				
VE, *L/M BTPS*	20.8	43.9	55.4	83.4
RR, *breaths/min*	21	26	34	34
Vt, *L BTPS*	1	1.72	2.13	2.45
V_{O_2}, *L/M STPD*	0.31	0.5	0.63	0.85
V_{O_2}, *mL/kg/M STPD*	3.9	6.2	7.9	10.6
V_{CO_2}, *L/M STPD*	0.27	0.48	0.59	0.84
R	0.86	0.97	0.93	0.99
VE/V_{O_2}	67.4	88.5	87.3	98.5
VE/V_{CO_2}	78.2	91.1	93.5	99.4
Vd, *L BTPS*	0.41	—	—	1.41
Vd/Vt, %	41	—	—	58

*Patient age, 35 years; height, 179 cm; weight 79.8 kg.

FIGURE 7-14. Rest and exercise arterial blood gas determination. Virtually all patients with CTEPH, even those normoxic at rest, have a decline in the arterial PO_2 with exercise. In this man, mild resting hypoxemia is accompanied by hypocapnia. Profound hypoxemia occurs with minimal exercise. Minute ventilation is dramatically elevated as a result of increased dead space ventilation (Vd/Vt). Vd/Vt is increased at rest and paradoxically worsens with exercise. The multiple inert gas technique has demonstrated that hypoxemia in this disorder is the consequence of moderate ventilation-perfusion inequality and a limited cardiac output, which depresses mixed venous PO_2 [28]. Desaturation during exercise is probably related to further depression of the mixed venous PO_2 and, in certain patients, to right-to-left shunting through a patent foramen ovale. $P(A-a)O_2$—alveolar-arterial gradient; R—respiratory quotient; RR—respiratory rate; VE—minute ventilation; Vt—tidal volume.

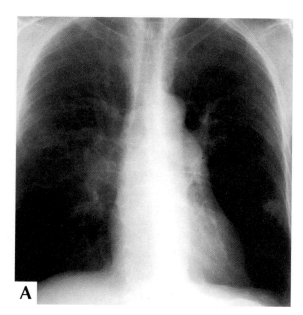

A

FIGURE 7-15. Chest radiographic findings. Chest radiography in a patient with CTEPH is often normal. However, close examination may demonstrate findings suggestive of the diagnosis. Areas of hypoperfusion and hyperperfusion with asymmetry in the size of the central pulmonary arteries or enlargement of both main pulmonary arteries may be present. There also may be evidence of old unilateral or bilateral pleural disease. The cardiac silhouette may reflect obvious right atrial or right ventricular enlargement; more often, right ventricular hypertrophy and enlargement are suggested only on the lateral film by encroachment on the normally empty retrosternal space.

A, Chest radiograph demonstrating marked enlargement of the right pulmonary artery and the apparent absence of the descending left pulmonary artery. The left lower lobe appears oligemic compared with the right. A pleural-based scar, representing an area of prior infarction, is present in the left mid-lung field. *(continued)*

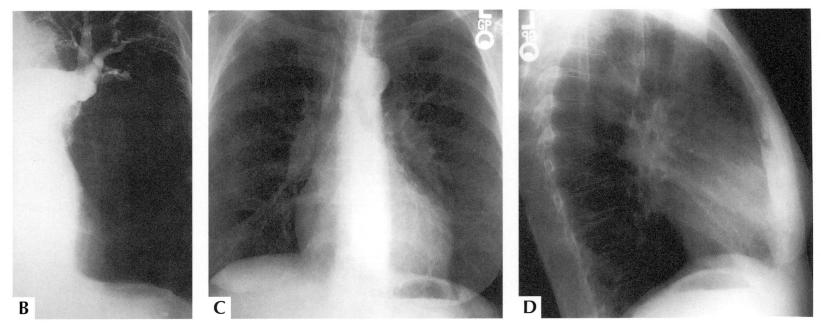

FIGURE 7-15. (*continued*) **B,** Pulmonary angiogram in the same patient demonstrating proximal occlusion of the descending left pulmonary artery with absence of flow to the lingula and left lower lobe. Chest radiographs of another patient demonstrating enlargement of the main pulmonary arteries and right ventricular prominence on both the anterior (**C**) and lateral (**D**) views.

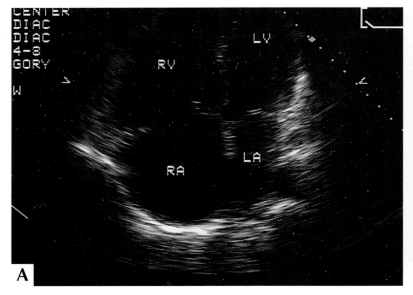

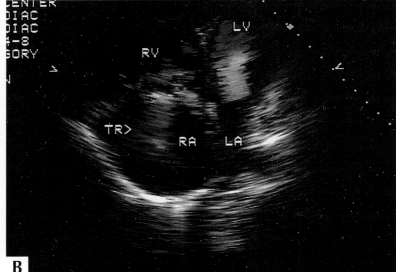

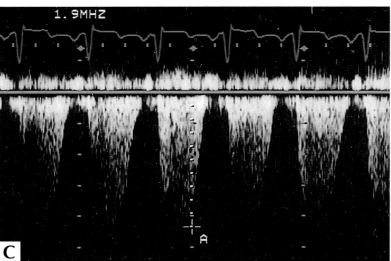

FIGURE 7-16. A, Characteristic echocardiogram of a patient with CTEPH. The typical echocardiogram in pulmonary hypertension demonstrates enlargement of the right atrium (RA) and right ventricle (RV). The normal shape of the RV is crescent, curving in front of and concave toward the left ventricle (LV). With RV volume overload, flattening of the interventricular septum is seen, transforming the RV crescentic shape into a more cylindric configuration.

B, Color flow echocardiogram demonstrating a tricuspid regurgitant jet.

C, Doppler ultrasound assessment of the tricuspid regurgitant jet. Using the Bernoulli equation, pulmonary artery (PA) systolic pressure can be estimated from the peak flow velocity of the tricuspid regurgitant jet (using the relationship that 4 times the peak velocity squared is equal to the transvalvular pressure gradient). Addition of the estimated or measured RA pressure to transvalvular pressure results in an estimated peak PA systolic pressure. In the illustrated case, PA systolic pressure = $4(4.35)^2$ + RA, or 76 mm Hg + RA.

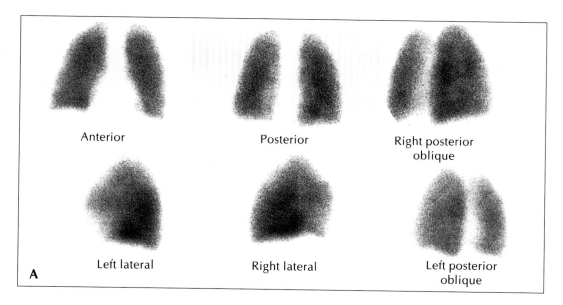

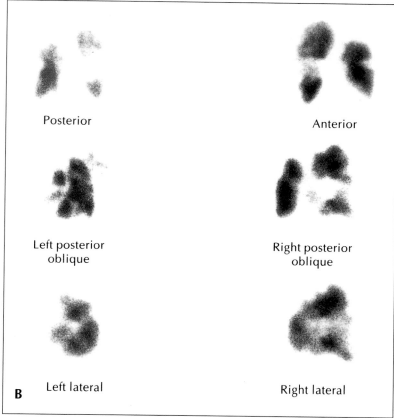

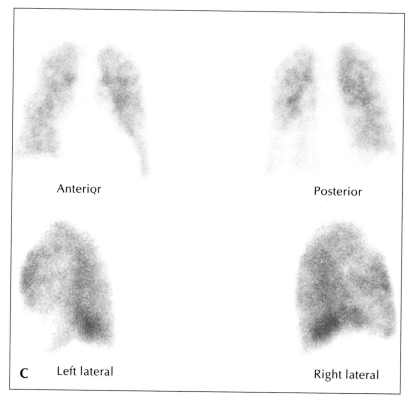

FIGURE 7-17. A, Normal six-view perfusion lung scan.
B, Perfusion lung scan in a patient with CTEPH. Ventilation scan was normal.
C, Perfusion lung scan in primary pulmonary hypertension. Ventilation-perfusion lung scanning provides an excellent, low-risk, noninvasive means of distinguishing between pulmonary hypertension due to potentially operable CTEPH and obliterative, small-vessel pulmonary hypertension [29–32]. In chronic thromboembolic disease, at least one (and, more commonly, several) segmental or larger mismatched defect is present. In primary pulmonary hypertension, the perfusion scan is either normal or has a mottled appearance consisting of patchy, subsegmental abnormalities. Although the ventilation-perfusion lung scan can suggest the diagnosis of CTEPH, it is incapable of confirming the diagnosis or establishing surgical feasibility. Any process that occludes major pulmonary arteries, either through external compression (fibrosing mediastinitis, mediastinal tumors) or intraluminal obstruction (thrombus, tumor), will result in similar defects.

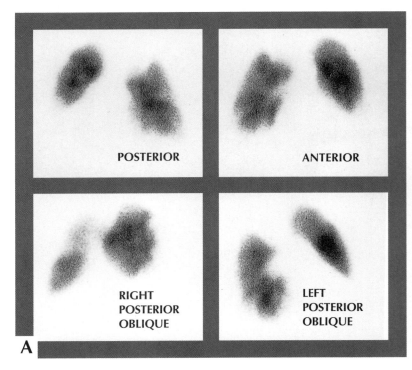

POSTERIOR

ANTERIOR

RIGHT
POSTERIOR
OBLIQUE

LEFT
POSTERIOR
OBLIQUE

A

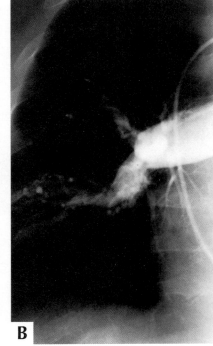

B

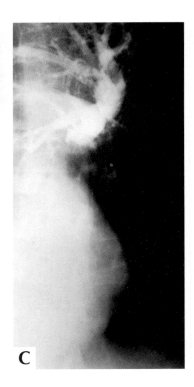

C

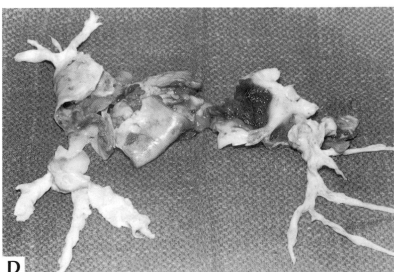

D

FIGURE 7-18. Although capable of suggesting the diagnosis of chronic thromboembolic disease, perfusion scanning often significantly understates the actual extent of chronic thromboembolic obstruction [33]. **A,** Perfusion scan in a patient with CTEPH. **B,** Right-sided angiogram in the same patient. **C,** Left-sided angiogram in the same patient. **D,** Chronic thromboembolic material obtained at the time of pulmonary thromboendarterectomy.

The perfusion scan, although clearly abnormal, does not provide an accurate estimation of the actual extent of central chronic thromboembolic obstruction. In CTEPH, the extent of perfusion defects cannot be used to predict with any reliability the severity of central vessel obstruction as defined either by angiography or by hemodynamic measurements. In patients with suspected pulmonary hypertension, a scan demonstrating segmental perfusion defects should raise the suspicion of CTEPH and lead to consideration of right heart catheterization and pulmonary angiography.

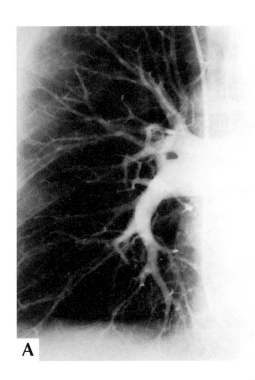

A

B

FIGURE 7-19. Normal right (**A**) and left (**B**) pulmonary angiograms. The appearance of the normal pulmonary vasculature is one of smoothly tapering branches that extend to the periphery of the lung fields. The principal function of the pulmonary arteries is the exchange of oxygen and carbon dioxide between alveolar air and blood in the pulmonary capillaries. By virtue of a separate blood supply via systemic bronchial arteries, usually arising from intercostal arteries on the right and the thoracic aorta on the left, and the presence of bronchopulmonary arterial anastomoses, even extensive thromboembolic pulmonary artery occlusion does not lead to necrosis of intrapulmonary structures.

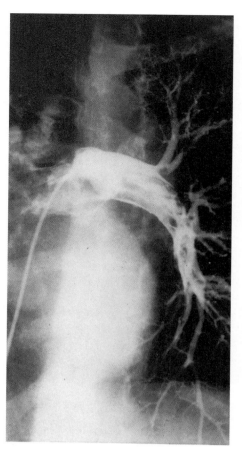

FIGURE 7-20. Pulmonary angiogram in acute pulmonary embolism. Left-sided pulmonary angiography demonstrates sharply defined, intraluminal defects consistent with acute pulmonary embolism. Pulmonary angiography has long been recognized as the diagnostic standard of reference for acute pulmonary embolism, and the diagnostic criteria of acute embolism have been well defined. The variable location, extent, organization, and pattern of recanalization of chronic thromboembolic pulmonary artery obstruction, however, leads to angiographic patterns that bear little resemblance to those encountered in acute embolism.

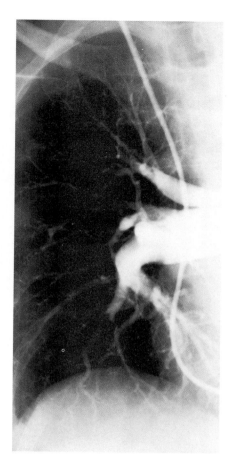

FIGURE 7-21. Pulmonary angiogram in primary pulmonary hypertension. The pulmonary angiogram in primary pulmonary hypertension usually demonstrates dilatation of the main pulmonary arteries, which then taper rapidly. There is a paucity and pruning of peripheral vessels. As opposed to surgically accessible CTEPH, in which the source of increased pulmonary vascular resistance is in the main, lobar, or segmental pulmonary arteries, increased pulmonary vascular resistance in primary pulmonary hypertension arises from small, muscular pulmonary arteries.

ANGIOGRAPHIC PATTERNS

"Pouch" defects involving segmental, lobar, or main pulmonary arteries

Pulmonary arterial webs or bands

Intimal irregularity

Abrupt narrowing of major pulmonary vessels

Obstruction of lobar vessels at their point of origin

FIGURE 7-22. Pulmonary angiographic findings in CTEPH. A properly performed and interpreted pulmonary angiogram plays a pivotal role in defining the location, extent, and surgical accessibility of the obstructing thrombotic lesions [34]. The complex patterns of organization and recanalization that occur in chronic thromboembolic disease result in an angiographic appearance that bears little resemblance to that seen in acute pulmonary embolism. Several of these angiographic findings are often present in each patient with operable chronic thromboembolic disease.

Despite concerns regarding the safety of pulmonary angiography in patients with pulmonary hypertension, the procedure can be performed with minimal complications by taking appropriate precautionary measures [35]. These include catheterization via the arm or neck to avoid inducing or dislodging lower extremity venous thrombi; a single injection of nonionic contrast media into the right and left main pulmonary arteries; modification of contrast volume and infusion rate; careful patient monitoring and oxygen administration during the procedure; and avoidance of repeated, selective injections.

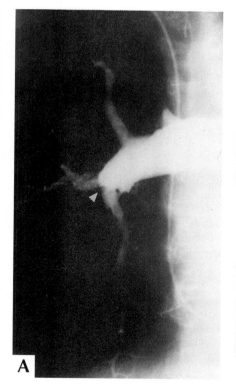

A

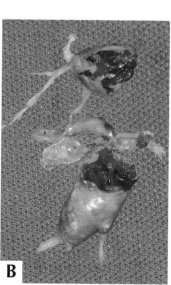

B

FIGURE 7-23. A, Pouch defect involving the proximal descending right pulmonary artery (*arrowhead*). Early in the angiographic sequence, contrast material may opacify this pouch; on subsequent angiograms, this apparent termination can slowly give rise to more distal vessels or can actually represent complete vascular obstruction. **B,** Specimens obtained at the time of pulmonary thromboendarterectomy.

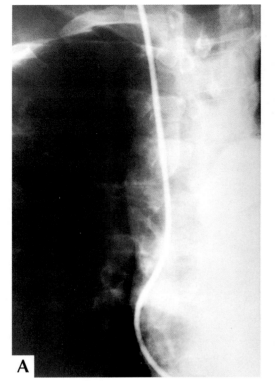

A

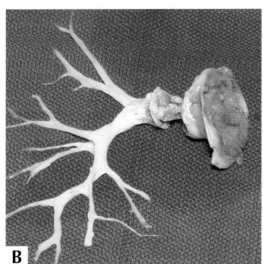

B

FIGURE 7-24. **A,** Pouch defect involving the proximal right main pulmonary artery. The smooth outline of the main pulmonary artery can be seen with no evidence of any vascular structure arising from the right side of the pulmonary artery. This angiographic finding can suggest the possibility of unilateral pulmonary artery agenesis [36]. Prior to anticipated surgical intervention, it is essential to make the differentiation between CTEPH and agenesis. Pulmonary angioscopy can be useful in making such a distinction. Other collateral clues, such as prior chest radiographic appearance, computed tomographic findings, the presence of flow murmurs over the contralateral lung, the presence of perfusion defects or pulmonary angiographic abnormalities in the contralateral lung, and a prior history of venous thromboembolism, can help differentiate the two conditions. **B,** Occluding thrombus removed at the time of pulmonary thromboendarterectomy.

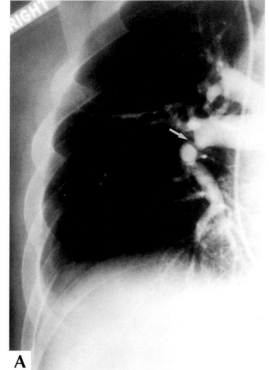

A

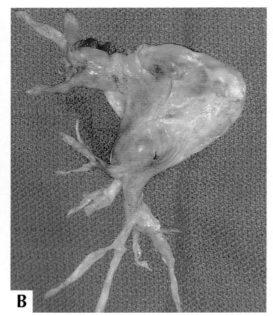

B

FIGURE 7-25. **A,** Classic web in descending right pulmonary artery with poststenotic dilatation *(arrow)*. *Pulmonary artery webs* or *bands* refer to lines with decreased opacity that traverse the width of the pulmonary vessel, usually at the lobar or segmental level. These findings are often associated with vessel narrowing and distal poststenotic dilatation. These bands persist throughout the angiographic sequence and should not be confused with a confluence of overlying shadows. **B,** Thrombus removed at the time of pulmonary thromboendarterectomy.

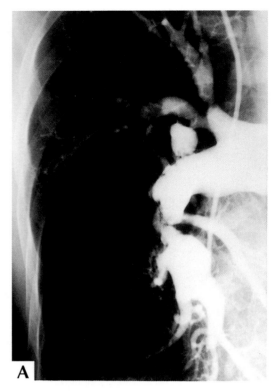

A

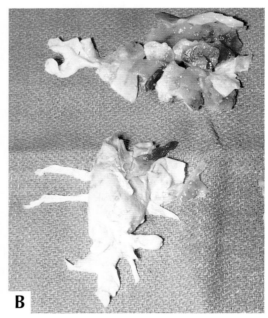

B

FIGURE 7-26. **A,** Angiogram demonstrating intimal irregularity involving the right main and descending pulmonary arteries. Webs are also apparent in the upper and lower lobe vessels. Intimal irregularity that gives a scalloped appearance to the pulmonary arterial wall is another common finding in chronic thromboembolic disease. At surgery, this abnormality has been associated with a chronic, irregularly organized thrombus that lines the vessel wall. Other findings in this angiogram include a pouch defect, web, and poststenotic dilatation lesions in the right upper lobe branches, and a pouch defect with subsequent flow in the right descending pulmonary artery.

B, Chronic thromboembolic material obtained at the time of pulmonary thromboendarterectomy.

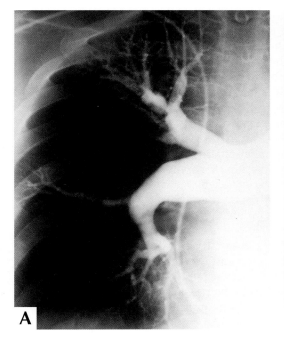

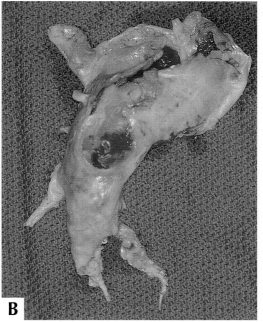

FIGURE 7-27. A, Right-sided pulmonary angiogram demonstrating abrupt narrowing of the descending right pulmonary artery immediately below a completely occluded anterior segment right upper lobe branch. The normal, gentle tapering of vessel size is replaced by a more abrupt decrease in the diameter of the opacified lumen. This narrowing is related to three potential findings at surgery: recanalization within a large thrombus; narrowing of the arterial lumen by concentric organized thrombus that lines the arterial wall; and actual contraction of the artery by organized thrombus. In the first two instances, there is often a discrepancy between the apparent outer edge of the vessel wall seen on chest radiographs or scout films and the outer edge of the column of contrast material seen at angiography.

B, Occluding thrombus removed at the time of thromboendarterectomy.

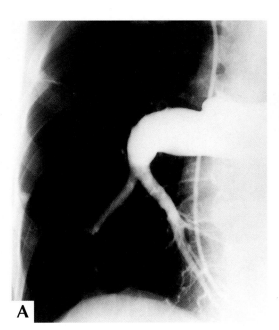

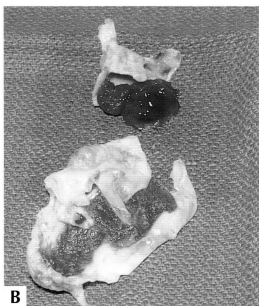

FIGURE 7-28. A, Right-sided pulmonary angiogram demonstrating obstruction of the right upper and middle lobe arteries at their point of origin from the main pulmonary artery. This finding is often associated with the presence of subtle intimal irregularities or with an abnormally straight border of the vessel wall. Vessels that should normally emerge from this region are not visualized. **B,** Specimens obtained at the time of pulmonary thromboendarterectomy.

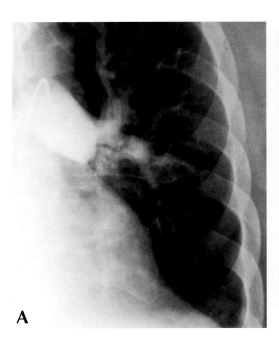

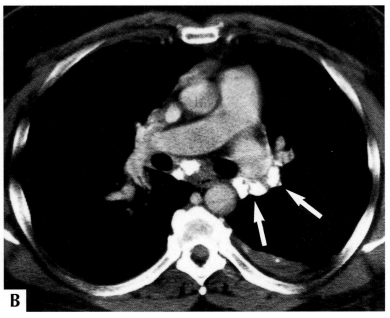

FIGURE 7-29.
A, Pulmonary angiogram in a patient with fibrosing mediastinitis demonstrating its similarity in appearance to chronic thromboembolic disease.

B, Chest computed tomographic (CT) scan demonstrating dense calcification (*arrows*) within the mediastinum and surrounding the left pulmonary artery. (*continued*)

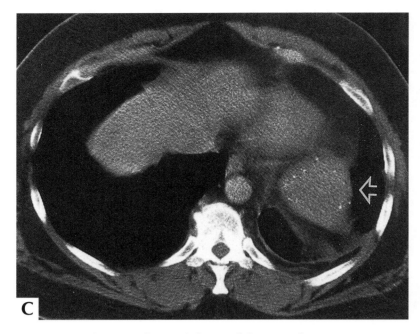

indicated. Although angiographic findings are highly suggestive of CTEPH, competing diagnoses do exist [34]. Pulmonary arterial webs and bands, originally described as angiographic evidence of chronic thrombi, can be found in other disease entities. Congenital stenotic lesions of the pulmonary arteries and a certain form of large-vessel arteritis (Takayasu's arteritis) may present a similar angiographic appearance. Total obstruction of major pulmonary arteries occurs in a number of other disorders, including carcinoma (vascular or primary lung), extrinsic compression from mediastinal lymphadenopathy, fibrosing mediastinitis, and pulmonary artery agenesis. Virtually the same differential diagnosis should be considered when abrupt narrowing of major pulmonary vessels is seen at angiography.

The pulmonary angiogram in CTEPH almost invariably demonstrates the bilateral presence of several of the angiographic abnormalities described. Pulmonary angioscopy may be necessary to confirm the diagnosis and to establish whether surgical intervention is feasible [37]. CT scanning of the chest to evaluate the mediastinum can exclude the possibility of fibrosing mediastinitis or extrinsic compression of the pulmonary arteries by mediastinal lymphadenopathy. Arch aortography may be indicated if a vasculitis is being considered. Neither bronchial arteriography nor intravascular ultrasonography has proven useful in determining surgical accessibility.

Figure 7-29. (*continued*) **C,** Abdominal CT scan demonstrating splenic calcifications (*arrow*). While the pulmonary angiogram usually completes the diagnostic sequence, other studies may be

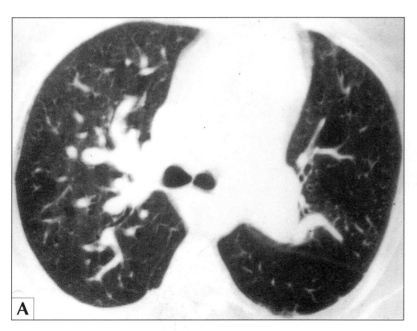

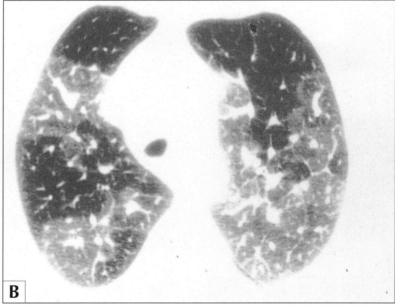

FIGURE 7-30. Chest computed tomography (CT) is of limited usefulness in evaluating patients with CTEPH other than in excluding suspected competing diagnoses such as fibrosing mediastinitis and other causes of extrinsic vascular compression. However, a number of nonspecific CT findings have been identified in certain patients with chronic thromboembolic disease.

A, Chest CT scan in a patient with chronic thromboembolic disease demonstrating variation in the size of the peripheral pulmonary vasculature.

B, Chest CT scan in a patient with chronic thromboembolic disease demonstrating a mosaic pattern of perfusion. This finding is probably a result of regional differences in perfusion due to central chronic thromboembolic obstruction. The normal lung demonstrates a faint homogenous pattern of perfusion.

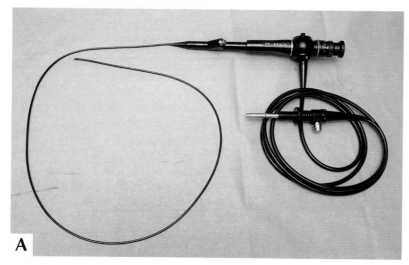

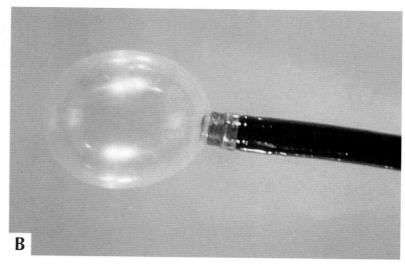

FIGURE 7-31. A, The pulmonary angioscope is a fiberoptic device that allows visualization of the pulmonary arteries to the segmental level. Pulmonary angioscopy poses a different set of problems from angioscopy of the coronary bed or peripheral vessels, including the wide variation in vessel size (particularly in patients with pulmonary hypertension), the degree of vessel branching, and the large volume of the pulmonary vascular bed. The current prototype is 120 cm long with an external diameter of 3 mm. The distal tip is capable of being moved through 90° of deflection. The instrument can be easily inserted through an 11F introducing sheath placed in the internal jugular vein, preferably the right. Under fluoroscopic guidance, the angioscope is advanced to the right atrium without balloon inflation. With the tip fully flexed, the tricuspid valve and right ventricular chamber are carefully traversed. Balloon inflation often assists passage across the pulmonic valve. Using fluoroscopic guidance, balloon inflation, and distal tip deflection, a complete examination of the pulmonary arteries to the segmental level can be achieved in a timely fashion.

B, Angioscope tip with the balloon inflated. Nonthrombogenic materials are used in balloon construction. The balloon is inflated with carbon dioxide to avoid air embolism in the event of balloon rupture. The balloon is secured to the tip of the angioscope under sterile conditions prior to the procedure with repetitive wrappings of fine (6/0) braided thread. Once in the pulmonary artery, the balloon is gradually inflated until an image appears. Complete occlusion is not always necessary for adequate visualization of the vascular wall. The balloon itself does not provide any significant resistance to moving the angioscope and usually has no adverse hemodynamic consequences when carefully inflated.

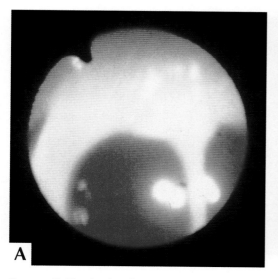

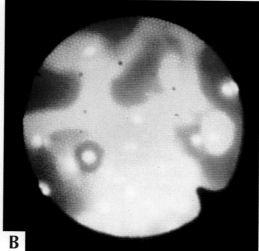

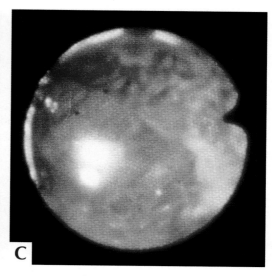

FIGURE 7-32. A, Angioscopic appearance of a normal pulmonary artery, which has a round or oval contour with a smooth, pale, glistening appearance to the intima, and bright red blood filling the lumen.

B, Angioscopic appearance of recanalization, demonstrating channels through an occluding thrombus.

C, Angioscopic appearance of a pitted mass of chronic thromboembolic material. The finding of atherosclerotic plaques is a nonspecific finding commonly seen in other forms of pulmonary hypertension.

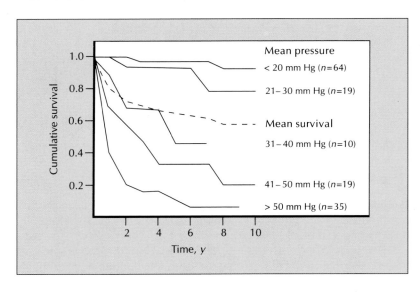

FIGURE 7-33. Cumulative survival curves in patients with CTEPH according to the initial mean pulmonary artery pressure [20]. The natural history of CTEPH beyond the time of symptom onset has not yet been firmly resolved. Part of this uncertainty arises from the evolving nature of the diagnostic and therapeutic approach to patients with this disease entity. It also arises from the disparate extent of hemodynamic compromise, degree of pulmonary vascular obstruction, and period of diagnostic delay at the time of initial presentation. Our own assessment, obtained primarily from a small cohort of patients who have been referred but have not been operated on for a variety of reasons, indicates that the median survival from the time of initial diagnosis until death is in the vicinity of 2 to 3 years, a finding similar to that of Riedel *et al.* [20]. It is also similar to the duration of survival reported in patients with primary pulmonary hypertension. The *dotted lines* represent predicted survival among men 40 to 50 years of age. (*Adapted from* Riedel and coworkers [20]; with permission.)

INDICATIONS FOR PULMONARY THROMBOENDARTERECTOMY

Pulmonary vascular resistance (PVR) >300 dynes/s/cm^{-5}, **OR**

Ventilatory impairment at rest or with exercise

Thrombus accessible to surgical removal

Consideration of comorbid conditions that might affect outcome

Willingness of the patient to assume the procedural risk

FIGURE 7-34. Indications for pulmonary thromboendarterectomy. The decision to proceed to operation is based on a number of objective and subjective factors. First, the chronic thromboemboli must be surgically accessible as determined by angiography or angioscopy. Present surgical techniques allow the removal of chronic thromboemboli from main, lobar, and segmental arteries. Those that begin more distally are not subject to endarterectomy. This determination is critical since failure to remove obstruction and to lower PVR at the time of surgery is associated with an adverse outcome. Second, the presence of vascular obstruction should be responsible for hemodynamic or ventilatory impairment at rest or with exercise.

Given the broad spectrum of the disease, it is clear that not all patients who have chronic thromboembolic obstruction require surgical correction. The overwhelming majority of operated patients have a PVR in excess of 300 dynes/s/cm^{-5}. However, occasional patients, especially those with involvement of one main pulmonary artery, have significant exercise limitation as a result of increased dead space ventilation and extraordinary minute ventilation demands during exercise despite normal or minimally abnormal pulmonary hemodynamics.

Third, the status of the right ventricle and the presence of comorbid disease must be considered since these influence operative risk and long-term outcome. Predictive factors include: NYHA class IV; age over 70 years; PVR exceeding 1000 dynes/s/cm^{-5}; right ventricular failure as manifested by an elevated right atrial pressure; and significant hepatic, renal, or pulmonary parenchymal disease. Finally, the patient must be willing to accept the mortal and morbid risks of the procedure. Age in itself is not a contraindication. Patients up to age 80, who were otherwise fit, have undergone successful pulmonary thromboendarterectomy.

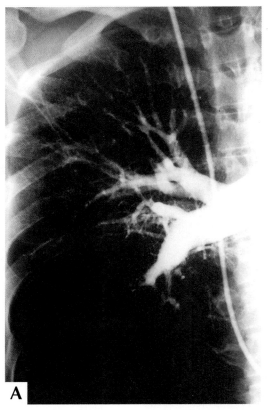

A

FIGURE 7-35. Example of the discordance between the degree of pulmonary vascular obstruction and the extent of functional and hemodynamic impairment. The extent of chronic thromboembolic pulmonary artery obstruction represents only one factor in defining an individual patient's symptomatic status. Although 40% to 50% of the pulmonary vascular bed must be obstructed for pulmonary hypertension to develop at rest, right ventricular response is also dependent on the status of the peripheral vascular bed and on right ventricular compensatory mechanisms. Pulmonary angiography demonstrates extensive chronic thromboembolic obstruction. **A,** Right anterior view. (*continued*)

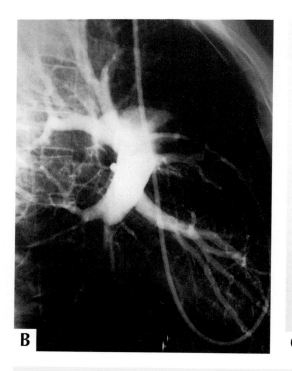 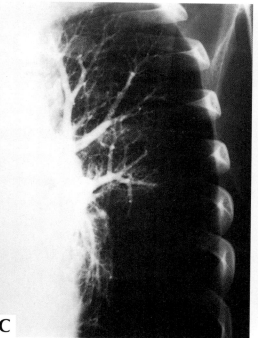 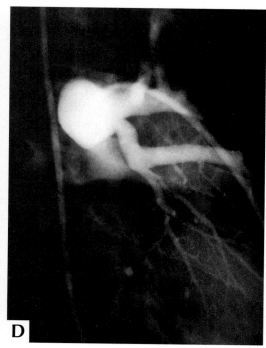

B

C

D

E. PREOPERATIVE PULMONARY HEMODYNAMICS

	REST	EXERCISE
RA	4	—
Pulmonary artery pressure	37/15 (20)	45/23 (30)
Cardiac output, *L/min*	4.8	8.3
PCWP	11	7
PVR, dynes/s/cm^{-5}	150	222

FIGURE 7-35. (*continued*) **B,** Right lateral view. **C,** Left anterior view. **D,** Left lateral view. Despite obstruction of greater than 50% of the pulmonary vascular bed, the patient was able to engage in long-distance swimming and running, although at a level considerably less intense than that prior to the embolic event.

E, Preoperative pulmonary hemodynamics. Based on the patient's subjective complaints as well as concerns regarding her cardiopulmonary status during anticipated future pregnancies, a pulmonary thromboendarterectomy was performed. Reperfusion of both lower lobes was established, postoperative pulmonary vascular resistance was less than 100 dynes/s/cm^{-5}, and the patient's functional status returned to normal.

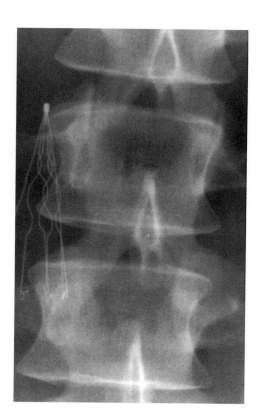

FIGURE 7-36. Greenfield filter in place in an infrarenal position. In our view, it is important that the patient be protected against embolic occurrence from the lower extremities, both in the high-risk perioperative period when full-dose anticoagulation is contraindicated and over the long term. A Greenfield filter is routinely placed into the inferior vena cava before surgery unless an obvious source of embolism, which does not involve the lower extremities or pelvis, is apparent. In some patients, indwelling cardiac pacing wires or other chronic intravenous devices have been the embolic source.

Two options exist if the filter cannot be placed by way of a percutaneous, femoral approach: one option is to place the filter from the internal jugular vein; the other option is to place the filter under direct observation through the right atrium at the time of surgery. Coronary angiography, performed at the time of right heart catheterization and pulmonary angiography, is performed in all patients with surgically accessible chronic thromboembolic disease who are over 35 years of age and who have significant coronary risk factors. Coincident coronary artery disease can be corrected by bypass graft at the time of the thromboendarterectomy.

SURGICAL TECHNIQUE AND POSTOPERATIVE COURSE
[SEE ALSO CHAPTER 8]

SURGICAL TECHNIQUE FOR PULMONARY THROMBOENDARTERECTOMY

Median sternotomy (not thoracotomy)

Cardiopulmonary bypass

Hypothermic circulatory arrest

Bilateral thromboendarterectomy

True endarterectomy (not embolectomy)

Exploration of interatrial septum

POSTOPERATIVE COMPLICATIONS AND CARE

"Usual" post-pump, open heart problems

Diaphragmatic paresis

Supraventricular arrhythmias

Pericardial effusion

Postoperative delirium

Pulmonary artery steal

Reperfusion lung injury

FIGURE 7-37. Two separate surgical procedures are available for CTEPH: thoracotomy or sternotomy with cardiopulmonary bypass [5–10]. In our judgment, sternotomy with cardiopulmonary bypass is the procedure of choice. The most critical need for sternotomy arises from the bilateral nature of the disease process. Sternotomy allows access to both pulmonary arteries and assures more complete removal of the chronically obstructing material. The use of cardiopulmonary bypass also allows periods of hypothermic circulatory arrest, which provides the bloodless operative field that is essential for meticulous lobar and segmental dissection. Furthermore, the need to traverse bronchial arterial collateral vessels and pleural adhesions makes a transthoracic approach potentially dangerous.

Thromboendarterectomy bears no resemblance to acute pulmonary embolectomy. The neointima is deceptive and is not easily recognizable as chronic thrombus to a surgeon inexperienced with the procedure. The procedure is a true endarterectomy, which requires careful dissection of chronic endothelialized material from the native intima to restore pulmonary arterial patency.

The changes in surgical approach over the past 20 years have been evolutionary [7–10]. The problem of phrenic nerve injury, diaphragmatic paralysis, and the need for prolonged ventilatory support in the postoperative period has been eliminated by the use of a cooling jacket rather than cold saline-slush for myocardial protection [8]. Circulatory arrest times have been shortened with a subsequent decrease in the incidence of postoperative delirium. Changes in surgical technique have been initiated to improve exposure of left lower lobe thrombi and to assure more secure suture lines. Recognition that thromboendarterectomy results in improvement or normalization of right atrial and ventricular chamber size, with reestablishment of tricuspid valve competence, has obviated the need for tricuspid annuloplasty. The performance of two or three thromboendarterectomies per week by the same surgeon has conferred benefits in terms of recognition of the varied expressions of chronic thrombosis and of special dissection variations for optimally dealing with them [10].

FIGURE 7-38. In addition to common complications in patients undergoing open heart procedures, patients undergoing thromboendarterectomy are at potential risk for several unique complications that can result in substantial morbidity, extension of intensive care unit and hospital stay, or death. Increasing experience with this unique patient population has resulted in the development of a critical care team consisting of physicians, nurses, respiratory therapists, pharmacists, and other ancillary personnel, who have developed the expertise to anticipate these complications, to understand their pathophysiology, and to intervene in a manner that optimizes patient outcome.

The need for a coordinated, multidisciplinary approach to the patient with CTEPH cannot be emphasized too strongly. The postoperative management of patients undergoing pulmonary thromboendarterectomy has evolved along with the surgical procedure over the past 20 years. Administration of prostaglandin E_1 has become routine in the early postoperative period to guard against immediate postpump pulmonary vasoconstriction and the potential for postprocedure in situ rethrombosis. The problem of postoperative supraventricular arrhythmias, most commonly sinus bradycardia and atrial flutter, resulted in the standard intraoperative placement of temporary atrial and ventricular pacing wires and improved strategies for postoperative pharmacologic management. Postoperative pericardial effusions have been managed effectively with the routine intraoperative placement of temporary pericardial catheters.

The incidence of postoperative delirium was demonstrated to be strongly associated with deep hypothermia and the duration of total circulatory arrest [38]. Increased surgical experience had led to a significant decline in circulatory arrest times, resulting in a decreased incidence of delirium [10]. When delirium occurs, improved strategies for effective sedation have been devised and implemented. The recognition that patients with anticardiolipin antibodies have a high incidence of heparin-associated thrombocytopenia has resulted in protocols that allow stabilization of platelets during cardiopulmonary bypass and during the early postoperative period [39].

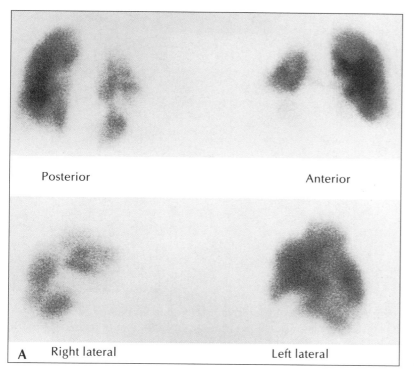

Posterior   Anterior

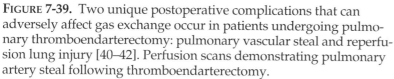

A Right lateral   Left lateral

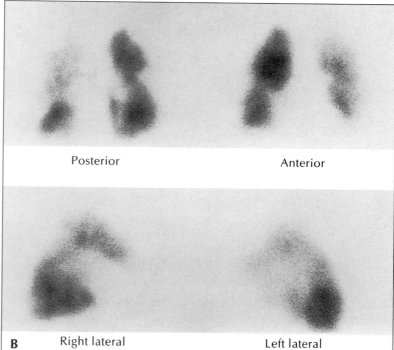

Posterior   Anterior

B Right lateral   Left lateral

FIGURE 7-39. Two unique postoperative complications that can adversely affect gas exchange occur in patients undergoing pulmonary thromboendarterectomy: pulmonary vascular steal and reperfusion lung injury [40–42]. Perfusion scans demonstrating pulmonary artery steal following thromboendarterectomy.

Preoperative scan (**A**) demonstrates multiple defects with minimal perfusion to the right lung. Postoperative scan (**B**) demonstrates almost complete reversal of pulmonary blood flow.

Pulmonary vascular steal represents a redistribution of pulmonary blood flow away from previously well-perfused segments and into the newly endarterectomized segments [40]. Although the basis for this phenomenon remains speculative, it is probably related to the temporary development of differential resistances in the pulmonary vascular bed following thromboendarterectomy: a low-resistance

circuit in the newly endarterectomized segments and a high-resistance circuit in the previously open segments resulting from small-vessel changes. An alternate explanation is that surgical disruption of the pulmonary vascular endothelium might induce a state of nonresponsive vasodilatation in the endarterectomized segments. The most clinically relevant observations regarding steal are that it occurs rather commonly following pulmonary thromboendarterectomy and that, if it is encountered after a successful procedure in which the involved vessels were not entered, rethrombosis or recurrent pulmonary embolism are unlikely causes.

Long-term follow-up has demonstrated that pulmonary vascular steal improves in the overwhelming majority of patients [41], suggesting that remodeling of the small-vessel changes in the previously open pulmonary vascular bed may occur over time.

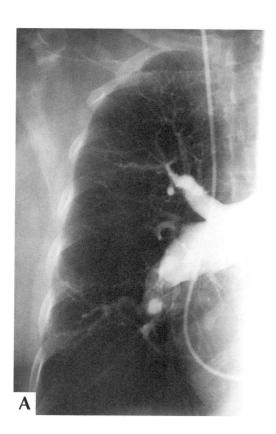

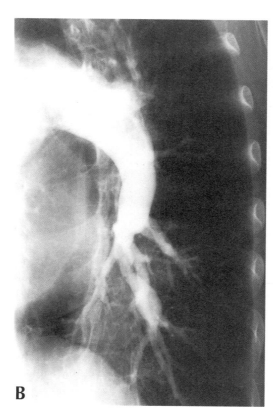

A   **B**

FIGURE 7-40. Reperfusion pulmonary edema sparing the upper lobes in a patient with predominantly lower lobe thromboendarterectomy. **A**, Preoperative right pulmonary angiogram. Note normal right upper lobe perfusion. **B**, Preoperative left pulmonary angiogram. (*continued*)

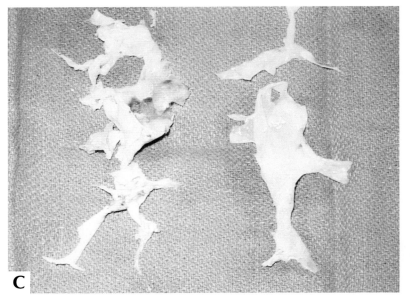

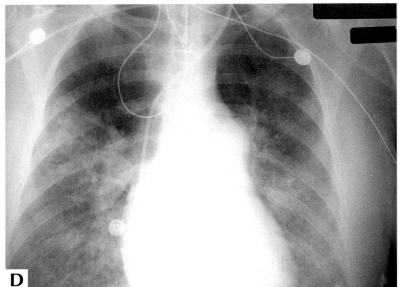

C

D

FIGURE 7-40. (*continued*) **C,** Surgical specimens obtained at the time of thromboendarterectomy. **D,** Postoperative chest radiograph demonstrating diffuse infiltrates with sparing of the upper lobes.

Although its exact pathophysiologic basis remains uncertain, reperfusion pulmonary edema, biochemically and clinically, appears to represent a focal form of acute lung injury (adult respiratory distress syndrome) that is limited radiographically to those areas of the lung from which proximal vascular obstruction has been removed [42]. It is highly variable in severity, ranging from acute, hemorrhagic, and potentially fatal complications to a mild

form resulting in postoperative hypoxemia. In its severe form, it represents a significant postoperative challenge in terms of ventilator management since pulmonary blood flow is shunted into edematous, noncompliant areas of lung that are poorly ventilated and thereby participate poorly in gas exchange. The extent and severity of reperfusion edema appear to have been moderated in recent years by the immediate postoperative administration of a large bolus of corticosteroids. The role of other agents that moderate the inflammatory response at different levels is currently under investigation.

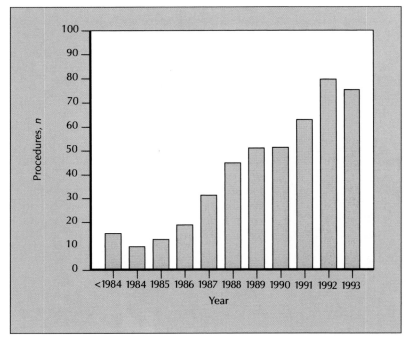

FIGURE 7-41. Annual number of pulmonary thromboendarterectomy procedures performed at the University of California at San Diego Medical Center. An increasing number of patients, from both national and international sites, have been referred over the past decade. Over 600 patients with presumed CTEPH have been evaluated by members of this program. By the end of 1993, 471 patients from 46 states, Canada, Australia, Great Britain, Spain, Saudi Arabia, Italy, Israel, Belgium, Austria, Taiwan, Mexico, and the Philippines had undergone thromboendarterectomy at this center. This increased pattern of referral probably represents an enhanced recognition of CTEPH as a potentially reversible form of pulmonary hypertension rather than reflecting an actual increase in the prevalence of the disease.

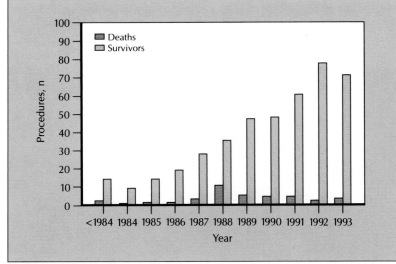

FIGURE 7-42. Perioperative mortality in patients undergoing pulmonary thromboendarterectomy at the University of California at San Diego Medical Center. The decrease in perioperative mortality has been related to improved methods of preoperative evaluation, including the use of angioscopy, increased surgical experience and improvement in surgical techniques, and advances in postoperative care. A vital aspect of the program has been the presence of an experienced and highly interactive medical-surgical team involving physicians and other health care workers such as program coordinators, nurses, pharmacists, and respiratory therapists. The preoperative evaluation, surgical technique, and postoperative care of these patients can be challenging, and an experienced team approach to these patients is essential for success.

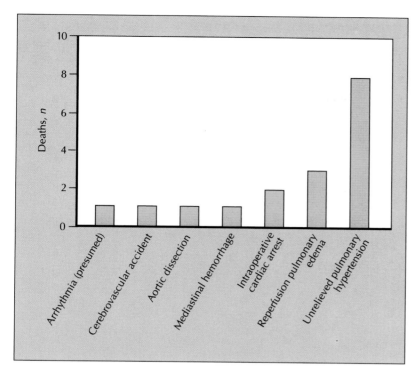

FIGURE 7-43. Cause of death in 17 (6.2%) of the 275 patients who underwent pulmonary thromboendarterectomy at the University of California at San Diego Medical Center between 1990 and 1993. At present, only two significant residual causes of mortality remain: the inability to remove sufficient thrombotic material at the time of operation, resulting in persistent postoperative pulmonary hypertension and right ventricular dysfunction; and severe reperfusion lung injury. Six deaths were the result of residual postoperative pulmonary hypertension and right ventricular failure in patients in whom pulmonary thromboendarterectomy failed to achieve substantial improvement in pulmonary hemodynamics. Two additional intraoperative deaths occurred in patients in whom an adequate thromboendarterectomy could not be performed and in whom weaning from cardiopulmonary bypass could not be achieved. Three patients died directly as a result of severe reperfusion lung injury. One patient died suddenly (presumed arrhythmia) after discharge from the intensive care unit. One death resulted from mediastinal hemorrhage after removal of a left atrial line while another patient died within the first postoperative week from an aortic dissection. Two patients operated on after being brought to the operating room in extremis and undergoing cardiac massage, had irreversible cerebral injury. One patient suffered an intraoperative cerebrovascular accident and died on the 26th postoperative day without regaining consciousness.

A. PULMONARY HEMODYNAMICS

	PREOPERATIVE	POSTOPERATIVE
PA mean pressure, *mm Hg*	46±12	28±9*
PA systolic pressure, *mm Hg*	76±21	47±16*
Cardiac output, *L/min*	3.7±1.1	5.7±1.2*
PVR, *dynes/s/cm⁻⁵*	901±467	261±163*

*$P<0.001$ vs preoperative value.

B. PULMONARY HEMODYNAMICS

	PREOPERATIVE	POSTOPERATIVE	FOLLOW-UP
PA mean pressure, *mm Hg*	48±12	27±8*	24±10
PA systolic pressure, *mm Hg*	80±21	44±15*	39±17†
Cardiac output, *L/min*	3.7±1.2	6.0±1.1*	4.8±1.0‡
PVR, *dynes/s/cm⁻⁵*	971±551	232±111*	282±251

*$P<0.001$ vs preoperative value. †$P<0.0015$ vs postoperative value. ‡$P<0.0001$ vs postoperative value.

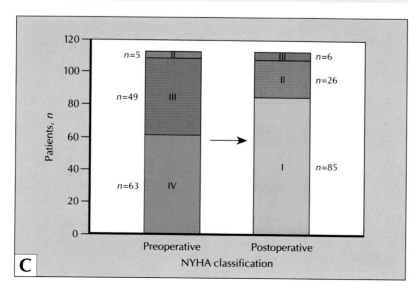

FIGURE 7-44. A, Pulmonary hemodynamics in 128 of 150 patients in whom postoperative values were obtained 48 to 72 hours after admission to the intensive care unit. Patients were off all vasoactive drugs.

B, Pulmonary hemodynamics obtained in 47 of the first 150 patients who returned for follow-up catheterization 6 to 24 months after surgery. Among survivors of thromboendarterectomy, the immediate hemodynamic improvement has been dramatic, with marked reductions in pulmonary artery (PA) pressures and pulmonary vascular resistance (PVR) [1–4]. The long-term hemodynamic outcome has also been dramatic [1–4]. Return of a severely compromised right ventricle to normal size and function has been well documented by echocardiography [43,44], an observation that has implications in the decision to perform heart-lung versus lung transplantation in other conditions. Many patients have now returned for follow-up evaluation, including repeat heart catheterization and pulmonary angiography. Results of this evaluation reflect the maintenance of the pulmonary hemodynamic improvement noted in the early postoperative period.

C, Perhaps the most important measure of long-term outcome has been the change in New York Heart Association (NYHA) functional class of these patients at 1 year after surgery. Most patients report steady improvement in their functional state over 3 to 9 months after hospital discharge. The majority return to class I functional status within the first year. The long-term postoperative management of these patients is relatively simple. Lifelong anticoagulant therapy is advised, despite the usual presence of the caval filter. This recommendation is based on the potential of venous thromboembolism recurrence with filter occlusion and on concerns about in situ rethrombosis of the pulmonary arteries. With a return to normal hemodynamic status, no restrictions are placed on a patient's level of activity.

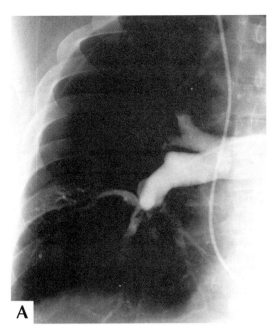 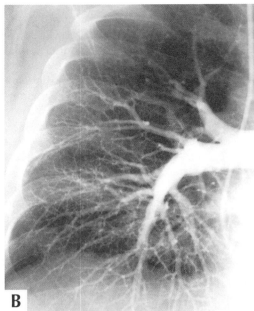

FIGURE 7-45. A, Preoperative right-sided pulmonary angiogram demonstrating pouch defects in the right upper and lower lobes with minimal right-sided perfusion.

B, Postoperative right-sided pulmonary angiogram demonstrating near normalization of perfusion. Angiographic improvement was accompanied by equally dramatic hemodynamic and functional improvement.

FUTURE INITIATIVES

Understanding of the pathophysiologic basis for failure or thrombus resolution

Improved application of preoperative evaluative techniques, including angioscopy

Ability to partition central from peripheral pulmonary vascular resistance

Methods to prevent or treat reperfusion pulmonary edema

Promotion of early diagnosis and management

FIGURE 7-46. Pulmonary thromboendarterectomy offers patients with CTEPH an opportunity for highly satisfactory improvement in their hemodynamic and functional status. Advances in diagnostic techniques, surgical selection and technique, and postoperative management have allowed recovery from this previously fatal form of pulmonary hypertension. The need for a coordinated, interactive, multidisciplinary team dedicated to the critical details of the complex problems these patients experience cannot be emphasized too strongly.

Each phase—evaluative, surgical, and postoperative—is characterized by a steep learning curve. Despite the dramatic improvement in perioperative mortality, a great deal still needs to be accomplished. The basis for failure of normal thromboembolic resolution has not been established and remains under active investigation. The differentiation of those patients with hemodynamically insignificant thromboembolic residua from those who will ultimately develop CTEPH will help to identify better the most appropriate time for surgical intervention. In patients with longstanding disease, the ability to partition the central, surgically accessible component of their increased pulmonary vascular disease from the secondary, small-vessel component will help to better define surgical indications and improve both operative and long-term postoperative outcomes.

The ability to preoperatively identify those patients who have developed potentially reversible small-vessel disease in their open pulmonary vascular bed may define those who will benefit from pharmacologic intervention in the postoperative period. Investigations are underway to determine the basis for reperfusion lung injury and to find effective means of prevention or therapy. Finally, educational efforts to assure early recognition are ongoing. Intervention, before right ventricular failure or fixed small-vessel pulmonary hypertensive changes occur, should result in improved mortality and long-term outcome.

REFERENCES

1. Moser KM, Auger WR, Fedullo PF: Chronic major-vessel thromboembolic pulmonary hypertension. *Circulation* 1990, 81:1735–1743.

2. Moser KM, Auger WR, Fedullo PF, *et al.*: Chronic thromboembolic pulmonary hypertension: clinical picture and surgical treatment. *Eur Respir J* 1992, 5:334–342.

3. Moser KM, Spragg RG, Utley J, *et al.*: Chronic thrombotic obstruction of major pulmonary arteries: results of thromboendarterectomy in 15 patients. *Ann Intern Med* 1983, 99:299–305.

4. Moser KM, Daily PO, Peterson K, *et al.*: Thromboendarterectomy for chronic major-vessel thromboembolic pulmonary hypertension: immediate and long-term results in 42 patients. *Ann Intern Med* 1987, 107:560–565.

5. Chitwood WR, Sabiston DC, Wechsler AS: Surgical treatment of chronic unresolved pulmonary embolism. *Clin Chest Med* 1984, 5:507–536.

6. Rich S, Levitsky S, Brundage BH: Pulmonary hypertension from chronic pulmonary thromboembolism. *Ann Intern Med* 1988, 108:425–434.

7. Utley JR, Spragg RG, Long WB, *et al.*: Pulmonary endarterectomy for chronic thromboembolic obstruction: recent surgical experience. *Surgery* 1982, 92:1096–1102.

8. Daily PO, Dembitsky WP, Peterson KL, *et al.*: Modifications of techniques and early results of pulmonary thromboendarterectomy for chronic pulmonary embolism. *J Thorac Cardiovasc Surg* 1987, 93:221–233.

9. Daily PO, Dembitsky WP, Iversen S, *et al.*: Risk factors for pulmonary thromboendarterectomy. *J Thorac Cardiovasc Surg* 1990, 99:670–678.

10. Jamieson SW, Auger WR, Fedullo PF, *et al.*: Experience and results with 150 pulmonary thromboendarterectomy operations over a 29-month period. *J Thorac Cardiovasc Surg* 1993, 106:116–127.

11. Rubin LJ: Primary Pulmonary Hypertension: ACCP Consensus Statement. *Chest* 1993, 104:236–250.

12. Rich S: Primary pulmonary hypertension. *Prog Cardiovasc Dis* 1988, 31:205–238.

13. World Health Organization: *Primary Pulmonary Hypertension.* Edited by Hatano S, Strasser T. Geneva: World Health Organization; 1975:7–45.

14. Benotti JR, Dalen JE: The natural history of pulmonary embolism. *Clin Chest Med* 1984, 5:403–410.

15. Hall RJC, Sutton GC, Kerr IH: Long-term prognosis of treated acute massive pulmonary embolism. *Br Heart J* 1977, 39:1128–1134.

16. Sutton GC, Hall RJC, Kerr IH: Clinical course and late prognosis of treated subacute massive, acute minor, and chronic pulmonary thromboembolism. *Br Heart J* 1977, 39:1135–1142.

17. Dalen JE, Banas JS, Brooks HL, *et al.*: Resolution rates of acute pulmonary embolism. *N Engl J Med* 1969, 280:1194–1199.

18. DeSoyza NB, Murphy ML: Persistent post-embolic pulmonary hypertension. *Chest* 1972, 6:665–668.

19. Tilkinian AG, Schroeder JS, Robin ED: Chronic thromboembolic occlusion of main pulmonary artery or primary branches. *Am J Med* 1976, 60:563–570.

20. Riedel M, Staned V, Widimsky J, *et al.*: Long-term follow-up of patients with pulmonary thromboembolism: late prognosis and evolution of hemodynamic and respiratory data. *Chest* 1982, 81:151–158.

21. Huisman MV, Buller HR, ten Cate JW, *et al.*: Unexpected high prevalence of silent pulmonary embolism in patients with deep venous thrombosis. *Chest* 1989, 95:498–502.

22. Dalen JE, Alpert JS: Natural history of pulmonary embolism. *Prog Cardiovasc Dis* 1975:259–270.

23. Olman MA, Marsh JJ, Lang IM, *et al.*: Endogenous fibrinolytic system in chronic large-vessel thromboembolic pulmonary hypertension. *Circulation* 1992, 86:1241–1248.

24. Moser KM, Bloor CM: Pulmonary vascular lesions occurring in patients with chronic major vessel thromboembolic pulmonary hypertension. *Chest* 1993, 103:685–692.

25. Fedullo PF, Auger WR, Moser KM, *et al.*: Hemodynamic response to exercise in patients with chronic, major vessel thromboembolic pulmonary hypertension. *Am Rev Respir Dis* 1990, 141:A-890.

26. Auger WR, Moser KM: Pulmonary flow murmurs: a distinctive physical sign found in chronic pulmonary thromboembolic disease. *Clin Res* 1989, 37:145A.

27. Horn M, Ries A, Neveu C, *et al.*: Restrictive ventilatory pattern in precapillary pulmonary hypertension. *Am Rev Respir Dis* 1983, 128:163–165.

28. Kapitan KS, Buchbinder M, Wagner PD, *et al.*: Mechanisms of hypoxemia in chronic thromboembolic pulmonary hypertension. *Am Rev Respir Dis* 1989, 139:1149–1154.

29. Fishmann AJ, Moser KM, Fedullo PF: Perfusion lung scans vs pulmonary angiography in evaluation of suspected primary pulmonary hypertension. *Chest* 1983, 84:679–683.

30. Moser KM, Page GT, Ashburn WL, *et al.*: Perfusion lung scans provide a guide to which patients with apparent primary pulmonary hypertension merit angiography. *West J Med* 1988, 148:167–170.

31. D'Alonzo GE, Bower JS, Dantzker DR: Differentiation of patients with primary and thromboembolic pulmonary hypertension. *Chest* 1984, 85:457–461.

32. Lisbona R, Kreisman H, Novales-Diaz J, *et al.*: Perfusion lung scanning: differentiation of primary from thromboembolic pulmonary hypertension. *AJR Am J Roentgenol* 1985, 144:27–30.

33. Ryan KL, Fedullo PF, Davis GB, *et al.*: Perfusion scan findings understate the severity of angiographic and hemodynamic compromise in chronic thromboembolic pulmonary hypertension. *Chest* 1988, 93:1180–1185.

34. Auger WR, Fedullo PF, Moser KM, *et al.*: Chronic major-vessel thromboembolic pulmonary artery obstruction: appearance at angiography. *Radiology* 1992, 182:393–398.

35. Nicod P, Peterson K, Levine M, *et al.*: Pulmonary angiography in severe chronic pulmonary hypertension. *Ann Intern Med* 1987, 107:565–568.

36. Moser KM, Olson LK, Schlusselberg M, *et al.*: Chronic thromboembolic occlusion in the adult can mimic pulmonary artery agenesis. *Chest* 1989, 95:503–508.

37. Shure D, Gregoratos G, Moser KM: Fiberoptic angioscopy: role in the diagnosis of chronic pulmonary arterial obstruction. *Ann Intern Med* 1985, 103:844–850.

38. Wragg RE, Dimsdale JE, Moser KM, *et al.*: Operative predictors of delirium after pulmonary thromboendarterectomy: a model for postcardiotomy delirium? *J Thorac Cardiovasc Surg* 1988, 96:529.

39. Auger WR, Moser KM, Fedullo PF, *et al.*: The association of heparin-induced thrombocytopenia and the lupus anticoagulant in patients with chronic thromboembolic pulmonary hypertension. *Am Rev Respir Dis* 1991, 143:A-803.

40. Olman MA, Auger WR, Fedullo PF, *et al.*: Pulmonary vascular steal in chronic thromboembolic pulmonary hypertension. *Chest* 1990, 98:1430–1434.

41. Moser KM, Metersky ML, Auger WR, *et al.*: Resolution of vascular steal after pulmonary thromboendarterectomy. *Chest* 1993, 104:1441–1444.

42. Levinson R, Shure D, Moser KM: Reperfusion pulmonary edema after pulmonary artery thromboendarterectomy. *Am Rev Respir Dis* 1986, 134:1241–1245.

43. Chow LC, Dittrich HC, Hoit BO: Doppler assessment of changes in right-sided cardiac hemodynamics after pulmonary thromboendarterectomy. *Am J Cardiol* 1988, 61:1092–1097.

44. Dittrich HC, Nicod PH, Chow LC: Early changes of right heart geometry after pulmonary thromboendarterectomy. *J Am Cell Cardiol* 1988, 11:937–943.

PULMONARY THROMBOENDARTERECTOMY

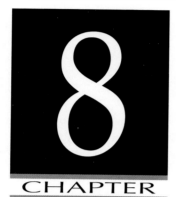

CHAPTER

Pat O. Daily

Chronic pulmonary hypertension due to unresolved major vessel pulmonary emboli occurs infrequently but is extremely debilitating [1]. It may be associated with deficiencies in proteins C and S as well as antithrombin III, and occasionally a lupus anticoagulant is detected. Furthermore, the embolic material may be highly organized and thus resistant to fibrinolysis. A defect in the fibrinolytic system may also play a role in unresolved pulmonary emboli [2]. Several embolic episodes may be necessary to cause chronic pulmonary vascular obstruction.

The possibility of chronic pulmonary embolism should be considered in patients who present with chronic pulmonary hypertension. Pulmonary artery catheterization and echocardiography can readily confirm the presence of pulmonary hypertension. The diagnosis of chronic pulmonary embolism may be suggested by pulmonary flow scanning. However, the definitive diagnosis depends on pulmonary arteriography. When pulmonary arteriography confirms the presence of proximally located major vascular obstruction, significant functional disability and pulmonary vascular resistance of at least 300 dynes-s-cm^{-5} are prerequisites for surgical consideration.

Features of pulmonary thromboendarterectomy include median sternotomy, cardiopulmonary bypass with deep hypothermia and circulatory arrest, distal exposure of the orifices of all the bronchopulmonary segmental arteries, and endarterectomy for areas of obstruction. Endarterectomy techniques are necessary because ingrowth of collagen, and elastic tissue causes the organizing embolic material to adhere firmly to the pulmonary arterial wall within several weeks after acute embolization.

Hospital mortality for pulmonary thromboendarterectomy is about 10%. Major postoperative morbidity is associated with ventilator dependency due to reperfusion pulmonary edema; this occurs in one third of patients. Patients with pulmonary vascular resistance reduced to less than 300 dynes-s-cm^{-5}, however, have an excellent long-term outlook according to a study by Reidel *et al.* [3]. Pulmonary thromboendarterectomy is less risky than lung or heart-lung transplantation. Current data on pulmonary transplantation indicate a 5-year survival of 42% for heart-lung transplantation, a 2-year survival of 51% for transplantation of both lungs, and a 2-year survival of 62.5% for transplantation of one lung [4]. This, in addition to the ever-present problems of infection and rejection in survivors, makes it clear that pulmonary thromboendarterectomy should be the primary therapeutic modality for chronic pulmonary embolism, if the indications for surgery are met.

A. RATIONALE FOR PULMONARY THROMBOENDARTERECTOMY

<1% of patients develop chronic pulmonary vascular resistance elevation after acute pulmonary embolism

For those who do, the 5-y survival without treatment is 50% if the mean pulmonary artery pressure is ≥30 mm Hg and 10% or less if ≥50 mm Hg

Within several weeks unresolved emboli become attached firmly to the pulmonary arterial wall, necessitating endarterectomy techniques for their removal

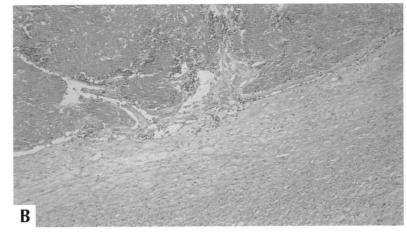

B

FIGURE 8-1. A, Rationale for pulmonary thromboendarterectomy. If resolution of pulmonary emboli does not occur shortly after acute pulmonary embolism, the emboli become firmly attached to the wall of the pulmonary artery through ingrowth of collagen and elastic tissue. Although significantly increased elevation in pulmonary vascular resistance caused by chronic pulmonary embolism occurs infrequently, the natural history of chronic pulmonary embolism becomes more dismal as the pulmonary artery pressure increases [3]. Consequently, relief of pulmonary vascular obstruction is necessary to ameliorate the otherwise grim outlook when pulmonary vascular resistance is 300 dynes-s-cm^{-5} or greater.

B, Embolus with ingrowth of fibrous tissue. Cross-section of a pulmonary artery stained with hematoxylin and eosin approximately 1 week after embolization. Build-up of collagen and elastic tissue precludes simple embolectomy and necessitates thromboendarterectomy techniques to remove all of the intima and a portion of the media of the pulmonary artery. (*Adapted from* Daily [5]; with permission.)

DIAGNOSTIC CONSIDERATIONS

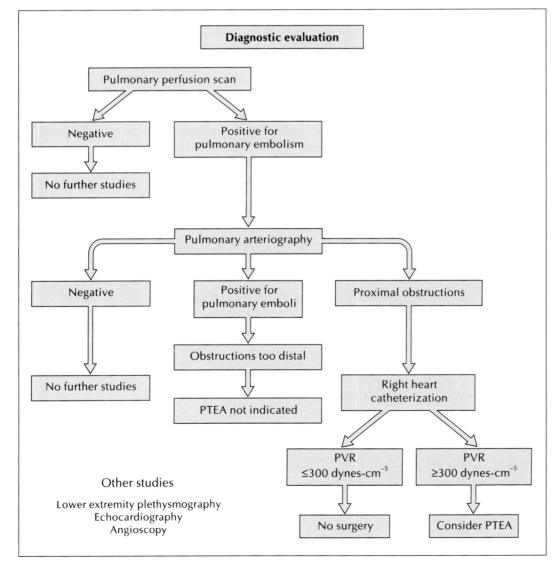

FIGURE 8-2. The pulmonary perfusion scan in patients with severe chronic pulmonary embolism can demonstrate multiple large perfusion deficits throughout both lung fields; however, it should be emphasized that perfusion scans typically underestimate the degree of pulmonary vascular obstruction [6]. Pulmonary arteriography, as described by Nicod *et al.* [7] and Auger *et al.* [8], is the definitive diagnostic modality. Typical findings are proximal high-grade obstructions of most of the right and left broncho-pulmonary segmental arteries. If pulmonary arteriography demonstrates significant proximal obstruction, the decision to perform surgery is based on an assessment of symptoms and whether pulmonary vascular resistance (PVR) is 300 dynes-s-cm^{-5} or greater, as determined by right heart catheterization.

Complete occlusion of either pulmonary artery may be confused with agenesis. Similarly, atrial septal defect and pulmonary artery occlusion with Eisenmenger's physiology may be misdiagnosed as chronic, organized pulmonary embolism [9,10]. Pulmonary angioscopy may be helpful in determining whether obstructions of the pulmonary artery are embolic in nature [11]. Lung biopsy does not allow distinction between primary pulmonary hypertension and chronic pulmonary embolism because plexiform lesions may be seen in both conditions [12]. Additional information can be obtained by lower extremity venous ultrasonography and echocardiography [13]. PTEA—pulmonary thromboendarterectomy.

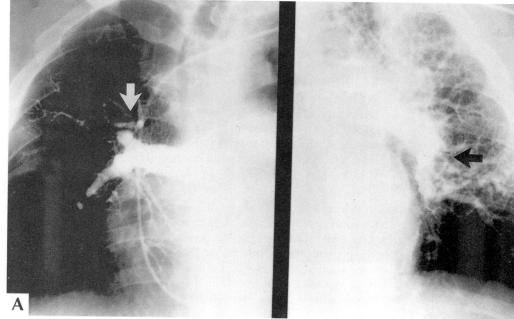

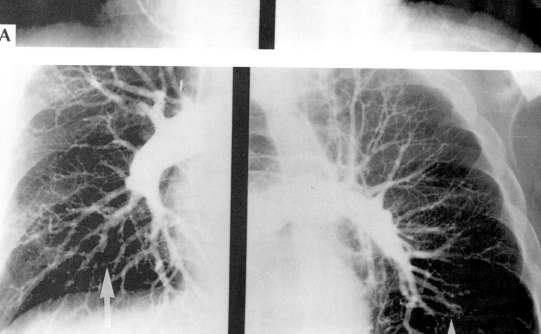

FIGURE 8-3. **A,** A representative preoperative pulmonary arteriogram of a patient with major pulmonary artery obstruction. More than 60% of the pulmonary vasculature is completely obstructed, although blood flow to the left upper lobe and the lingula is preserved (*arrows*). As demonstrated in this figure, there is usually relatively little blood flow to any of the bronchopulmonary segmental arteries of the entire right lung. **B,** At follow-up 8 months after pulmonary thromboendarterectomy, significantly increased pulmonary artery perfusion is noted, especially in the right pulmonary artery system and the left lower lobe (*arrows*). There is, however, some persistence of bronchopulmonary segmental artery defects. In this patient, the mean pulmonary artery pressure decreased from 65 mm Hg to 16 mm Hg, and the pulmonary vascular resistance decreased from 1892 dynes-s-cm^{-5} to 101 dynes-s-cm^{5} at the time of follow-up. (*Adapted from* Daily and coworkers [14]; with permission.)

SURGICAL ASPECTS

SURGICAL INDICATIONS

Chronicity of symptoms ≥3–6 mo

Significant functional disability (New York Heart Association functional classification III or IV)

Pulmonary vascular resistance at least 300 dynes-s-cm^{-5}

Pulmonary arteriography demonstrating at least 50% obstruction of the pulmonary arterial vasculature with the obstructions at least as proximal as the lobar level

FIGURE 8-4. Surgical indications. Although patients may have numerous symptoms after an episode of acute massive pulmonary embolism, significant improvement can occur over a 3- to 6-month period. Thus, only patients who have had chronic symptoms should be considered for pulmonary thromboendarterectomy. Candidates should also be disabled and have a New York Heart Association (NYHA) functional classification of III or IV. Based on a natural history study by Reidel *et al.* [3], patients should have an elevated pulmonary vascular resistance of at least 300 dynes-s-cm^{-5} and a mean pulmonary artery pressure of at least 30 mm Hg. Finally, the pulmonary arteriogram should ordinarily demonstrate obstruction of 50% or greater of pulmonary artery vasculature, with obstructions at least as proximal as the lobar level. With obstructions that begin at the bronchopulmonary segmental artery, surgical results are often suboptimal.

CONTRAINDICATIONS TO SURGERY

Advanced hepatic failure with ascites

Metastatic neoplasm

Chronic renal failure requiring dialysis

Distal location of chronic obstructions at bronchopulmonary artery level or beyond

Advanced, severe diabetes mellitus

Severe left ventricular dysfunction

FIGURE 8-5. Surgical contraindications. In general, associated diseases of an irreversible nature represent contraindications to surgery. Such entities include advanced hepatic failure with ascites or, particularly, anasarca, metastatic neoplasia, and chronic renal failure requiring dialysis. Severe left ventricular dysfunction is a lesser contraindication, as is advanced, severe diabetes mellitus. Age per se is *not* a contraindication for pulmonary thromboendarterectomy. In a series of 149 patients, subjects ranged in age from 20 to 82 years with a mean age of 51±15 years [15]. Obstruction of the distal pulmonary arteries at the bronchopulmonary segmental artery or beyond will usually contraindicate the procedure because of the likely inadequate removal of obstructive material.

SURGICAL CONSIDERATIONS

Insert vena cava filter preoperatively or intraoperatively if lower extremity venous disease is present

Confine dissection of the pulmonary arteries to the mediastinum and hilar tissues

Use a cooling jacket to optimize myocardial hypothermia of the right ventricle

Systemic deep hypothermia (16°C to 20°C) with periods of circulatory arrest limited to 20 minutes

Inspect the right atrium, interatrial septum, tricuspid valve, and right ventricle

Treat cardiac lesions such as atrial septal and valvular defects and coronary artery stenoses

FIGURE 8-6. Important surgical considerations. If lower extremity venous thrombosis is documented, a filter is placed in the vena cava to minimize the probability of repeat embolization after pulmonary thromboendarterectomy. Collection of blood and fluid in the pleural space is minimized by confinement of pulmonary artery dissection to the mediastinal and hilar tissues. To optimize myocardial protection, myocardial hypothermia is maintained at a temperature of approximately 10°C. The use of saline slush for myocardial hypothermia is associated with unacceptably high incidence of phrenic nerve paresis [14]. Therefore, a cooling jacket is used. Chronic hypoxemia causes bronchial artery hyperplasia and subsequent severe bronchial back bleeding; as a result, periods of circulatory arrest are necessary to maintain adequate visualization of the operative field [16,17]. If periods of circulatory arrest are limited to 20 minutes, several periods of arrest can be obtained without causing irreversible neurologic deficits [18,19]. Other defects must also be considered and surgically corrected when encountered [15,20]. Specifically, if atrial septal defects are not closed, they may result in postoperative hypoxemia by causing right-to-left shunting or embolization. It is also important to ensure that no residual thrombi or emboli are present in the right atrium, right ventricle, or proximal pulmonary artery. Such cardiac problems as valvular defects and coronary artery stenosis can be corrected during cooling or rewarming.

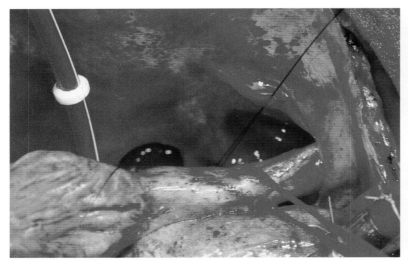

FIGURE 8-7. Mobilization of the superior vena cava. The patient's head is to the viewer's right. The superior vena cava has been mobilized to allow access to the right pulmonary artery. Dissection of the superior vena is carried out in a superior direction as far as the azygous vein posteriorly and the innominate vein anteriorly. In an inferior direction, dissection is performed to the junction of the superior vena cava and the right atrium. The superior vena cava can then be moved either to the patient's left or right to maximize exposure of the right pulmonary artery and the right pulmonary arteriotomies. (*Adapted from* Daily and coworkers [14]; with permission.)

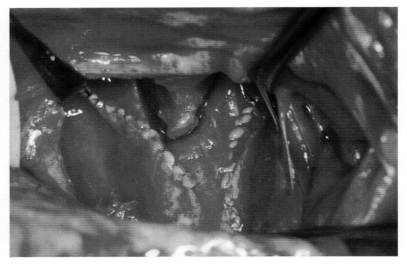

FIGURE 8-8. Exposure of the right pulmonary artery. The patient's head is to the viewer's right. Both the upper lobe and the intermediate branch of the right pulmonary artery can be visualized. The first incision is made in the right pulmonary artery approximately 1.5 cm proximal and inferior to the origin of the right branch of the upper lobe. This incision is extended into the intermediate branch. If necessary, another incision is started in the right pulmonary artery, also about 1 to 2 cm proximal to the origin of the right upper lobe. This incision is extended distally to the trifurcation of the right upper lobe and allows visualization of the three bronchopulmonary segmental arteries of this lobe. Additional distal extension can be obtained by mobilization and anterior and inferior retraction of the right superior pulmonary vein. The incisions are then closed with two rows of continuous 6.0 polypropylene suture; incision closure is typically done during reperfusion, which occurs between periods of circulatory arrest. (*Adapted from* Daily and coworkers [14]; with permission.)

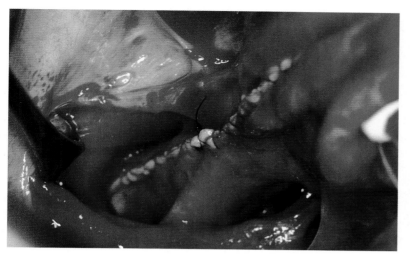

FIGURE 8-9. Exposure of the left pulmonary artery. The patient's head is to the viewer's right. On the left side, the incision in the pulmonary artery is started 3 to 4 cm proximal to the pericardial reflection and is extended beyond the pericardial reflection and distally to the point where the left superior bronchus crosses the pulmonary artery, which limits distal extension of the incision. It is possible to visualize all of the bronchopulmonary segmental arteries through this incision except, occasionally, the anterior-medial segment. As before, the incision is closed with two rows of continuous 6.0 polypropylene suture. Care should be taken to avoid inadvertently extending the incision into the lingular branch of the pulmonary artery, which is located in the lower central portion of this illustration. (*Adapted from* Daily and coworkers [14]; with permission.)

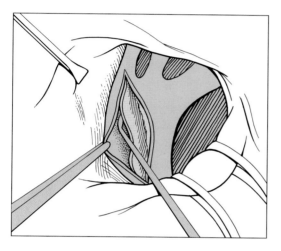

FIGURE 8-10. Endarterectomy plane. The patient's head is to the viewer's right. The incision described in Fig. 8-8 has been performed. When bronchopulmonary segmental arteries of the middle lobe arise from the lower lobe, sufficient exposure for endarterectomy is provided. The critical consideration is identification of the correct plane between the arterial wall and the embolized but organized material that is incorporated into the arterial wall. In order to facilitate identification of the plane, outer layers of the arterial wall are grasped gently with vascular forceps, and dissection is started with a spatula and continued with an aspirating dissector [21]. The aspirating dissector allows simultaneous dissection and removal of blood, thereby minimizing periods of circulatory arrest. Some continued back bleeding will occur during dissection, despite circulatory arrest. (*Adapted from* Daily and coworkers [19]; with permission.)

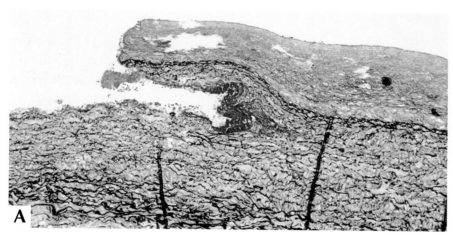

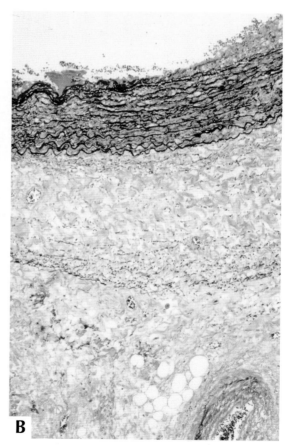

FIGURE 8-11. Microscopic endarterectomy plane. **A,** Dissection plane. The lumen of this partially endarterectomized pulmonary artery is the space at the top of the illustration. The organized embolus can be seen adhering densely to the intima of the pulmonary artery; the embolic material consists of elastic and collagen tissue. Because of this dense adherence, endarterectomy results in removal of the intima as well as a small portion of the media. The dissection plane can be seen clearly toward the center of the figure; in this particular example, the dissection plane was terminated, thereby demonstrating accurately where the plane of dissection occurs during pulmonary thromboendarterectomy.

B, Dissected pulmonary artery demonstrating complete endarterectomy of a pulmonary arterial branch. The intima and the innermost layer of media have been removed, causing the pulmonary arterial lumen to become lined by pulmonary arterial media. In the lower right-hand corner of the illustration, pulmonary parenchymal tissue can be visualized. As demonstrated in this illustration, the pulmonary arterial wall lining consists only of the medial layer after pulmonary thromboendarterectomy. (*Adapted from* Daily [22]; with permission.)

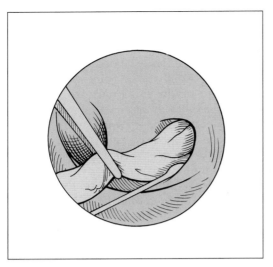

FIGURE 8-12. Endoscopic view of endarterectomy. An endoscope has been passed through the pulmonary arteriotomy to demonstrate the appearance of the endarterectomy. A vascular forceps is used to grasp material obstructing the bronchopulmonary segmental artery, and an aspirating dissector is passed in a distal direction 360 degrees circumferentially. The specimen is then grasped in a more distal direction, and the process is repeated. It is necessary to use a hand-over-hand technique, with forceps alternating with aspirating dissector to remove the material completely. (*Adapted from* Daily and coworkers [19]; with permission.)

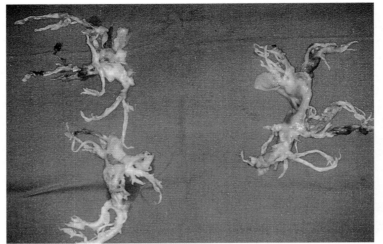

FIGURE 8-13. A representative surgical specimen obtained when all of the bronchopulmonary segmental arteries in both lungs have been endarterectomized. In essence, the specimen is a cast of all bronchopulmonary segmental arteries and their subsegmental branches. The right pulmonary artery specimen is to the viewer's left. (*Adapted from* Daily [23]; with permission.)

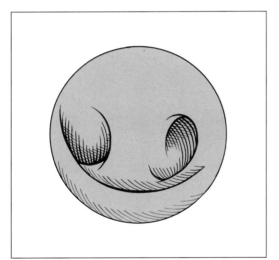

FIGURE 8-14. Endoscopic view of endarterectomized pulmonary arteries. An endoscopic view of the site shown in Fig. 8-12 after endarterectomy reveals the glistening, smooth wall of the bronchopulmonary segmental arterial branch. To the viewer's left, a previously endarterectomized branch can also be seen. (*Adapted from* Daily and coworkers [19]; with permission.)

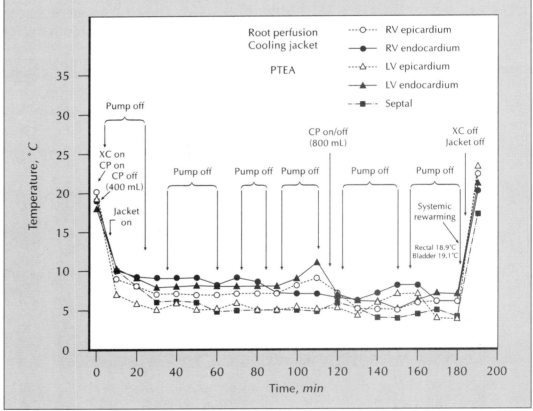

FIGURE 8-15. Myocardial temperature curves. In this patient, the aortic cross clamp time was 186 minutes; this time was the longest of the series, which included 149 patients. Throughout the period of aortic cross clamping, all myocardial temperatures were maintained at less than 10°C. Maintaining this temperature is necessary to optimize myocardial protection because there may be some residual elevation of pulmonary vascular resistance; however, saline slush is contraindicated because it often causes phrenic nerve paresis. Six periods of circulatory arrest occurred in this patient, for a total of 120 minutes of circulatory arrest—also the longest in the series. No neurologic sequelae occurred. CP—cardioplegia; LV—left ventricular; PTEA—pulmonary thromboendarterectomy; RV—right ventricular. (*Adapted from* Daily and coworkers [14]; with permission.)

A. PREOPERATIVE PATIENT DESCRIPTORS

Age, y	Mean: 51±15	Range: 20–82
Gender, n(%)	Male: 94(63.1)	Female: 55(36.9)
Duration of symptoms, mo	Mean: 61.1±66.3	Range: 1–432

New York Heart Association functional class, n(%)

I	1 (0.7)
II	13 (8.7)
III	66 (44.3)
IV	69 (46.3)

B. PREOPERATIVE PATIENT DESCRIPTORS

Other diseases, n(%)	41(27.5)
Coronary artery disease	17(11.4)
Previous myocardial infarction	6/17(4.0)
Renal failure	8(5.4)
Peripheral vascular disease	13(8.7)
Diabetes (insulin dependent)	3(2.0)
Ascites, n(%)	13(8.7)
PaO$_2$ at rest on room air, mm Hg	Mean: 68±19 Range: 29–104
Mean pulmonary artery pressure, mm Hg	Mean: 45.9±13.8 Range: 18–105
Pulmonary vascular resistance, dynes-s-cm^{-5}	Mean: 806±348 Range: 170–2000

FIGURE 8-16. Preoperative patient descriptors. **A,** In this group of 149 patients, age range was 20 to 82 years, with a mean of 51 years. Approximately two thirds of the patients were male, and symptoms had been present for a mean of 61 months. More than 90% of the patients were in the New York Heart Association functional classes of III or IV.

B, The most common concurrent disorder was coronary artery disease; such disease occurred in 17 patients, six of whom had previous myocardial infarctions. There was significant elevation of pulmonary vascular resistance, as evidenced by a mean pulmonary artery pressure of 45.9±13.8 mm Hg and a mean pulmonary vascular resistance of 806±348 dynes-s-cm^{-5}.

POSTOPERATIVE COMPLICATIONS (n=124)

Average time on ventilator, d	4.7±5.7 (1–35)
	n(%)
New myocardial infarction	2(1.6)
Reintubation	12(9.7)
Tracheostomy	6(4.8)
Phrenic nerve paresis (transient)	1(0.8)
Pneumonia (+culture)	19(15.3)
Sternal wound infection	6(4.8)
Sepsis (+blood culture)	9(7.3)
Bleeding requiring reoperation	7(5.6)
Postoperative low cardiac output (cardiac index <2.0 >6 h)	6(4.8)
Focal cerebral deficit	5(4.0)
Requiring dialysis	5(4.0)
Days in hospital (hospital survivors)	19.8±12.5(2–71)

FIGURE 8-17. Postoperative complications (excluding intraoperative deaths). Although the average number of postoperative days on the ventilator for this series of patients was 4.7±5.7, only 39 of 124 patients (31.6%) required ventilatory support for 5 or more days; these patients were arbitrarily classified as ventilator dependent [24]. Although focal cerebral deficits occurred in five of the 124 patients, these deficits were not permanent. By comparison with most procedures involving cardiopulmonary bypass, such as coronary artery bypass grafting and valve replacement, the in-hospital postoperative period for this group of patients was substantially longer than average (19.8±12.5 days).

POSTOPERATIVE PATIENT DESCRIPTORS (*n*=146)

Associated procedures	n(%)
Coronary artery bypass	13(8.9)
Coronary artery bypass/aortic valve replacement	1(0.7)
Coronary artery bypass/mitral valve replacement	1(0.7)
Tricuspid valve annuloplasty	4(2.7)
Aortic valve débridement	1(0.7)
Patent foramen ovale or atrial septal defect closure	41(28.1)
Caval procedure	23(15.4)
Reduction in pulmonary vascular resistance, %	67±28 (Range: 0–93)
Last pulmonary vascular resistance, *dynes-s-cm*$^{-5}$	236±139
Total cardiopulmonary bypass time, *min*	185±42 (Range: 113–344)
Total circulatory arrest time, *min*	58±21 (Range: 16–129)
Total aortic cross clamp time, *min*	115±33 (Range: 51–207)

FIGURE 8-18. Postoperative patient descriptors (excluding intraoperative deaths). The most commonly performed surgical procedure associated with thromboendarterectomy was closure of a patent foramen ovale or atrial septal defect; this was done in 28.1% of patients [15]. This high rate of associated atrial septal defects again emphasizes the importance of careful inspection of the atrial septum. In this group of patients, the aortic cross clamp was applied immediately before the first circulatory arrest period and was removed as rewarming was begun, unless other procedures were performed. Cardiopulmonary bypass times typically included 45 to 60 minutes of cooling to reach 20°C or less and 90 to 120 minutes for returning to normothermia. In most patients, a substantial reduction of pulmonary vascular resistance (mean of 67%) occurred. The mean pulmonary vascular resistance for the group at the time of the last measurement of cardiac output and pulmonary artery pressure before removal of the Swan-Ganz catheter was 236±139 dynes-s-cm^{-5}.

EARLY OUTCOMES

MULTIVARIATE ANALYSIS

VARIABLES	VENTILATOR DEPENDENCY		MORTALITY	
	ALL PATIENTS (*n*=39) *P* VALUE	HOSPITAL SURVIVORS (*n*=28) *P* VALUE	TOTAL MORTALITY (*n*=16) *P* VALUE	RESPIRATORY FAILURE (*n*=12) *P* VALUE
Ascites	0.0008	0.0002	—	—
Total CPB time	0.0342	0.0350	0.0015	—
>4 blood product units	0.0397	—	—	—
% Change in PVR ≤50%	0.0880	—	0.0001	0.0001
Preoperative PVR	—	0.0546	0.0016	0.0912

P value not listed if ≤0.20.

FIGURE 8-19. Multivariate analysis of postoperative complications for ventilator dependency and hospital mortality. In one study, independent predictors of ventilator dependency, arbitrarily defined as the need for postoperative ventilation for 5 days or longer, and hospital mortality were determined [24]. Increased cardiopulmonary bypass (CPB) times predicted both end points, and failure to achieve at least a 50% reduction in pulmonary vascular resistance (PVR) strongly predicted hospital mortality (*P*<0.0001). Other independent predictors of ventilator dependency were ascites and the need for four or more units of blood or blood products. Other predictors, although not reaching statistical significance, indicated that with a larger population base, old age, associated diseases, and a New York Heart Association (NYHA) functional classification of IV may predict both ventilator dependency and hospital mortality. Although not quite reaching statistical significance, higher preoperative levels of pulmonary vascular resistance (>865 dynes-s-cm^{-5}) may be associated with increased hospital mortality.

CAUSES OF DEATH

	DEATH, n(%)	POSTOPERATIVE DAYS BEFORE DEATH
Respiratory and multiorgan failure	10 (58.8)	19.9 (range; 4–47)
Pulmonary hemorrhage*	3 (17.6)	1 (range; 0–3)
Acute myocardial infarction	1 (5.9)	3
Right heart failure*	1 (5.9)	0
Pulmonary artery thrombosis	1 (5.9)	6
Late cardiac tamponade	1 (5.9)	17

FIGURE 8-20. Causes of death. By far, the most common cause of postoperative death was respiratory and multiorgan failure [15]. Although it occurred in only three patients, intraoperative pulmonary hemorrhage remains a problem because of lack of awareness of the causes as well as ineffective treatment. It appears that pulmonary hemorrhage occurs after a breakdown in the alveolar capillary membrane, which allows diffuse bronchial hemorrhage. Postmortem evaluation of pulmonary hemorrhage patients has demonstrated no apparent surgical defect in the pulmonary arterial walls. To date, the predictors and treatment of this disastrous complication have not been defined. It is possible that therapeutic attempts to decrease the formation of oxygen free radicals and chemical blockade of anaphylatoxins may be beneficial. The one death from late cardiac tamponade occurred 1 week after the patient was discharged from the hospital. *Asterisks* indicate intraoperative deaths.

HOSPITAL MORTALITY AND MORBIDITY RATES

	NUMBER OF CASES	HOSPITAL MORTALITY*, n(%)	PHRENIC NERVE PARESIS, n(%)	MEAN TIME ON RESPIRATOR, d
Group A	16	3 (18.7)	0 (0)	8.4
Group B	7	1 (14.3)	5 (71)	32.2
Group C	149	17 (11.4) } P=NS	2 (1.34)	4.5
Group D	150	13 (8.7) }	Unknown	2.0

Group A: 2/1/75 to 10/20/83.
Group B: 3/12/84 to 9/11/84.
Group C: 10/1/84 to 9/18/89.
Group D: after 1/90 to 3/92.

FIGURE 8-21. Hospital mortality and morbidity within 30 days or during hospitalization. Relatively few series of patients undergoing pulmonary thromboendarterectomy have been reported. By 1984, Chitwood *et al.* [25], in an extensive review of the literature, were able to identify only 85 patients, 22% of whom died perioperatively. Most had undergone unilateral thoracotomy. Another report of a significant group of patients who had undergone thromboendarterectomy was that of Jault and Cabrol [26]. In the authors' series, 33 patients had an operative mortality of 20%.

In group A, the pleural cavities were entered. This was avoided in group B; however, myocardial hypothermia was obtained by saline slush wrapped in a laparotomy pad, and this practice resulted in an unacceptably high incidence of phrenic nerve paresis. Beginning with group C (from October 1, 1984, to the present), the method of cardioplegia remained the same, but myocardial hypothermia was maintained with a cooling jacket placed around the right and left ventricles [27,28]. In addition, dissection is confined to the pericardial space and the mediastinum within the hilar tissues. Phrenic nerve paresis occurred in only two of 149 patients and was transient. In Group C, the mean period of ventilatory support was 4.5 days. Jamieson *et al.* [29] added 150 cases operated on from February 1990 to March 1992 (group D). This group had a hospital mortality of 8.7%, which was not significantly different from group C. Lateral rather than medial retraction of the superior vena cava was used exclusively in group D, whereas both lateral and medial retraction were used in group C.

REFERENCES

1. Moser KM, Auger WR, Fedullo PF: Chronic major-vessel thromboembolic pulmonary hypertension. *Circulation* 1990, 81:1735–1743.

2. Olman MA, Marsh JJ, Lang IM, *et al.*: Endogenous fibrinolytic system in chronic large-vessel thromboembolic pulmonary hypertension. *Circulation* 1992, 86:1241–1248.

3. Reidel M, Stanek V, Widimsky J, *et al.*: Long term follow-up of patients with pulmonary thromboembolism. Late prognosis and evolution of hemodynamic and respiratory data. *Chest* 1982, 81:151–158.

4. The Registry of the International Society for Heart and Lung Transplantation: Ninth official report. *J Heart Lung Transplant* 1992, 11:599–606.

5. Daily PO: Embolectomy for acute pulmonary embolism. In *Venous Disorders*. Edited by Bergan JJ, Yao JST. Philadelphia: WB Saunders Co; 1990:531–541.

6. Ryan KL, Fedullo PF, Davis GB, *et al.*: Perfusion scan findings understate the severity of angiographic and hemodynamic compromise in chronic thromboembolic pulmonary hypertension. *Chest* 1988, 93:1180–1185.

7. Nicod P, Peterson KM, Levine MS, *et al.*: Pulmonary angiography in severe chronic pulmonary hypertension. *Ann Intern Med* 1987, 107:565–568.

8. Auger WR, Fedullo PF, Moser KM, *et al.*: Chronic major vessel thromboembolic pulmonary artery obstruction: appearance at angiography. *Radiology* 1992, 182:393–398.

9. Schamroth CL, Sareli P, Pocock WA, *et al.*: Pulmonary arterial thrombosis in secundum atrial septal defect. *Am J Cardiol* 1987, 60:1152–1156.

10. Yamaki S, Horiuchi T, Miura M, *et al.*: Pulmonary vascular disease in secundum atrial septal defect with pulmonary hypertension. *Chest* 1986, 89:694–698.

11. Shure D, Gregoratos G, Moser KM: Fiberoptic angioscopy: role in the diagnosis of chronic pulmonary arterial obstruction. *Ann Intern Med* 1985, 103:844–850.

12. Moser KM, Bloor CM: Pulmonary vascular lesions occurring in patients with chronic major vessel thromboembolic pulmonary hypertension. *Chest* 1993, 103:685–692.

13. Moser KM, Auger WR, Fedullo PF, *et al.*: Chronic thromboembolic pulmonary hypertension: clinical picture and surgical treatment. *Eur J Respir Dis* 1992, 5:334–342.

14. Daily PO, Dembitsky WP, Peterson KL, *et al.*: Modifications of techniques and early results of pulmonary thromboendarterectomy for chronic pulmonary embolism. *J Thorac Cardiovasc Surg* 1987, 93:221–233.

15. Daily PO, Dembitsky WP, Iversen S, *et al.*: Current early results of pulmonary thromboendarterectomy for chronic pulmonary embolism. *Eur J Cardiothorac Surg* 1990, 4:117–123.

16. Moser KM, Kapitan KS, Channick R, *et al.*: Bronchial arterial blood flow in chronic thromboembolic pulmonary hypertension. *Circulation* 1991, 84(suppl II):1382.

17. Daily PO, Johnston GG, Simmons CJ, *et al.*: Surgical management of chronic pulmonary embolism. *J Thorac Cardiovasc Surg* 1980, 79:523–531.

18. Wragg RE, Dimsdale JE, Moser KM, *et al.*: Operative predictors of delirium after pulmonary thromboendarterectomy. A model for postcardiotomy delirium? *J Thorac Cardiovasc Surg* 1988, 96:524–529.

19. Daily PO, Dembitsky WP, Iversen S: Technique of pulmonary thromboendarterectomy for chronic pulmonary embolism. *J Cardiovasc Surg* 1989, 4:10–24.

20. Dittrich HC, Nicod PH, Chow LC, *et al.*: Early changes of right heart geometry after pulmonary thromboendarterectomy. *JACC* 1988, 11:937–943.

21. Daily PO, Dembitsky WP, Daily RP: Dissectors for pulmonary thromboendarterectomy. *Ann Thorac Surg* 1991, 51:842–843.

22. Daily PO: Chronic pulmonary embolism. In *Thoracic Surgery/Esophageal Surgery*. Edited by Pearson FG. New York: Churchill Livingstone; 1994, in press.

23. Daily PO: Surgical treatment of acute and chronic pulmonary embolism. In *Current Concepts in Vascular Surgery-II*. Edited by Ernst CB, Stanley JC. Philadelphia: BC Becker; 1990:1006–1010.

24. Daily PO, Dembitsky WP, Iversen S, *et al.*: Risk factors for pulmonary thromboendarterectomy. *J Thorac Cardiovasc Surg* 1990, 99:670–678.

25. Chitwood WR, Sabiston DC, Wechsler AS: Surgical treatment of chronic unresolved pulmonary embolism. *Clin Chest Med* 1984, 5:507–536.

26. Jault F, Cabrol C: Surgical treatment for chronic pulmonary thromboembolism. *Herz* 1989, 14:192–196.

27. Kinney TB, Daily PO, Pfeffer TA: Optimizing myocardial hypothermia: I. Temperature probe design and clinical inferences. *Ann Thorac Surg* 1991, 51:278–283.

28. Daily PO, Kinney TB: Optimizing myocardial hypothermia: II. Cooling jacket modifications and clinical results. *Ann Thorac Surg* 1991, 51:284–289.

29. Jamieson SW, Fedullo PF, Kriett JM, *et al.*: Experience and results with 150 pulmonary thromboendarterectomy patients over a 29-month period. *J Thorac Cardiovasc Surg* 1993, 106:116–127.

USE OF RIGHT VENTRICULAR CIRCULATORY SUPPORT IN CARDIAC SURGERY

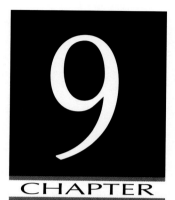

CHAPTER 9

John M. Armitage and Robert Kormos

The principal goal of mechanical circulatory support is to provide blood flow to the body's end organs in situations in which the natural heart fails to do so. Cardiac surgeons encounter the need for mechanical circulatory support in one of two settings: in patients with postcardiotomy failure and in patients facing hemodynamic deterioration while awaiting cardiac transplantation.

Despite improvements in surgical technique and perioperative myocardial preservation, a proportion of patients undergoing cardiac surgery are at risk of developing postoperative low output syndrome. Approximately 1% to 1.5% of patients undergoing cardiac surgery cannot be weaned from cardiopulmonary bypass despite adequate volume loading, metabolic stabilization, physiologic pacing, and full inotropic or intra-aortic balloon support. In addition, 10% to 15% of patients with acute myocardial infarction and subsequent cardiogenic shock, and up to 20% of patients awaiting cardiac transplantation, may be candidates for more extensive circulatory support. This support may be instituted for true ventricular "assistance" for postcardiotomy cardiogenic shock or as a "bridge" to cardiac transplantation when a donor heart is not immediately available. In the former case, the patient's ventricle is expected to recover, but in the latter it is not. Although mechanical circulatory support devices are used more frequently in patients with left ventricular failure, this chapter focuses on the management of intractable failure of the right ventricle.

PATHOPHYSIOLOGY OF VENTRICULAR DYSFUNCTION

IMBALANCE BETWEEN MYOCARDIAL
OXYGEN SUPPLY AND DEMAND

Inadequate myocardial protection
Metabolic abnormalities
Incomplete revascularization
Coronary spasm
Coronary embolism (air, fat,
  or particulate matter)

ISCHEMIC AND REPERFUSION INJURY

Increased cellular and interstitial edema
Decreased ventricular compliance

VENTRICULAR DYSFUNCTION

Ventricular dilatation
Increased peak wall stress
Increased oxygen demand

FIGURE 9-1. The pathophysiologic elements leading to ventricular dysfunction are complex, interrelated, and cyclic. Once set in motion they are self-perpetuating in the absence of interventional therapy.

CONVENTIONAL INTRAOPERATIVE THERAPY OF RIGHT VENTRICULAR FAILURE

Optimal volume loading
  (central venous pressure 18–22 mm Hg)
Increased reperfusion period
Inotropic support ± pulmonary vasodilator therapy
Atrioventricular pacing
Intra-aortic balloon pump support
Corrections of residual surgical defects
  (valve replacement ± coronary bypass)

FIGURE 9-2. The medical therapy of refractory ventricular failure after cardiac surgery involves correction of electrolyte, acid-base, and metabolic abnormalities; adequate volume loading; treatment of dysrhythmias; and atrioventricular sequential (physiologic) pacing. While these corrections are being made, a 10- to 20-minute period of reperfusion on cardiopulmonary bypass is advisable and often may permit weaning from bypass. Although inotropic agents such as calcium, epinephrine, dopamine, or dobutamine may be required, they may induce a ventricular irritability. Finally, the presence of residual, surgically correctable abnormalities, such as incomplete revascularization, valvular defects, or septal defects, should be corrected.

INDICATIONS FOR RIGHT VENTRICULAR ASSISTANCE FOR INTRACTABLE RIGHT VENTRICULAR FAILURE

PRIMARY (INDEPENDENT RIGHT VENTRICULAR FAILURE)

Pulmonary embolism
Pulmonary hypertension (reactive established)
Volume overload
Congenital heart disease
Cardiomyopathy

SECONDARY

Predominantly right-sided
  Associated with surgery for tricuspid valve disease
  Inadequate right ventricular myocardial protection
  Myocardial contusion
Associated with left ventricular failure
  Following cardiac surgery for acquired heart disease
  Right ventricular infarction secondary to coronary
    artery disease
  Following complications of myocardial infarction
    (ventricular septal defect or mitral valve insufficiency)
  In patients awaiting cardiac transplantation

FIGURE 9-3. Indications for right ventricular assistance. Right ventricular failure occurs either primarily, as a result of poor myocardial protection during cardiopulmonary bypass or incomplete myocardial revascularization, or secondary to severe left ventricular failure. Occasionally, right ventricular failure may occur during left ventricular support and is characterized by an inability to provide adequate left ventricular assist device flow because of low left atrial filling pressure in association with a high central venous pressure.

The treatment options leading to right ventricular support are similar to those for left ventricular support and include treatment of associated left ventricular failure, volume loading, physiologic pacing, inotrope support, and intra-aortic balloon counterpulsation, which reduces pulmonary artery pressure indirectly by reducing left atrial pressure. In addition, counterpulsation improves right ventricular function by improving coronary perfusion. In some patients, isoproterenol reduces pulmonary vascular resistance and increases right ventricular contractility. Severe reactive pulmonary vascular hypertension may be reduced by prostaglandin E_1. More recently, a pulmonary artery balloon developed for counterpulsation has been shown experimentally to be efficacious in the treatment of severe right ventricular failure; unfortunately, it has been slow to gain clinical acceptance.

Two major categories of ventricular assist device systems have been used clinically with significant success in the United States: extracorporeal bypass pump systems (roller pump, centrifugal pump, and membrane oxygenator systems) and pneumatic or electrically driven paracorporeal or implantable systems.

CRITERIA FOR RIGHT VENTRICULAR ASSISTANCE

Cardiac index <1.8 L/min/M²
Systolic blood pressure <90 mm Hg (mean, 60 mm Hg)
Central venous pressure >25 mm Hg
Left atrial pressure <10 mm Hg

FIGURE 9-4. Isolated right ventricular failure is unusual but can be characterized by four main criteria. The physician in such cases is unable to raise the left atrial pressure above 10 to 15 mm Hg with volume, despite an elevated central venous pressure (25 to 30 mm Hg). The medical therapy of isolated right ventricular failure is usually limited because of the dysrhythmias (including tachycardia) secondary to high doses of inotropic agents. Patients on left ventricular support who fulfill the above criteria will be considered candidates for additional right ventricular support.

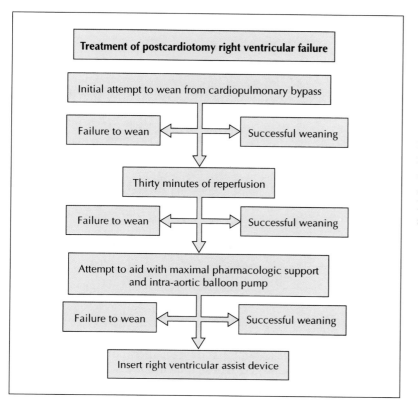

FIGURE 9-5. Treatment of postcardiotomy right ventricular failure. In general, patients are candidates for mechanical circulatory support following postcardiotomy failure if they satisfy the following criteria: they have undergone technically successful cardiac surgery; they fail traditional methods to wean from cardiopulmonary bypass; they fulfill specific hemodynamic or clinical criteria; and they have had no more than 4 to 5 hours of cardiopulmonary bypass. At the end of cardiac surgery, several distinct interventions should be carried out if there is a problem in weaning the patient from cardiopulmonary bypass and before the decision to insert a ventricular assist device is made. A circulatory support system should be implanted as soon as the failure to wean is detected by traditional means. However, the surgeon should not deviate from the normal progression of less invasive therapies that are available.

CONTRAINDICATIONS TO RIGHT VENTRICULAR ASSISTANCE

Active infection or sepsis
Hepatic failure
Renal failure
Coagulopathy
Cerebrovascular hemorrhage or accident
Metastatic cancer
Recent (6 wk) primary infarction

FIGURE 9-6. Contraindications to ventricular assistance. Although many potential candidates are assessed for circulatory support, most are not suitable for the rigors of long-term ventricular bypass. The successful use of a ventricular assist device depends on careful patient selection. In general, any patient who would not be considered a candidate for cardiac transplantation should not be placed on a circulatory support system. Patients who are over 70 years of age, have had technically unsuccessful surgery, are suffering from an uncontrolled bleeding diathesis, have active sepsis or fever, or have other major chronic debilitating diseases should be excluded from mechanical circulatory support.

PHYSIOLOGIC PRINCIPLES OF RIGHT VENTRICULAR ASSISTANCE

DIRECT PHYSIOLOGIC EFFECT
Decreases right ventricular preload and afterload
Decreases right ventricular end-diastolic pressure
Decreases right ventricular wall tension
Decreases oxygen demand
Allows for recovery of depleted ATP stores

HEMODYNAMIC EFFECTS
Increases cardiac output
Increases left ventricular filling
Increases pulmonary blood flow leading to better
    arterial oxygenation
Increases mean arterial pressure, thereby increasing
    coronary blood flow

FIGURE 9-7. The direct physiologic and hemodynamic effects of right ventricular assistance. The right ventricular assist device thus sets the stage for recovery of right ventricular function [1,2].

RESULTS OF THE INTERNATIONAL REGISTRY FOR CIRCULATORY SUPPORT RIGHT VENTRICULAR ASSIST DEVICES

	PATIENTS, n	PATIENTS WEANED OR TRANSPLANTED, n (%)	PATIENTS DISCHARGED, n (%)
Postcardiotomy pump failure	142	54 (38)	32 (22) (59% of patients weaned)
Acute myocardial infarction and postcardiotomy pump failure	37	17 (46)	9 (24) (53% of patients weaned)
Bridge to transplantation	9	4 (44)	2 (22) (50% of patients weaned)
Total	188	75 (40)	43 (23) (57% of patients weaned) and about one quarter survive and are discharged.

FIGURE 9-8. The results of right ventricular support appear to be influenced by several factors. A delay in the insertion of the device once ventricular failure is identified, the presence or development of biventricular failure, and the presence of completed myocardial infarction at the time of insertion of the device result in increased mortality. About half the patients can be weaned from a ventricular assist device, and about one quarter survive and are discharged. These data are the same whether pneumatic systems or centrifugal pumps are used. Data were taken from the International Registry for Circulatory Support Right Ventricular Assist Devices [3]. Average length of support was 4 days (range, 0 to 90 days).

COMPLICATIONS AND CAUSES OF DEATH IN VENTRICULAR ASSIST

COMPLICATION	COMPLICATION ONLY, %	CAUSE OF DEATH, %
Bleeding	34	18
Renal failure	32	26
Biventricular failure	24	—
Respiratory failure	17	16
Infection	14	10
Embolism	3	—
Mechanical failure	1	—
Embolus	—	5

FIGURE 9-9. The most common complications in patients undergoing ventricular assist. Death usually results from progressive multiorgan dysfunction in the setting of compromised flow. Other causes of death include bleeding, infection, and myocardial infarction after device removal. Failure of functional recovery of the heart while on circulatory support relates to the size of completed infarction of the ventricle. Myocardial necrosis diagnosed by biopsy at the time of implant of the device is present in 86% of patients who fail support and in only 25% of those who recover. It also appears that, in general, patients undergoing univentricular left or right support have little better overall survival than those undergoing biventricular support. Data was taken from the International Registry for Circulatory Support Right Ventricular Assist Devices [3].

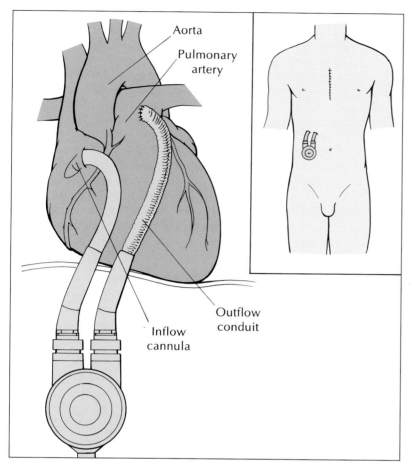

FIGURE 9-10. Pneumatic paracorporeal systems. The most common type of pneumatic paracorporeal system used for right ventricular assistance is the Pierce-Donachy type pump (Thoratec Laboratories, Berkeley, CA). This pump employs a pneumatically activated polyurethane pumping chamber and a polycarbonate housing. The chamber has Bjork-Shiley (Shiley, Inc., Irvine, CA) inlet and outlet valves and a stroke volume of 65 mL. It can operate at a fixed rate, which is determined by the user, a fill-to-empty mode by which the heart ejects when a switch is tripped by the pumping chamber being filled, or a mode synchronized to the R wave of the electrocardiogram.

This device lies outside the abdominal wall; two percutaneous cannulae drain the left atrium and return blood to the aorta (inset). The device can be used for left, right, or biventricular support with the use of two pumps. The inflow cannula to the pump is sewn directly to the left ventricular apex or right atrium, and arterial return is through a Dacron (Dupont, Wilmington, DE) conduit sewn in an end-to-side fashion to the ascending aorta or pulmonary artery. A second type of inflow cannula has been designed to be placed through the left or right atrial appendage. For most cases of postcardiotomy failure, the atrial cannula is chosen usually because of space considerations on the ascending aorta where venous grafts have been sewn.

These devices are Food and Drug Administration–regulated and expensive; therefore, they require a considerable amount of technical and engineering expertise. These more complex pumps have a larger role to play, both as investigational therapeutic tools and also as a bridge to cardiac transplantation [4,5].

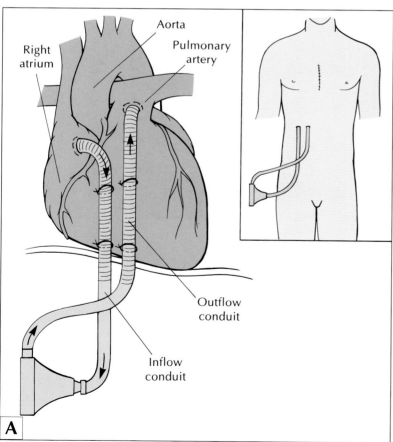

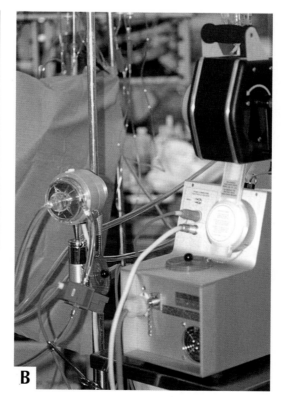

FIGURE 9-11. Centrifugal bypass system. **A,** Centrifugal right ventricular assist device (RVAD) showing the right atrial and pulmonary arterial cannulation sites. **Inset,** The patients's appearance following placement of the RVAD and closure of sternotomy with remote cannula exit sites. **B,** Bedside centrifugal bypass machine.

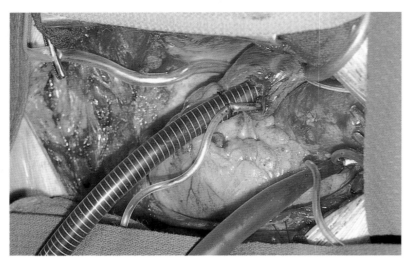

FIGURE 9-12. Operative cardiac cannulation. The Biomedicus centrifugal pump (Biomedicus Inc., Minnetonke, MI) requires $300 in disposable pump parts per case and is relatively simple to apply. This system has been used extensively by Magovern *et al.* [6] for patients

with both univentricular and biventricular failure. The Biomedicus pump consists of rotating cones that import a centrifugal force to the blood, moving it through a constrained vortex. Its nonocclusive nature is purported to result in less trauma to blood elements and tubing. Because of the unique shape and negative charge of the internal surfaces of the rotating cones, the pump has been used reportedly with minimal or no heparin. More recently, methods of bonding heparin to bypass pump tubing have been successfully used in these Biomedicus centrifugal pump heads.

One disadvantage to this system is that the pump head requires changing every 24 to 48 hours as dictated by the regulatory restrictions on its use. This is due not only to potential bearing wear and overheating, but also to the fact that even with anticoagulation, small amounts of thrombi are known to collect beneath the rotor and along its internal struts. Nevertheless, this device is attractive to many centers where patients with medically refractory low output syndromes require treatment. This is primarily because of its cost effectiveness and ease of implantation. The pump adjusts automatically by reducing its output in the presence of an increased afterload resulting from arterial outflow obstruction even though the pump continues to rotate. A reservoir and heat exchanger are not required.

FIGURE 9-13. Extracorporeal membrane oxygenation (ECMO) is a highly efficient system for support of both right and left ventricular function, as well as pulmonary function. The ECMO circuit includes an oxygenator and thus requires systemic heparinization. Its long-term use in adults is limited by the risks of bleeding and infection. Initiation of ECMO support immediately unloads the right ventricle and improves systemic oxygenation by virtue of the gas exchange that occurs within the circuit. ECMO is most efficient when short-term cardiac and pulmonary support are required and direct thoracic surgical intervention is not needed. The limitations of the ECMO system are its duration of support and the flow limitations inherent in size and placement of venous cannulation.

Labels in Figure 9-13: Right carotid artery; Alternate arterial inflow (pediatric); Aorta; Pulmonary artery; Right atrium; Right ventricle; Inferior vena cava; Femoral artery; Femoral vein

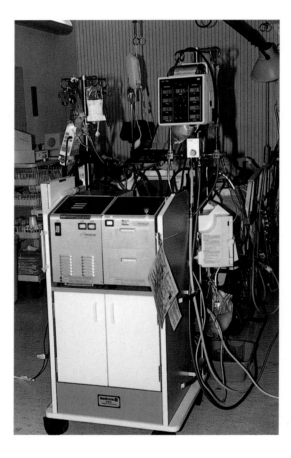

FIGURE 9-14. Extracorporeal membrane oxygenation system at a patient's bedside.

REFERENCES

1. Kormos RL, Gasior T, Antaki JF, *et al.*: Evaluation of right ventricular function during clinical left ventricular assistance. *Trans Am Soc Artif Intern Organs* 1989, 35:547–550.

2. Morita S, Kormos RL, Kawai A, *et al.*: Effect of left ventricular assistance on ventricular/arterial coupling and efficiency of energy transfer from pressure-volume area to external mechanical work of the right ventricle. In *Heart Replacement, Artificial Heart 4.* Edited by Akutsu T, Koyanagi H. Tokyo: Springer-Verlag; 1993:259–263.

3. Pae WE, Pierce WS: Combined registry for the clinical use of mechanical ventricular assist pumps and the total artificial heart. Hershey, PA: Department of Artificial Organs, Milton S. Hershey Medical Center; August 1989.

4. Kormos RL, Borovetz HS, Gasior T, *et al.*: Experience with univentricular support in mortally ill cardiac transplant candidates. *Ann Thorac Surg* 1990, 49:261–272.

5. Kormos RL, Borovetz HS, Armitage JM, *et al.*: Evolving experience with mechanical circulatory support. *Ann Surg* 1991, 214:471–477.

6. Magovern GJ Jr: The biopump and postoperative circulatory support. *Ann Thorac Surg* 1993, 55:245–249.

HEART-LUNG TRANSPLANTATION

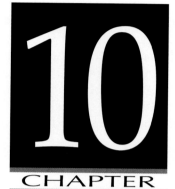

10

CHAPTER

David H. Adams

More than 1300 adult and pediatric patients have undergone heart-lung transplantation for a variety of diseases, including congenital heart disease with Eisenmenger's syndrome, primary pulmonary hypertension (PPH), cystic fibrosis (CF), and emphysema. The extension of single-lung transplantation to patients with pulmonary vascular diseases (*eg*, PPH) and the emergence of "bilateral sequential" lung transplantation in patients with septic lung disease requiring double-lung replacement (*eg*, CF) have diversified the choice of transplantation procedures for potential recipients. Because many patients traditionally managed by heart-lung replacement do not require heart replacement, the current application of heart-lung transplantation focuses predominantly on patients with Eisenmenger's syndrome or end-stage pulmonary disease associated with severe irreversible right heart failure.

The evolution of heart-lung transplantation as a safe and useful technique has involved increased understanding in several important areas. Careful recipient selection remains the single most important feature in the successful application of heart-lung transplantation. With the exception of their cardio-pulmonary disease, potential recipients should be generally healthy and should possess adequate physiologic reserve to survive the early postoperative period. Recipient exclusion criteria include age older than 65 years, severe hepatic or renal insufficiency, and advanced diabetes mellitus or peripheral vascular disease. Appropriate donor selection criteria have been equally well defined. Potential donors should be younger than 50 years of age with no prior history of cardiopulmonary disease. The potential donor's lungs are particularly scrutinized because pulmonary insufficiency is a major source of early morbidity following transplantation. There should be no evidence of significant parenchymal consolidation, and measured gas exchange should be normal.

Another important advance in the field of heart-lung transplantation involved the development of techniques to allow distant procurement of the heart-lung block while ensuring adequate organ preservation and early graft function. Common techniques currently employed include core cooling with cardiopulmonary bypass, the use of a modified autoperfusing Starling preparation, and pulmonary artery flush with simple topical hypothermia.

The operative principles resulting in successful heart-lung transplantation are now defined, allowing the application of heart-lung transplantation in selected patients who have undergone previous thoracotomies and even previous heart-lung transplantation. Refinements in postoperative immunosuppressive management continue to evolve and play an important role in the outcome, since heart-lung recipients are prone to the development of episodes of acute lung rejection and pulmonary infections, particularly during the first 3 months following transplantation. A three-drug regimen, which includes cyclosporine, azathioprine, and prednisone, is employed in the majority of centers today. Chronic rejection, manifested by the development of obliterative bronchiolitis, has emerged as the leading cause of late morbidity and mortality in heart-lung recipients. Despite aggressive augmentation of immunotherapy, approximately half of all patients who develop obliterative bronchiolitis develop terminal respiratory failure. Recent experience has suggested that repeat heart-lung transplantation or single-lung transplantation can result in successful rehabilitation in selected heart-lung recipients with obliterative bronchiolitis.

Several issues in heart-lung transplantation continue to evolve. Long-term follow-up of patients undergoing single-lung transplantation for selected diseases, which traditionally have been managed by heart-lung transplantation, will result in further definition of appropriate recipient categories. Further experience in the field of xenotransplantation may help to solve the significant problem of donor availability faced by every transplant center. Continued improvements in immunosuppressive therapy will decrease the incidence of infection as well as acute and chronic rejection and, therefore, ameliorate long-term outcome. Further understanding of the pathogenesis of obliterative bronchiolitis and its treatment will also improve long-term outcome. In this regard, a number of patients undergoing heart-lung transplantation will ultimately develop terminal obliterative bronchiolitis and require repeat transplantation, allowing further advances in this challenging area.

BACKGROUND AND EPIDEMIOLOGY

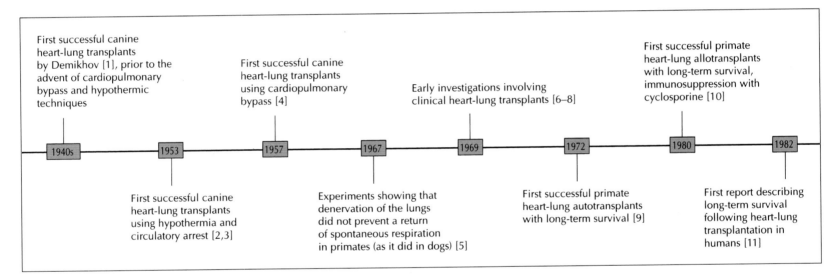

FIGURE 10-1. Major experimental and clinical milestones in the field of heart-lung transplantation.

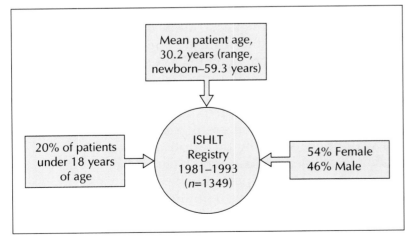

FIGURE 10-2. Epidemiologic characteristics of 1349 heart-lung transplant recipients. These data were collected from the International Society for Heart and Lung Transplantation (ISHLT) Registry between 1981 and 1993 [12]. Fifty-four percent of recipients were female and 46% male. The mean patient age was 30.2 years, with a range between newborn and 59.3 years. Twenty percent of heart-lung recipients were younger than 18 years of age.

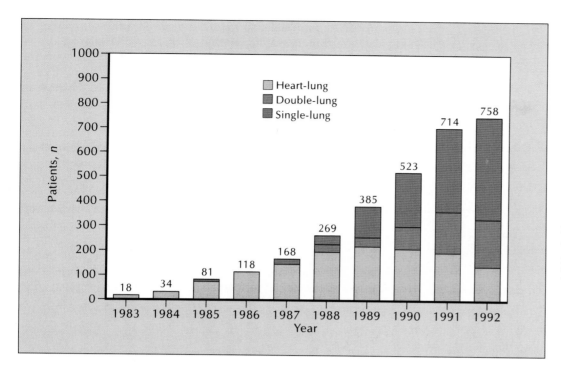

Figure 10-3. Numbers of patients who have undergone heart-lung, double-lung, or single-lung transplantations reported to the Registry of the International Society for Heart and Lung Transplantation (ISHLT) since 1983 [12]. The gradual decline in the number of heart-lung transplant procedures during the 1990s has been more than counterbalanced by a progressive increase in the number of single- and double-lung transplantations. In response to an insufficient heart-lung donor pool and the realization that many heart-lung recipients do not require heart replacement, single- and double-lung transplantation is now applied in many patients previously managed by heart-lung transplantation.

RECIPIENT AND DONOR SELECTION

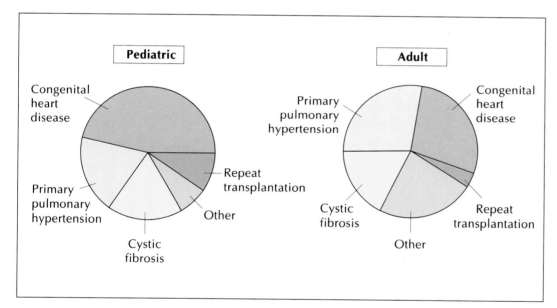

Figure 10-4. Indications for heart-lung transplantation in the 1349 patients reported to the International Society for Heart and Lung Transplantation (ISHLT) Registry since 1981 [12]. The most common diagnosis leading to heart-lung transplantation is congenital heart disease, usually complicated by Eisenmenger's syndrome; the next most common diagnosis is primary pulmonary hypertension [13,14]. Parenchymal lung diseases successfully treated by transplantation include emphysema, cystic fibrosis, pulmonary fibrosis, fibrosing alveolitis, eosinophilic granuloma, lymphangioleiomyomatosis, pulmonary sarcoidosis, and alveolar cell carcinoma [15,16]. Chronic rejection manifested by the development of obliterative bronchiolitis represents an emerging indication for retransplantation in heart-lung recipients [17].

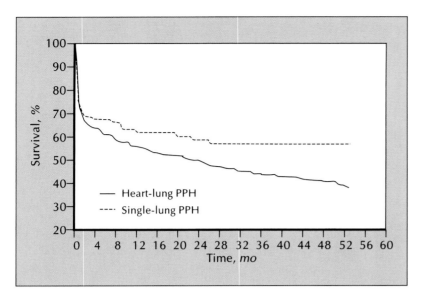

FIGURE 10-5. Kaplan-Meier survival curves comparing survival in patients with primary pulmonary hypertension (PPH) managed by heart-lung transplantation or single-lung transplantation, demonstrating the successful application of single-lung transplantation for this disease process (M. Kaye, MD, personal communication). The extension of single-lung transplantation to many pulmonary diseases (*eg*, chronic obstructive pulmonary disease, pulmonary vascular disease), and the emergence of "bilateral sequential" double-lung procedures in the management of patients requiring double-lung replacement (*eg*, cystic fibrosis), have diversified the choice of transplant procedures for potential recipients (*see* Fig. 10-3) [18–20]. Limitations of suitable heart-lung blocks, replacement of a "normal" heart in some recipients, and the use of three donor organs for one recipient are the primary reasons that most heart-lung recipients in the future will have Eisenmenger's syndrome or end-stage pulmonary disease with concurrent irreparable primary cardiac disease [21]. In cases of heart-lung transplantation for end-stage pulmonary disease without primary cardiac disease, "domino" transplantation of the recipient's heart is usually warranted [22].

A. RECIPIENT INCLUSION CRITERIA

End-stage irreversible cardiopulmonary disease
Age: neonate to 60 years
NYHA class III–IV; 1- to 2-y life expectancy
Stable psychosocial status

B. RECIPIENT EXCLUSION CRITERIA

ABSOLUTE

Brittle diabetes mellitus
Advanced peripheral vascular disease
Hepatic insufficiency, bilirubin >2.5 mg/dL
Renal insufficiency, creatine clearance <50 mL/min/m²
Active infection

RELATIVE

Steroid dependency
Previous thoracotomy

C. DONOR SELECTION CRITERIA

CARDIAC

Normal electrocardiogram and echocardiogram
Normal chamber pressures and cardiac output
Minimal inotropic support

PULMONARY

Absence of significant parenchymal consolidation
Nonpurulent endotracheal secretions
Adequate gas exchange (PaO$_2$>300 on F$_I$O$_2$=1.0)

GENERAL

Age <50 y
Negative cardiopulmonary history

Cyclosporine nephrotoxicity predictably is problematic in patients with poor renal function prior to transplantation. Similarly, patients with active bacterial or viral infections are not appropriate transplant candidates. Patients on chronic steroid therapy should be considered on a case-by-case basis, with a goal to wean prednisone dosages to 20 mg or less on alternating days [23]. Extensive previous cardiac or thoracic surgery is clearly associated with increased morbidity and mortality, and such patients should also be reviewed on a case-by-case basis [24].

C, Donor selection criteria in heart-lung transplantation. Although criteria may vary among transplant centers, there is general agreement that potential donors should be younger than 50 years of age and have a negative cardiopulmonary history including recent trauma. Cardiac function should be satisfactory with no evidence of infarction or significant ischemia on electrocardiography with normal wall motion and absent significant valvular pathology by echocardiography. Typically, a Swan-Ganz catheter is used to measure right heart pressures and cardiac output, which should reflect normal cardiac function with minimal inotropic support (usually dopamine, <10 µg/kg/min).

FIGURE 10-6. Recipient and donor selection. **A,** Recipient inclusion criteria for heart-lung candidates. Patients should be younger than 60 years of age with end-stage cardiopulmonary disease not amenable to medical or surgical therapy. They have New York Heart Association (NYHA) class III or IV symptoms with a 1- to 2-year life expectancy without transplantation. Patients must also have an adequate psychosocial support system available.

B, Recipient exclusion criteria for heart-lung candidates. Patients with advanced systemic processes such as brittle diabetes or severe peripheral vascular disease are not appropriate candidates. Heart-lung transplantation in patients with liver and renal dysfunction is also contraindicated. Reversible liver compromise on the basis of passive congestion secondary to right-heart failure may respond to diuretic therapy, and as a rule liver enzymes should be normal with a bilirubin of 2.5 mg/dL or less.

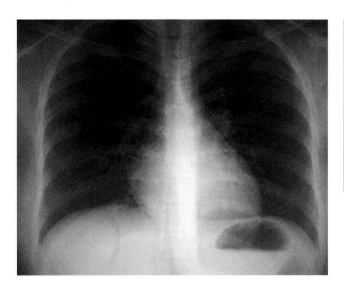

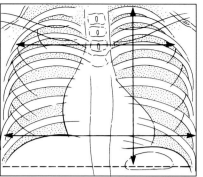

FIGURE 10-7. Measurements used to assess the chest size of potential heart-lung donors and recipients [25]. The transverse diameter of the chest is measured at the level of the aortic knob and its widest dimension measured at the top of the diaphragm. The vertical dimension, measured from the acromion notch to the level of the costophrenic angle, is also noted. The donor and recipient chest sizes should be matched similarly to avoid postoperative problems such as pulmonary atelectasis or persistent pleural effusion. Ideally, the donor chest should be slightly smaller than that of the recipient.

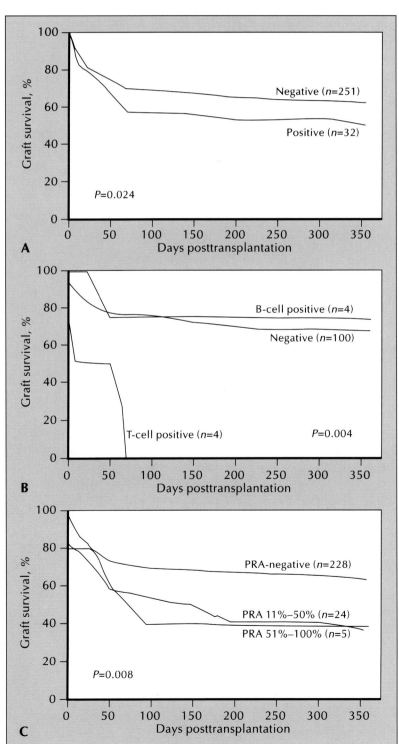

FIGURE 10-8. Donor recipient immunologic matching. ABO blood group compatibility between donor and recipient is essential. Data from 283 heart-lung transplantations performed at Harefield Hospital (Middlesex, UK) were analyzed recently to determine the importance of the lymphocytotoxic cross-match result and the panel-reactive antibody (PRA) status on graft survival [26].

A, Donor-reactive cross-matching was performed for 283 heart-lung recipients. One-year actuarial survival for a negative cross-match was 61% compared with 50% in patients with a positive cross-match.

B, Discrimination of T- and B-cell cross-matches increases the sensitivity of the cross-match. T- and B-cell cross-match results for 108 heart-lung recipients also showed good correlation with 1-year graft survival: 68% for patients with a negative cross-match, 75% for patients with a B-cell–positive cross-match, and 0% for patients with a T-cell–positive cross-match.

C, A significant correlation was also seen between PRA status and poor graft survival in heart-lung recipients. One-year actuarial survival for patients who were PRA-negative was 64%, compared with 37% in patients with a PRA frequency of 11% to 50%, and 40% in highly sensitized patients with a PRA greater than 51%. These authors also showed that PRA status was highly predictive of a positive cross-match result: 75% of highly sensitized cardiac transplant recipients exhibited a positive cross-match against respective donors, while in those patients with a PRA frequency of less than 11% there was a significant reduction in the number of positive cross-matches to 4.5% (data not shown). The PRA test can be used to identify patients who have donor-reactive antibodies. These patients should undergo preoperative testing with a lymphocytotoxic T-cell cross-match. If the T-cell cross-match is positive, heart-lung transplantation should not be undertaken. (*Adapted from* Smith and coworkers [26]; with permission.)

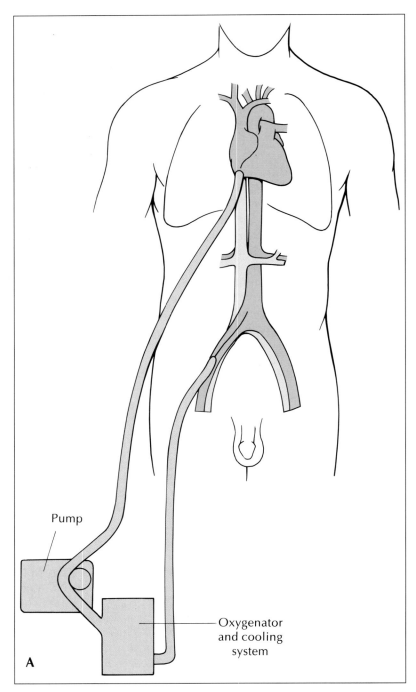

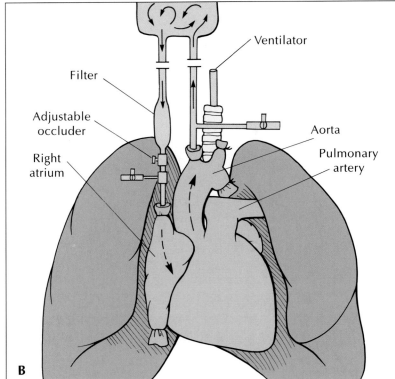

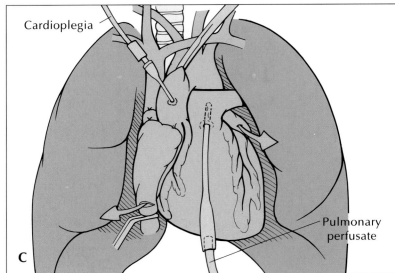

FIGURE 10-9. Techniques employed to allow distant procurement of the heart-lung block to ensure adequate organ preservation and early graft function. The lung is particularly sensitive to prolonged ischemia [27] and these techniques are designed to maximize lung preservation and prevent postimplantation alveolar-capillary barrier membrane dysfunction. **A,** Yacoub introduced core cooling of the donor to less than 10°C by establishing cardiopulmonary bypass as a technique to allow distant heart-lung retrieval, thereby allowing for safe ischemic times up to approximately 5 hours [28]. This technique is used at Harefield Hospital in the United Kingdom and elsewhere [25]. **B,** Griffith *et al.* [14] and Hardesty and Griffith [29] reported the use of a modified autoperfusing Starling preparation to provide continued pulmonary and coronary blood flow in order to extend the period of preservation of the heart-lung block to 4 to 6 hours. **C,** Other groups have achieved excellent results in heart-lung preservation by giving prostaglandin-E$_1$ to ensure pulmonary vasodilation followed by cold pulmonary artery flush and simple topical hypothermia [30,31].

OPERATIVE PRINCIPLES

Median sternotomy or clam-shell thoracosternotomy

Careful takedown of pleural adhesions

Cardiopulmonary bypass with aortic, caval cannulation

Donor cardiectomy followed by lung removal

Avoid injury to phrenic, recurrent laryngeal, vagus nerves

Meticulous attention to hemostasis prior to placement of heart-lung block

Tracheal, aortic, right atrial anastomoses

FIGURE 10-10. The operative principles leading to successful heart-lung transplantation have been outlined previously [23,28,32]. Most patients are approached via a median sternotomy. A subgroup of patients likely to have dense pleural adhesions (*eg*, cystic fibrosis, previous thoracotomy), who are not at increased risk for excessive postoperative bleeding, can alternatively be approached via a clam-shell thoracosternotomy. Cardiopulmonary bypass with aortic and bicaval cannulation precedes donor cardiectomy and then lung removal (either separately or as a block). Care should be taken to identify and protect the phrenic, recurrent laryngeal, and vagus nerves. After removal of the recipient heart and lungs, hemostasis of the posterior mediastinum is meticulously assured, since these areas are poorly seen following heart-lung replacement. The donor heart-lung block is placed in its orthotopic position and anastomoses are created joining the donor and recipient trachea, right atrium, and aorta. If the recipient heart is used in a domino procedure, the donor implantation requires separate superior and inferior vena caval anastomoses [22].

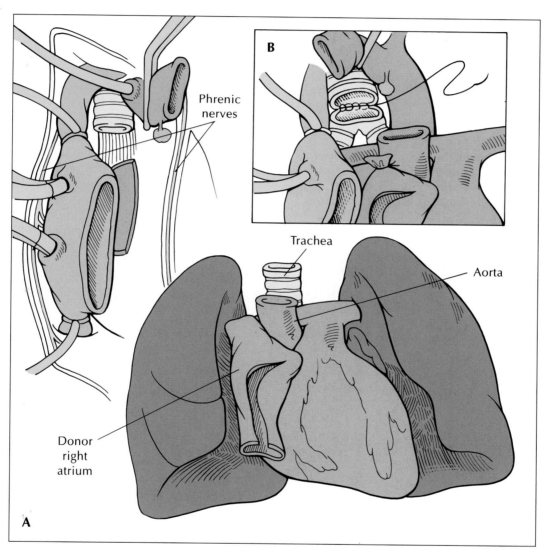

FIGURE 10-11. Surgical technique of heart-lung transplantation. **A,** The donor heart-lung block is positioned by placement of the right lung below the recipient right atrial cuff and phrenic pedicle and the left lung beneath the left phrenic pedicle, thereby placing the heart in its orthotopic position. **B,** The tracheal anastomosis is first performed using a running suture. (*continued*)

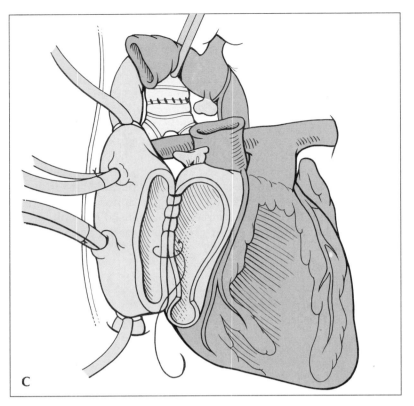

C

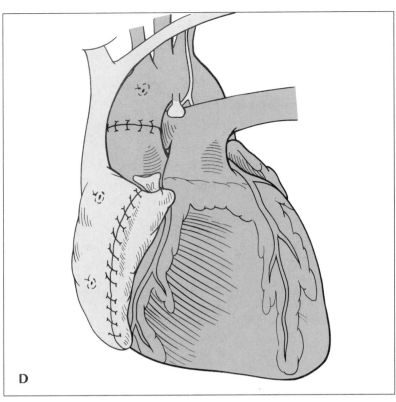

D

FIGURE 10-11. (*continued*) **C,** The donor right atrium is prepared in a manner similar to that for standard cardiac transplantation, and the right atrial anastomosis is then created using a running technique. (In the case of a domino transplantation, direct caval anastomoses would be performed instead of atrial anastomoses.)

D, The aortic anastomosis is performed in an end-to-end fashion with a running suture. Illustrated here is the completed procedure with all cannulas removed. (Parts A, C, and D *adapted from* Reitz [25]; part B *adapted from* Jamieson and coworkers [32]; with permission.)

POSTOPERATIVE CARE

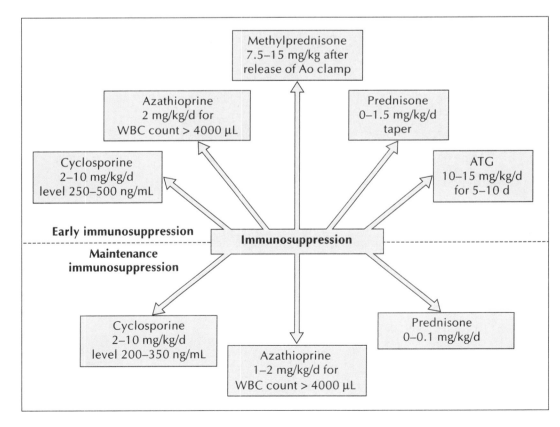

FIGURE 10-12. Immunosuppression protocol for heart-lung transplant recipients. Several immunosuppressive protocols have been used and they remain center-dependent. The majority of centers base immunosuppression on a three-drug protocol including cyclosporine, azathioprine, and corticosteroids, although the Harefield group continues to employ a steroid-free maintenance protocol [16]. Induction therapy with antithymocyte globulin (ATG) is practiced in the majority of centers. The cyclosporine dose is adjusted according to the blood level and the recipient's renal function. Azathioprine is administered typically at a dose of 2 mg/kg/d provided the white blood cell (WBC) count is over 4000 µL. Methylprednisone, 7.5 to 15 mg/kg, is given intravenously during the procedure after the release of the aortic cross-clamp. Some centers delay beginning oral corticosteroids for 1 to 2 weeks because of a concern regarding impaired tracheal healing. In a majority of centers, patients are maintained on a low dose of oral prednisone.

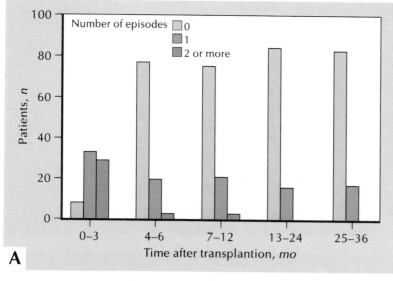

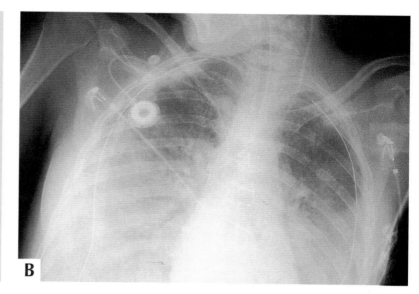

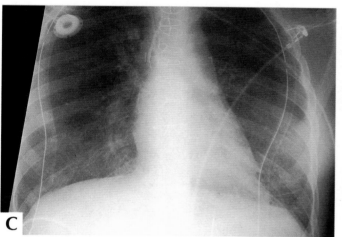

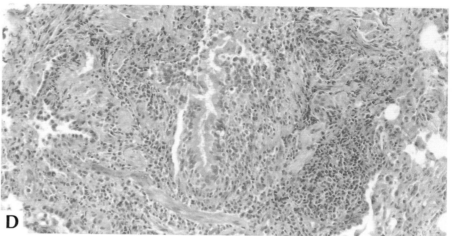

FIGURE 10-13. Acute rejection after heart-lung transplantation.

A, The number of acute rejection episodes occurring in heart-lung transplant recipients at Harefield Hospital between 1984 and 1991 [33]. Seventy-nine patients underwent the procedure for cystic fibrosis. Approximately 90% of patients developed one or more episodes of acute rejection during the first 3 postoperative months. Thereafter, acute rejection episodes were much less common (approximately 20% of patients had one episode per year). There were no episodes of acute rejection in patients surviving longer than 36 months. Acute cardiac rejection is less common after heart-lung transplantation

compared with isolated heart transplantation [34]. Isolated pulmonary rejection or synchronous rejection of the heart and lungs can occur [35].

B, Acute pulmonary rejection presents with fever, malaise, shortness of breath, and a reduction in arterial oxygen saturation. This chest radiograph of a heart-lung recipient with acute rejection demonstrates the typical appearance of a diffuse interstitial infiltrate.

C, Note prompt regression of the infiltrate following intravenous steroid therapy.

D, Lung biopsy specimen demonstrating acute airway rejection. (Part A *adapted from* Madden and coworkers [33]; with permission.)

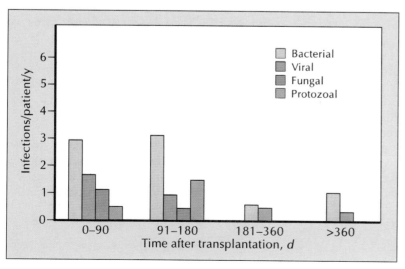

FIGURE 10-14. Infection rates over time and the pathogens involved following heart-lung transplantation. Infectious complications result in serious morbidity and mortality following heart-

lung transplantation. Heart-lung recipients are at a greater risk for infection compared with heart recipients. This figure summarizes the occurrence of infection in 18 heart-lung recipients cared for in the University of Pittsburgh Transplant Program between 1981 and 1985.

Bacterial pathogens are responsible for the majority of infections [36]. Appropriate perioperative antibiotic therapy and an aggressive approach (*eg,* bronchoscopy, lavage, biopsy) to identify involved strains and sensitivities are crucial. Cytomegalovirus (CMV) is the pathogen responsible for the majority of severe opportunistic viral respiratory infections. Infected patients are treated with gancyclovir in combination with intravenous hyperimmune globulin. A majority of transplant centers now avoid transplantation between CMV-positive donors and CMV-negative recipients [37]. *Pneumocystis carinii* is the most commonly identified protozoal pathogen, although the incidence of *P. carinii* pneumonia has been diminished by the routine administration of prophylactic low-dose cotrimoxazole [33]. Fungal superinfections usually accompany established bacterial infections and are often difficult to eradicate. (*Adapted from* Dummer and coworkers [36]; with permission.)

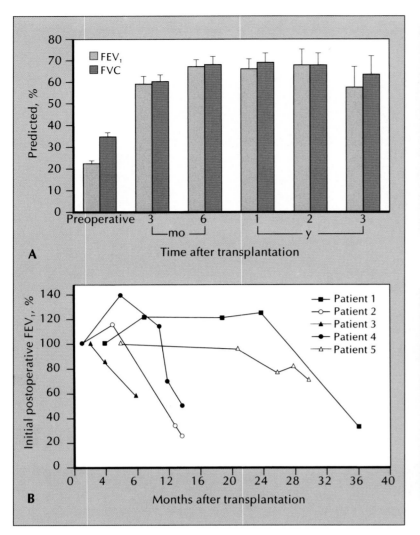

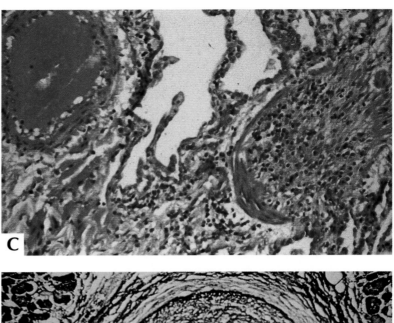

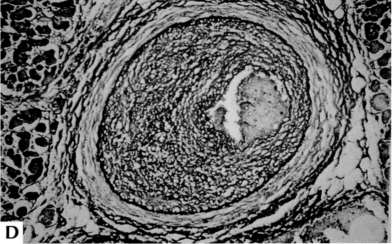

FIGURE 10-15. Chronic rejection following heart-lung transplantation. **A,** Pulmonary function improves dramatically in a majority of patients following heart-lung transplantation, as is demonstrated by these data from 79 patients following heart-lung transplantation for cystic fibrosis [33]. FEV_1—forced expiratory volume at 1 second; FVC—forced vital capacity. **B,** Late deterioration in lung function usually results from the development of obliterative bronchiolitis. Patients usually present with insidious symptoms including dry cough and breathlessness. Spirometric studies in five patients who developed obliterative bronchiolitis after heart-lung transplanta-

tion are plotted, and demonstrate the gradual fall in FEV_1 typically observed [38]. **C,** Obliterative bronchiolitis following heart-lung transplantation. The bronchiolar lumen is obliterated by fibrous and inflammatory tissue, with partial destruction of the bronchial wall. **D,** Cardiac graft arteriosclerosis following heart-lung transplantation. Concentric intimal sclerosis severely narrows the lumen. Although recognized to occur in heart-lung recipients [39], severe disease is much less prevalent compared with heart transplant recipients [28]. (Part A *adapted from* Madden and coworkers [33]; part B *adapted from* Burke and coworkers [38]; with permission.)

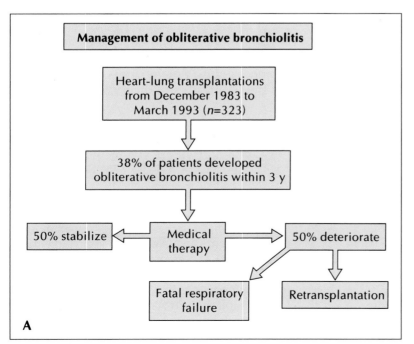

FIGURE 10-16. The role of retransplantation in obliterative bronchiolitis. **A,** Current management of heart-lung recipients with obliterative bronchiolitis [17]. Three hundred twenty-three patients underwent heart-lung transplantation at Harefield Hospital between December 1983 and March 1993. The cumulative probability of developing obliterative bronchiolitis in this group of patients was 38% within the first 3 postoperative years [16]. Lung function stabilized in 50% of patients with aggressive augmentation of immunosuppression, generally involving intravenous methylprednisone pulsing followed by the addition of high-dose steroids (1 to 2 mg/kg/d for 1 month) to standard cyclosporine-azathioprine maintenance therapy. The remaining 50% of patients developed terminal respiratory failure, leaving retransplantation as the only potential effective option. *(continued)*

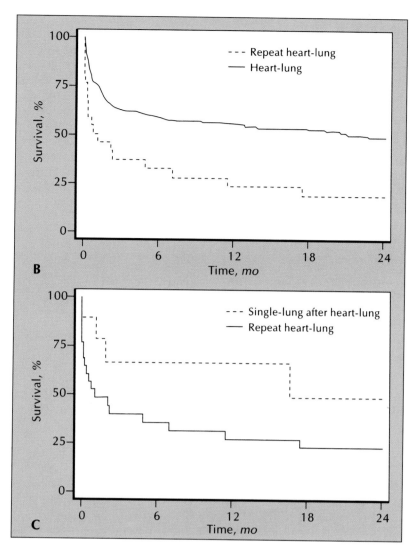

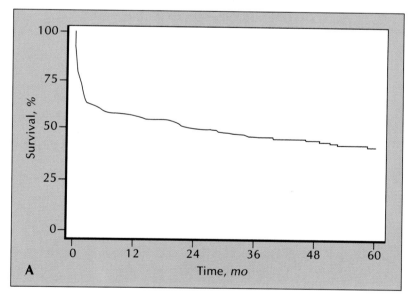

FIGURE 10-16. (*continued*) **B,** Between October 1986 and August 1990, 25 patients underwent repeat heart-lung transplantation (mean interval between transplants, 21±3 months; range, 7 to 61 months; 83% ventilator-dependent) [17]. Kaplan-Meier survival for patients undergoing retransplantation was 50%, 25%, and 25% at 1, 12, and 24 months, respectively, which was significantly worse than the 75%, 57%, and 51% survival rates at similar time intervals in 292 first-time heart-lung recipients at Harefield Hospital (*P*<0.05) [17]. Bleeding was the major complication in this group and was associated with early death in eight patients (32%). Interestingly, the development of recurrent obliterative bronchiolitis resulted in terminal graft failure in three patients following repeat heart-lung transplantation.

C, Adams *et al.* [17] have also explored the role of single-lung retransplantation in nine heart-lung recipients with terminal obliterative bronchiolitis (mean interval between transplants, 36±8 months; range, 9 to 83 months; 88% ventilator-dependent). Kaplan-Meier survival for recipients managed by single-lung retransplantation was 89%, 67%, and 50% at 1, 12, and 24 months, respectively, compared with 50%, 25%, and 20% at similar time intervals in the repeat heart-lung group. Bleeding was not a significant problem in the single-lung retransplantation group (no deaths, one reoperation for bleeding), and this certainly contributed to improved early survival. These data suggest that single-lung retransplantation appears to be the preferred option in carefully selected heart-lung recipients with terminal obliterative bronchiolitis. (Parts B and C *adapted from* Adams and coworkers [17]; with permission.)

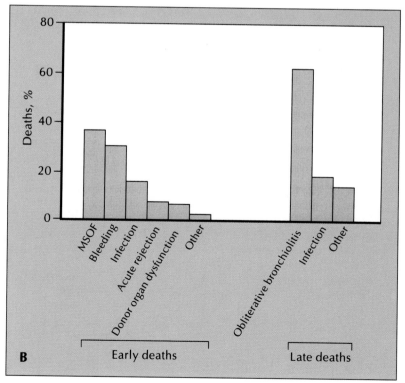

FIGURE 10-17. Late results following heart-lung transplantation. **A,** Five-year Kaplan-Meier survival curve for 290 patients undergoing heart-lung transplantation at Harefield Hospital [17]. The overall survival rates following heart-lung transplantation at 1, 3, and 5 years were 57%, 47%, and 43%, respectively.

B, The major causes of early (<1 month) and late (≥1 month) deaths occurring in 303 patients who underwent heart-lung transplantation at Harefield Hospital between December 1983 and May 1991 [16]. Sixty-eight percent (*n*=91) of the total deaths (*n*=134) occurred during the first postoperative month. Most early deaths were associated with perioperative problems, including multisystem organ failure (MSOF), bleeding, and donor organ dysfunc-

tion. Infection and acute rejection accounted for the majority of the other early deaths observed. Thirty-two percent (*n*=43) of the total deaths occurred after the first month (range, 3 to 84 months; mean, 40 months). Obliterative bronchiolitis (63%) and infection (19%) were responsible for the majority of deaths occurring in heart-lung recipients surviving at least 1 month posttransplantation.

FUTURE CONSIDERATIONS

Further define recipient categories

Solve donor shortage (xenotransplantation)

Improve immunosuppressive therapy

Resolve the pathogenesis of obliterative bronchiolitis

Further experience with retransplantation

FIGURE 10-18. Future considerations in the field of heart-lung transplantation. Continued follow-up of patients undergoing single-lung transplantation for selected diseases traditionally managed by heart-lung transplantation (*eg*, primary pulmonary hypertension, cystic fibrosis) should allow further definition of appropriate recipient categories in the future. Donor availability continues to represent a major limitation in the application of heart-lung transplantation, perhaps ultimately to be solved by xenotransplantation. Continued improvements in immunosuppressive therapy should diminish the impact of infection as well as acute and chronic rejection on long-term outcome. Obliterative bronchiolitis has emerged as the leading cause of death in long-term surviving heart-lung recipients, and further definition of its pathogenesis and therapy remains crucial. In this regard, a number of previously transplanted heart-lung recipients ultimately will develop terminal obliterative bronchiolitis and require repeat transplantation, allowing further advances in this challenging area.

REFERENCES

1. Demikhov VP: Experimental Transplantation of Vital Organs. New York: Consultants Bureau; 1962.

2. Neptune WB, Cookson BA, Bailey CP, *et al.*: Complete homologous heart transplantation. *Arch Surg* 1953, 66:174–178.

3. Marcus E, Wong SNT, Luisada AA: Homologous heart grafts. *Arch Surg* 1953, 66:179–191.

4. Watts R, Howard HS: Cardio-pulmonary transplantation. *Surg Forum* 1957, 8:313–317.

5. Nakae S, Webb WR, Theodorides T, *et al.*: Respiratory function following cardiopulmonary denervation in dog, cat and monkey. *Surg Gynecol Obstet* 1967, 125:1285–1292.

6. Cooley DA, Bloodwell RD, Hallman GL, *et al.*: Organ transplantation for advanced cardiopulmonary disease. *Ann Thorac Surg* 1969, 8:30–46.

7. Wildevuur CR, Benfield JR: A review of 23 human lung transplantations by 20 surgeons. *Ann Thorac Surg* 1970, 9:489–515.

8. Losman JG, Campbell CD, Replogle RL, *et al.*: Joint transplantation of heart and lungs: past experience and present potentials. *J Cardiovasc Surg* 1982, 23:440–452.

9. Castaneda AR, Zamora R, Schmidt-Habelmann, *et al.*: Cardiopulmonary autotransplantation in primates (baboons): late functional results. *Surgery* 1972, 72:1064–1070.

10. Reitz BA, Burton NA, Jamieson SW, *et al.*: Heart-lung transplantation, autotransplantation and allotransplantation in primates with extended survival. *J Thorac Cardiovasc Surg* 1980, 80:360–372.

11. Reitz BA, Wallwork JL, Hunt SA, *et al.*: Heart-lung transplantation: successful therapy for patients with pulmonary vascular disease. *N Engl J Med* 1982, 306:557–564.

12. Kaye MP: The Registry of the International Society for Heart and Lung Transplantation: tenth official report—1993. *J Heart Lung Transplant* 1993, 12:541–548.

13. Jamieson SW, Stinson EB, Oyer PE, *et al.*: Heart-lung transplantation for irreversible pulmonary hypertension. *Ann Thorac Surg* 1984, 38:554–562.

14. Griffith BP, Hardesty RL, Trento A, *et al.*: Heart-lung transplantation: lessons learned and future hopes. *Ann Thorac Surg* 1987, 43:6–16.

15. Modry DL, Kaye MP: Heart-lung transplantation: the Canadian experience from December 1967 to September 1985. *Can J Surg* 1986, 29:275–279.

16. Madden D, Radley-Smith R, Hodson M, *et al.*: Medium term results of heart-lung transplantation. *J Heart Lung Transplant* 1992, 11:S241–S243.

17. Adams DH, Cochrane AD, Khaghani A, *et al.*: Re-transplantation in heart-lung recipients with obliterative bronchiolitis. *J Thorac Cardiovasc Surg* 1994, 107:450–459.

18. Levine SM, Gibbons WJ, Bryan CL, *et al.*: Single lung transplantation for primary pulmonary hypertension. *Chest* 1990, 98:1107–1115.

19. Pasque MK, Cooper JD, Kaiser LR, *et al.*: Improved technique for bilateral lung transplantation. *Ann Thorac Surg* 1990, 49:785–791.

20. Bisson A, Bonnette P: A new technique for double lung transplantation: bilateral single lung transplantation. *J Thorac Cardiovasc Surg* 1992, 103:40–46.

21. Trulock EP: Recipient selection. *Chest Surg Clin North Am* 1993, 3:1–18.

22. Yacoub MH, Banner NR, Khaghani A: Heart-lung transplantation for cystic fibrosis and subsequent domino heart transplantation. *J Heart Transplant* 1990, 9:459–467.

23. Starnes VA: Heart-lung transplantation: indications, technique, and result. *Chest Surg Clin North Am* 1993, 3:113–121.

24. Yacoub MH, Khaghani A, Banner N, *et al.*: Distant organ procurement for heart-lung transplantation. *Transplant Proc* 1989, 21:2548–2550.

25. Reitz BA: Heart-lung transplantation. In *Heart-Lung Transplantation*. Edited by Baumgartner WA, Reitz BA, Achuff SC. Philadelphia: WB Saunders Company; 1990:319–371.

26. Smith JD, Danskine AJ, Laylor RM, *et al.*: The effect of panel reactive antibodies and the donor specific crossmatch and graft survival after heart and heart-lung transplantation. *Transplant Immunol* 1993, 1:60.

27. Haverich A, Scott WC, Jamieson SW: Twenty years of lung preservation: a review. *J Heart Transplant* 1985, 4:234–240.

28. Yacoub MH, Banner NR: Recent developments in lung and heart-lung transplantation. *Transplant Rev* 1989, 3:1–29.

29. Hardesty RL, Griffith BP: Auto-perfusion of the heart and lungs for preservation during distant procurement. *J Thorac Cardiovasc Surg* 1987, 93:11–18.

30. Baldwin JC, Frist WH, Starkey TD, *et al.*: Distant graft procurement for combined heart-lung transplantation using pulmonary artery flush and simple topical hypothermia for graft preservation. *Ann Thorac Surg* 1987, 43:670–673.

31. Wallwork J, Jones K, Cavorocchi N, *et al.*: Distant procurement of organs for clinical heart-lung transplantation using a single flush technique. *Transplantation* 1987, 44:654–658.

32. Jamieson SW, Stinson EB, Oyer PE, *et al.*: Operative technique for heart-lung transplantation. *J Thorac Cardiovasc Surg* 1984, 87:930–935.

33. Madden BP, Hodson ME, Tsang V, *et al.*: Intermediate-term results of heart-lung transplantation for cystic fibrosis. *Lancet* 1992, 339:1583–1587.

34. Baldwin JC, Oyer PE, Stinson EB, *et al.*: Comparison of cardiac rejection in heart and heart-lung transplantation. *J Heart Transplant* 1987, 6:352–356.

35. Griffith BP, Hardesty RL, Trento A, *et al.*: A synchronous rejection of heart and lungs following cardiopulmonary transplantation. *Ann Thorac Surg* 1985, 40:448–493.

36. Dummer JS, Montero CG, Griffith BP, *et al.*: Infections in heart-lung transplant recipients. *Transplantation* 1986, 41:725–729.

37. Hutter JA, Scott J, Wreghitt T, *et al.*: The importance of cytomegalovirus in heart-lung transplant recipients. *Chest* 1989, 95:627–631.

38. Burke CM, Theodore J, Dawkins KD, *et al.*: Posttransplant obliterative bronchiolitis and other late sequelae in human heart-lung transplantation. *Chest* 1984, 86:824–829.

39. Tazelaar HD, Yousem SA: The pathology of combined heart-lung transplantation: an autopsy study. *Hum Pathol* 1988, 19:1403–1416.

Venous Thrombosis and Insufficiency

DIAGNOSIS OF VENOUS THROMBOSIS

Joseph F. Polak

Venous thrombosis is ubiquitous and often underdiagnosed. The spectrum of the disease is surprisingly wide, ranging from the most dramatic presentation of all, that of a fatal pulmonary embolism, to completely asymptomatic episodes from which the patient recovers with no untoward effects.

A complete understanding of venous thrombosis cannot be achieved solely by reviewing pathologic specimens. Its dynamic nature can be better understood by reviewing the appearance of thrombi as they are visualized by the various diagnostic imaging tests. Venography, still considered the gold standard for identifying venous thrombi, does not easily permit monitoring of the evolution of thrombi *in vivo*. Other techniques, mainly noninvasive, offer a better window to understanding the way this disease process evolves *in vivo*. For example, thrombi in formation have increased uptake of radiolabeled fibrinogen. External monitoring of this uptake has led to a more complete understanding of the origin and time course of early postoperative venous thrombosis [1]. Impedance plethysmography, a test based on the physiology of venous capacitance in the calf veins and drainage through the more proximal veins, has been used to identify patients with suspected venous thrombosis with a high risk of developing pulmonary embolism [2]. Serial application of this test in patients with deep vein thrombosis has shown that there may be improvement of venous drainage to the affected extremity by 6 months following an acute and extensive episode of venous thrombosis [3].

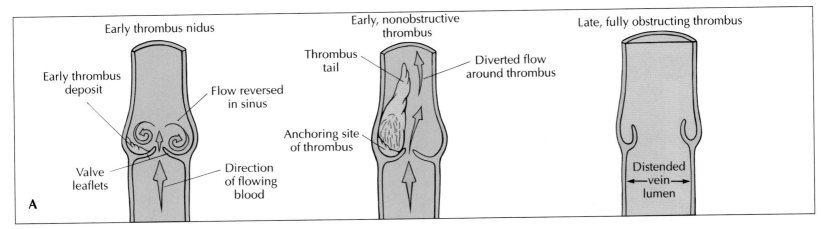

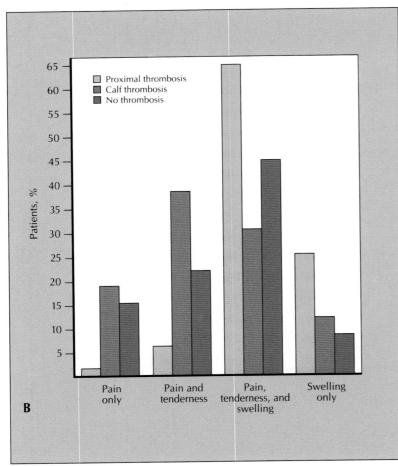

FIGURE 11-1. A, Different stages of thrombus formation. From pathologic studies, it is now understood that early thrombi deposit in areas of stagnant flow (*left*) [4]. This is typically seen at the vein valve sinus where there is relative stagnation and flow reversal. The inciting events responsible for early thrombus formation are not fully understood, but likely include an endothelial environment with a propensity to coagulate because of trauma, increased elaboration of coagulation factors, and stasis. Although the factors responsible for continued growth of thrombi cannot be defined specifically, the pathology of thrombus growth is basically elongation of the thrombus tail, as a fibrin network, from its anchoring point within the sinus of the vein valve (*middle*). Most thrombi likely do not evolve beyond this stage. The thrombus can grow to expand and occupy the full lumen of the vein (*right*). Because the volume occupied by the fibrin network is larger than that of the dissolved blood constituents, vein distention is commonly the end result. In obstructing thrombosis, symptoms are likely caused by local distention and activation of pain receptors in the vein wall and surrounding tissues. The finding of vein distention on venous sonography supports the diagnosis of obstructive venous thrombosis. In addition, localized edema or inflammatory changes can activate pain and stretch receptors in the contiguous tissues. Distal to the obstructing thrombus, the obstruction impairs venous return and causes an increase in hydrostatic pressure, resulting in the extravasation of fluid in the extracellular space. **B,** Frequency of symptoms of pain, tenderness, and swelling in patients with confirmed proximal and calf vein thrombosis versus those without thrombosis in whom the diagnosis is initially suspected. Clinically, edema and localized pain are not specific to the diagnosis of acute deep vein thrombosis. The diagnostic specificity of clinical findings of edema and the presence of symptoms is approximately 50% [5].

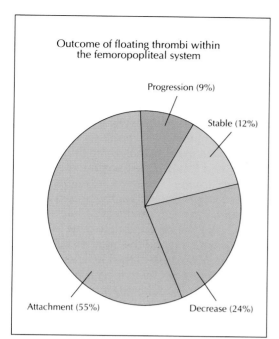

Outcome of floating thrombi within the femoropopliteal system

Progression (9%)

Stable (12%)

Attachment (55%)

Decrease (24%)

FIGURE 11-2. Outcome of floating thrombi within the femoropopliteal system. Venographic studies have shown that there is a high rate of resolution of early venous thrombi, possibly as a result of endogenous processes. A more recent sonographic study has shown that partly occlusive thrombi will often attach to the vein wall [6]. A large proportion of the remaining thrombi will not change in size or may actually decrease in size. Progression is seen in approximately 10% of cases even while heparin is being administered. It is as yet unknown whether progression is an indicator of impending pulmonary embolism.

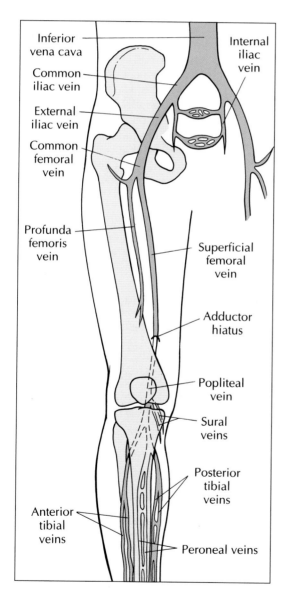

Inferior vena cava

Internal iliac vein

Common iliac vein

External iliac vein

Common femoral vein

Profunda femoris vein

Superficial femoral vein

Adductor hiatus

Popliteal vein

Sural veins

Posterior tibial veins

Anterior tibial veins

Peroneal veins

FIGURE 11-3. The major venous channels of the lower extremity. The inferior vena cava, which lies to the right of the aorta, branches into the common iliac veins. On the left, the common iliac vein crosses below the right iliac artery or the aorta. This causes relative compression of the vein and is likely the cause of slower venous flow in the left leg with respect to the right. It presumably accounts for the greater occurrence of venous thrombosis in the left leg with respect to the right leg in 55% to 60% of cases. The common iliac vein bifurcates into external and internal iliac veins. The internal iliac veins tend to be smaller in diameter and connect with the contralateral internal iliac veins. These are rarely the source of primary thrombi and, if thrombi do occur, they tend to be obstructive in nature with concurrent involvement of the external or common iliac branches.

As it progresses through the pelvis and crosses the inguinal ligament, the external iliac vein becomes the common femoral vein, which bifurcates into the profunda femoris and the true (superficial) femoral veins. Although the latter are often referred to as the superficial femoral veins, they are both deep veins. The profunda femoris vein is responsible for venous drainage of the proximal two thirds of the thigh. The true (superficial) femoral vein is responsible for venous drainage of the distal third of the thigh. As the femoral vein crosses through the adductor hiatus, defined by the adductor muscle in the lower thigh, it becomes the popliteal vein. The popliteal vein has major muscular branches to the gastrocnemius muscle. Approximately 6 cm below the knee joint, the popliteal vein sends off the anterior tibial veins that cross the interosseous membrane and then lie on top of it. Posteriorly, the tibioperoneal trunk branches into the true posterior tibial and peroneal veins. Below the popliteal vein, the deep vein system is almost always duplicated. Popliteal vein duplications are present in 30% to 35% of the population. More proximal duplications of the femoral vein are present in 20% to 25% of patients [7]. Duplications are extremely rare above this level.

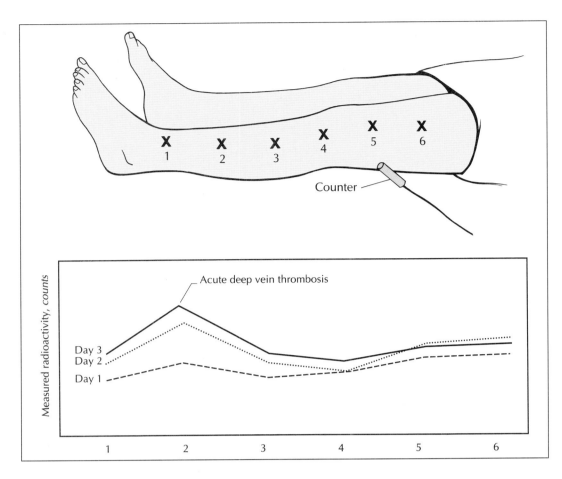

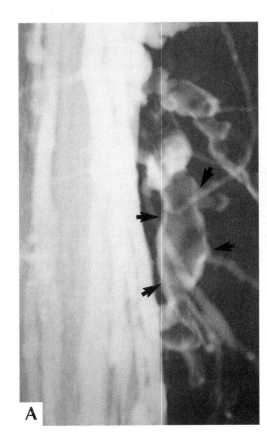

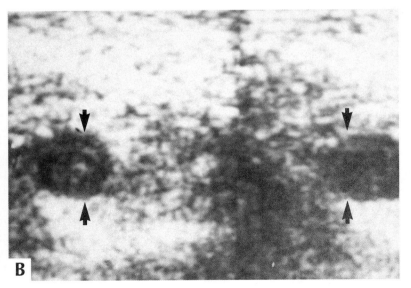

FIGURE 11-4. Iodine-125 fibrinogen scanning has been used extensively to study the natural history of venous thrombosis. Fibrinogen labeled with iodine-125 is given intravenously, and this complex accumulates in forming thrombi. The lower extremity is subsequently surveyed for the presence of accumulating radioactivity at 24-hour intervals. The technique accurately detects thrombi in both the calf and the more distal portion of the thigh. Because of the low energy of the Iodine-125 isotope, there is poor penetration in deeper tissues of the thigh, and the accuracy is poor in the proximal thigh. False-positive readings can be caused by cellulitis, wound healing, or reactive inflammation. When compared with adjacent points, persistent elevation of counts by at least 20% is considered diagnostic for the presence of forming venous thrombi. This elevation must persist for 24 hours. Increases of at least 20% at a given location when compared with the counts detected in previous days (normally after the first 24 hours) is also used as a diagnostic end-point. This diagnostic method was used in many of the original studies that established that calf vein thrombi spread more proximally to the popliteal vein in approximately 20% of patients [1].

FIGURE 11-5. A, This venogram shows the typical appearance of a calf vein thrombus in the soleal veins. The thrombus is outlined by contrast agent (*arrows*). This finding—a discrete filling defect—is one of the two criteria used for the diagnosis of acute deep vein thrombosis. The other criterion is the presence of a sharp cut-off in the contrast column.

B, The corresponding sonogram clearly depicts a noncompressible echogenic structure within the soleal vein (*arrows*).

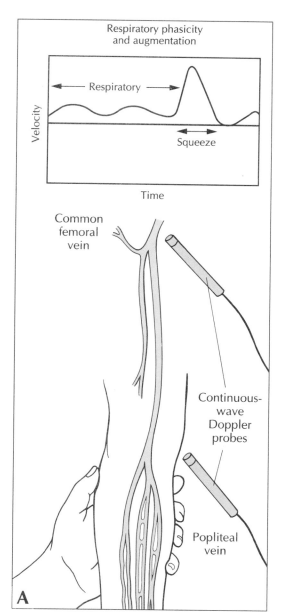

FIGURE 11-6. A, Obstructive venous thrombosis can be detected by analyzing flow signals within the veins with either continuous-wave Doppler or, more recently, pulsed-wave Doppler [8]. Both use a sound beam to interrogate blood flow velocity within the veins. Frequency shifts in the returning signals are caused by differences in the motion of erythrocytes within the vein. A typical example of the detected waveforms is shown in the top portion of the figure. During respiration, there is typically a cyclic variation in the velocity wave-form detected within the femoral vein (respiratory phase). This variation is slightly less pronounced at the popliteal vein and may be difficult to elicit at the calf. During inspiration, there is a relative decrease in blood flow because of the increase in intra-abdominal pressure. During expiration, flow velocity is increased. An ancillary maneuver used to exclude the presence of an obstructive process is flow augmentation, which is accomplished by emptying the venous blood pool within the calf veins. This can be achieved either by externally squeezing the calf and expelling the blood that will then flow into the popliteal femoral and ultimately the iliac veins or by having the patient dorsiflex and plantarflex the foot, which also expels blood from the calf veins. The end result is a marked increase in the velocity signals detected more proximally, within the popliteal and femoral veins (squeeze phase).

The finding of normal respiratory variation and a normal response to flow augmentation excludes the presence of significant venous obstruction caused either by an intrinsic process, such as venous thrombosis, or an extrinsic process, such as compression by a pelvic tumor. This physiologic principle also explains the mechanisms of action of the impedance plethysmogram, a well-recognized method for establishing the presence of obstructive venous thrombosis.

B, Doppler tracing of a normal response to inspiration (INS) with a decrease in the velocity of blood flow.

C, Doppler tracing of a decrease in the amplitude of the venous signals and loss in this response to respiratory variation. This finding suggests a proximal (iliac vein) obstruction to venous return. (*continued*)

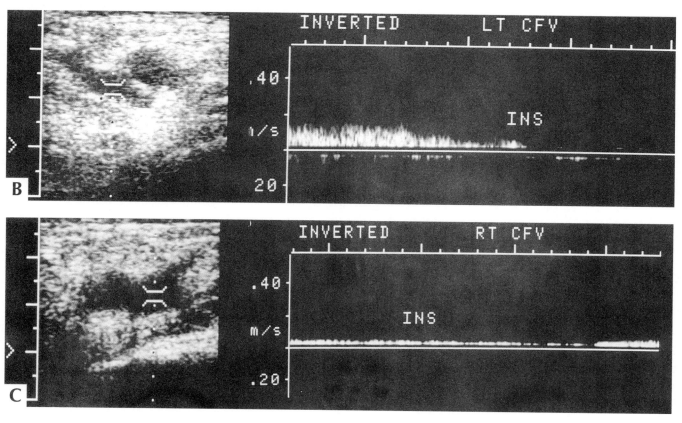

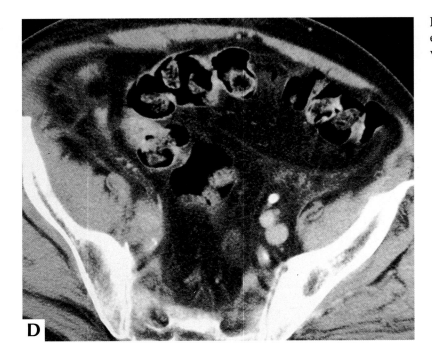

FIGURE 11-6. (*continued*) **D,** The findings are explained by an enlarged lymph node causing extrinsic compression of the iliac vein on the right.

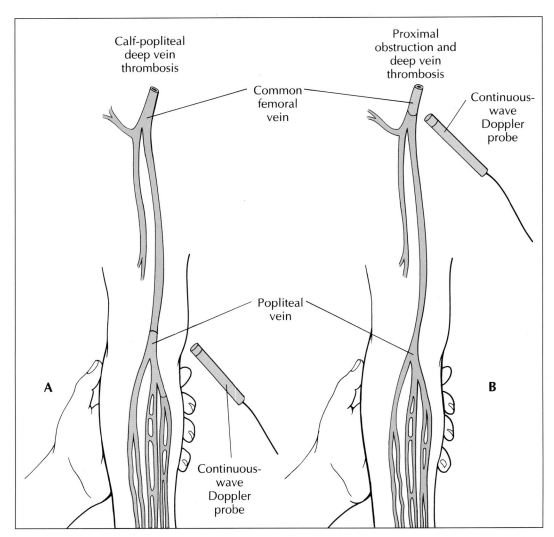

FIGURE 11-7. Respiratory phasicity and venous augmentation (*see* top of Fig. 11-6A) will typically be lost in the presence of obstructive venous thrombosis. **A,** No flow signals are detected within a vein containing a large amount of thrombus.

B, Flow signals are not detected in the vein below the level of an obstruction. Such an obstructive process may be located within the iliac vein and be responsible for marked limb swelling [9]. In the latter scenario, the diagnosis of an obstructive process is suggested, even though direct evidence of venous thrombosis is not obtained. A more complete examination, either by venography or contrast-enhanced pelvic computed tomography, can then be performed to better evaluate the iliac veins (*see* Fig. 11-6D).

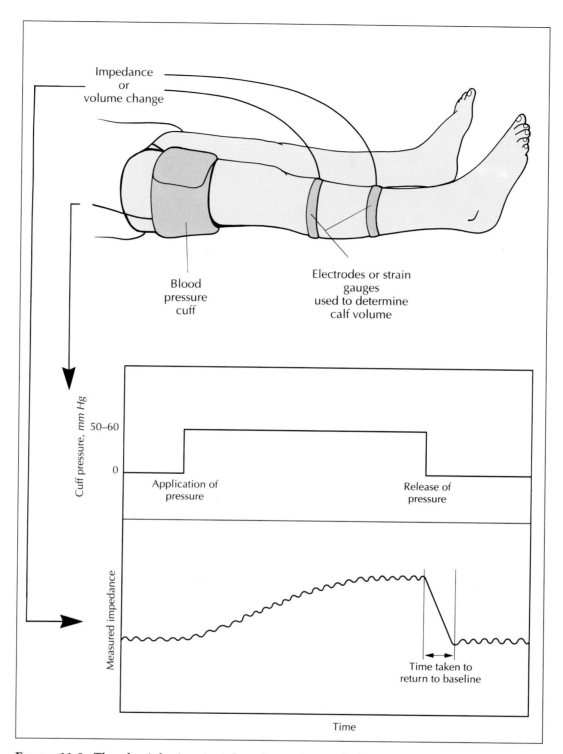

FIGURE 11-8. The physiologic principles of impedance plethysmography. This test
was the mainstay for the noninvasive evaluation of lower extremity venous thrombosis.
It can also help in the understanding of the pathophysiology of deep vein thrombosis.
The examination is performed by inflating (to about 40 mm Hg) and deflating a blood
pressure cuff placed over the proximal thigh, which obstructs venous return but does not
interfere with flow so that there is continued filling of the venous system. Following this
filling phase, release of the proximal pressure cuff results in rapid emptying of part of the
blood volume trapped within the calf and a return to baseline values. Volume changes
within the calf are measured simultaneously. An electric impedance method is shown
here. Other techniques to measure calf volume include pressure cuffs or strain gauges.

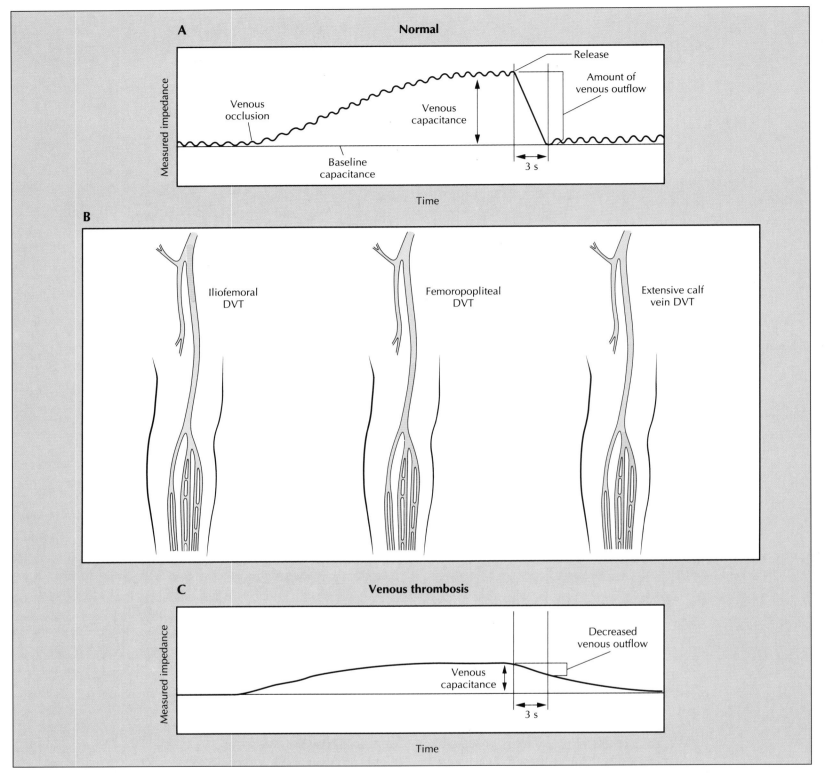

FIGURE 11-9. A, Normal response to the plethysmographic examination. The amount of blood accumulated during blood pressure cuff inflation, or venous capacitance, is measured when the impedance values have stabilized. Venous outflow is measured as the change in impedance value in the first 3 seconds following release of the blood pressure curve.

B, Situations in which venous thrombosis in the iliofemoral, the femoropopliteal, or, extensively in the calf veins affect the impedance plethysmogram.

C, Because of the space-occupying nature of the thrombus, the blood volume or venous capacitance of the calf is decreased.

Venous outflow is decreased because of the venous obstruction. In addition, the obstructive process may dampen the normal baseline phasic signals due to respiration. Serial impedance plethysmography has been very cost-effective in monitoring patients with suspected symptomatic, large obstructive venous thrombosis, although serial sonography may be more effective [2,10,11]. Impedance plethysography has performed poorly when asymptomatic postoperative patients were screened for the presence of deep vein thrombi [12]. This is mainly a reflection of the nonobstructive nature of venous thrombi in this latter patient population. DVT—deep vein thrombosis.

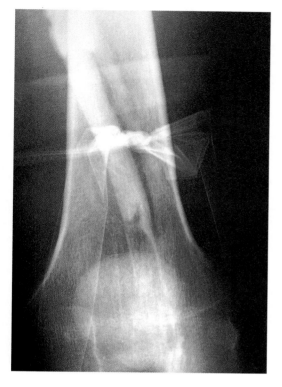

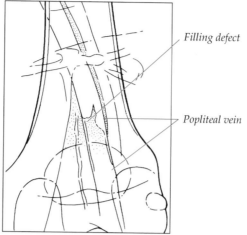

FIGURE 11-10. This venogram shows a discrete filling defect in the popliteal vein of a patient with a history of previous deep vein thrombosis (DVT). A duplicated and patent popliteal vein is seen to the side. This venogram is diagnostic of an acute DVT. There is no evidence of the previous DVT.

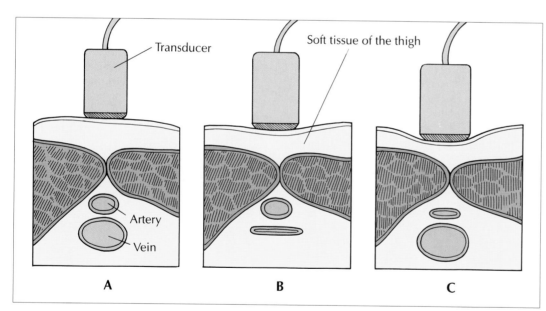

FIGURE 11-11. A primary diagnostic criterion used to establish the presence of deep vein thrombosis by sonography is the loss of vein compressibility [13–15]. **A**, Baseline. **B**, Normal compression. The vein will completely collapse when gentle pressure is applied to the skin overlying it. As a general rule, the applied pressure is kept below what is necessary to collapse the artery. The artery is not as affected because intra-arterial pressure is much greater than venous pressure, and the structure of the arterial wall is more resistant to the pressure deformation than the venous wall. **C**, Abnormal compression. The lumen of a vein containing either a fully obstructing or partly obstructing thrombus cannot be compressed. Associated with acute venous thrombi is passive dilation of the vein itself. In C, the arterial wall has been deformed by applying pressure aggressively.

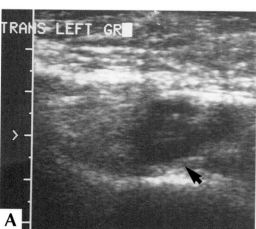

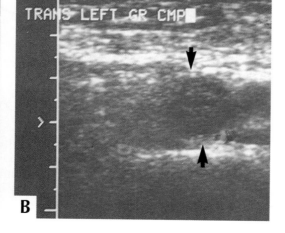

FIGURE 11-12. A, Sonogram at the level of the common femoral vein and artery shows an echogenic structure (*arrow*) within the common femoral vein [16]. **B,** Pressure has been applied to the skin. The common femoral vein lumen cannot be compressed (*arrows*), confirming the diagnosis of acute deep vein thrombosis.

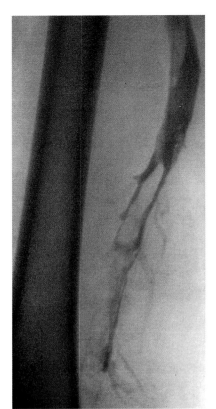

FIGURE 11-13.
This acute venous thrombus of the femoral vein shows the typical thrombus tail at the leading edge of a partly obstructed thrombus. This represents the more proximal extent of the developing thrombus. More distally, the thrombus is fully obstructive and therefore is not seen on the venogram.

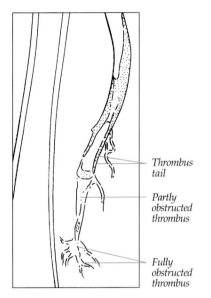

Thrombus tail

Partly obstructed thrombus

Fully obstructed thrombus

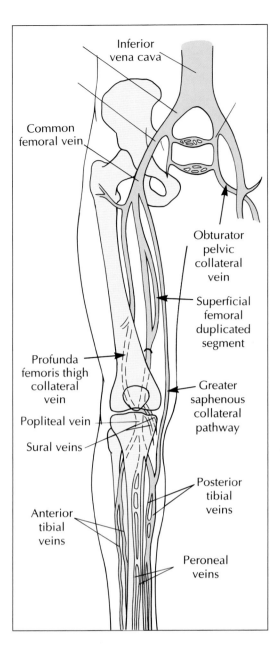

Inferior vena cava

Common femoral vein

Obturator pelvic collateral vein

Superficial femoral duplicated segment

Profunda femoris thigh collateral vein

Popliteal vein

Sural veins

Greater saphenous collateral pathway

Anterior tibial veins

Posterior tibial veins

Peroneal veins

FIGURE 11-14. Some of the major collateral pathways that can be seen in the presence of deep venous thrombosis. Quite often, involvement of the deep venous system results in reversal of the normal drainage through the perforating veins that connect the superficial to the deep venous system. There is then flow in the greater saphenous vein, which will serve as a major collateral pathway from the calf. At the level of the popliteal vein, there is often a communicating venous channel that joins the more peripheral branches of the profunda femoral vein. Another major collateral consists of duplicated femoral vein segments. The prevalence of duplicated venous segments is approximately 20% to 25% in the femoral vein and 30% to 35% in the popliteal vein [7]. Obstruction of one of the two parallel channels does not necessarily compromise flow in the other. In such a situation, symptoms may be minimal and swelling may not be present. Another common collateral pathway—the obturator vein—develops when proximal thrombosis involves the iliac vein. This collateral is seen following more extensive episodes of venous thrombosis. There are often cross-collateral connections through the internal iliac plexi to the contralateral internal iliac veins.

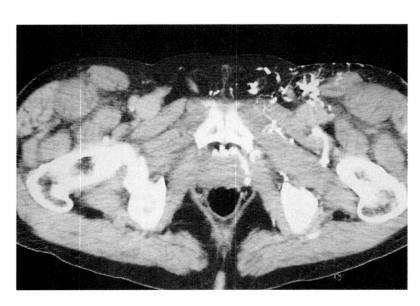

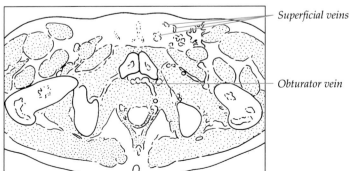

Superficial veins

Obturator vein

FIGURE 11-15. This patient with phlegmasia cerulea dolens had the diagnosis confirmed by computed tomography performed while contrast was injected into the left foot. The obturator vein and other internal iliac branches serve as major collateral pathways as do more superficial branches.

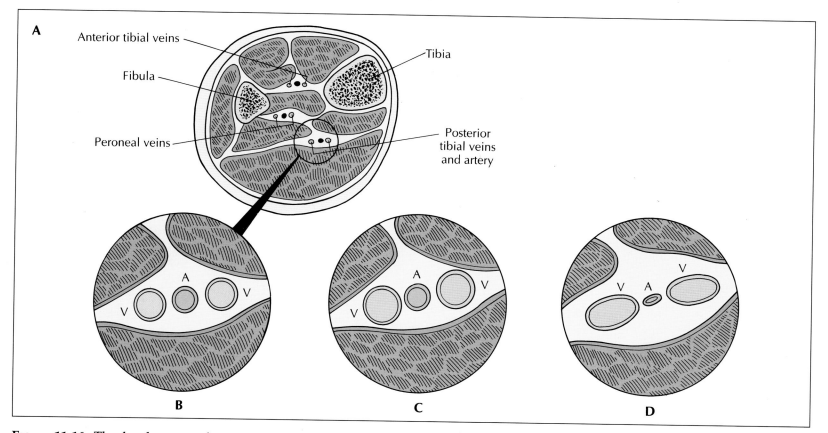

FIGURE 11-16. The development of severe venous obstruction. **A,** Cross-section at calf level at which sections are depicted. **B,** Normal resting diameter of posterior tibial artery and veins. **C,** In most instances of obstructive venous thrombosis, some edema is noted within the soft tissues. The veins are obstructed and appear enlarged, and the associated increases in interstitial pressures distend the fascial planes. **D,** In phlegmasia cerulea dolens, the most severe form of obstructive venous thrombosis, complete obstruction to venous return elicits massive edema within the distal soft tissues because of a marked increase in the interstitial pressures. This increased pressure can cause local compression of the vein and artery. This may compromise still patent veins and may be sufficient to obstruct arterial inflow, ultimately causing ischemia and muscle infarction. The presence of edema without evidence of impaired venous flow proximally suggests that deep vein thrombosis is not the cause of the edematous changes and that lymphatic obstruction or other systemic causes are to blame. A—artery; V—vein.

SUBACUTE AND CHRONIC DVT

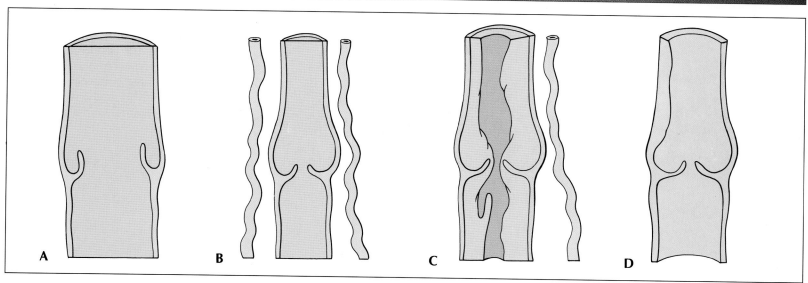

FIGURE 11-17. Possible scenarios in the natural history of obstructive venous thrombosis. Distended and obstructed vein segment involved with DVT (**A**). One possible scenario is failure to recanalize the native venous segment (**B**). In such a case, the vein will decrease in caliber over time and remain permanently obstructed. Flow will be reestablished through collaterals that tend to parallel the course of the native vein. In general, however, there is partial recanalization of the affected segment (**C**). The extent of vein distention decreases. Collaterals are also often seen. The flow channel within the recanalized vein tends to be irregular. On sonography, the walls are thickened. There is partial loss of compressibility of the vein lumen. Less commonly, there is almost complete resorption of the thrombus (**D**). Careful evaluation with sonography sometimes shows evidence of wall thickening in one portion of the previously affected vein.

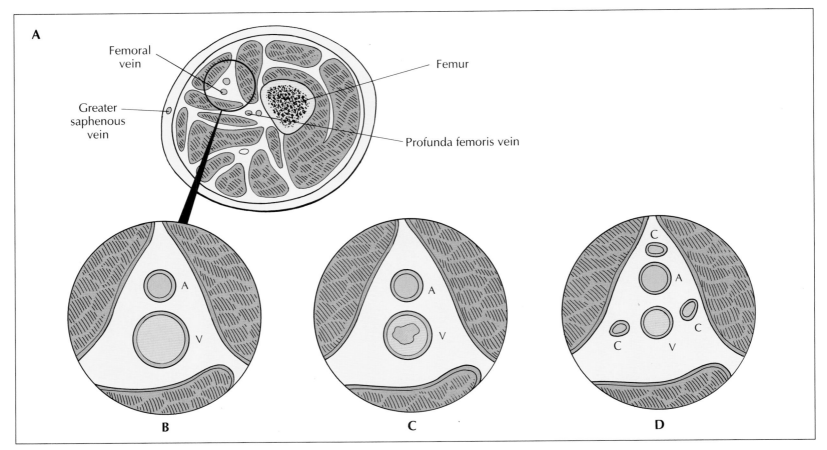

FIGURE 11-18. The evolution of venous thrombosis as seen by sonography.

A, Cross-section at which the sections are depicted. B, In the acute phase of obstructive symptomatic venous thrombosis there is marked distention of the vein as well as loss of compressibility (see Fig. 11-12). There tends not to be flow within the affected venous channel, or, in cases of partial obstruction, there is flow at the periphery of the vein (see Fig. 11-23).

C, Partial recanalization is the more common outcome (see Fig. 11-24),

and is associated with some decrease in the caliber of the vein. Flow persists principally in the center of the channel. With more extensive venous thrombosis, there is often failure to recanalize the vein segment.

D, Collaterals can become very prominent. In this case, the native femoral vein remains obstructed and with time decreases in caliber as fibroblasts replace the original fibrin and clot with a mixture of collagen, ground substance, and smooth muscle cells. The collaterals vary in their number and size. A—artery; C—collaterals; V—vein.

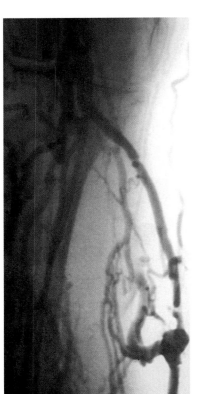

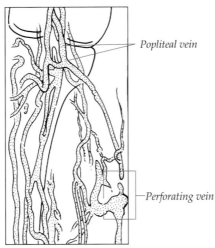

FIGURE 11-19. This venogram is typical of what is seen following obstructive venous thrombosis. The popliteal vein is occluded and a collateral channel can be seen. The posterior tibial vein is occluded and a large perforating vein has redirected flow into the superficial system.

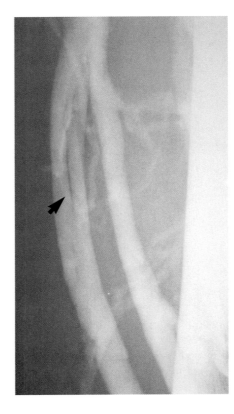

FIGURE 11-20. A common manifestation of chronic deep vein thrombosis is shown on this venogram. A synechia is present in one duplicated femoral vein. In addition, the wall of the femoral vein is irregular.

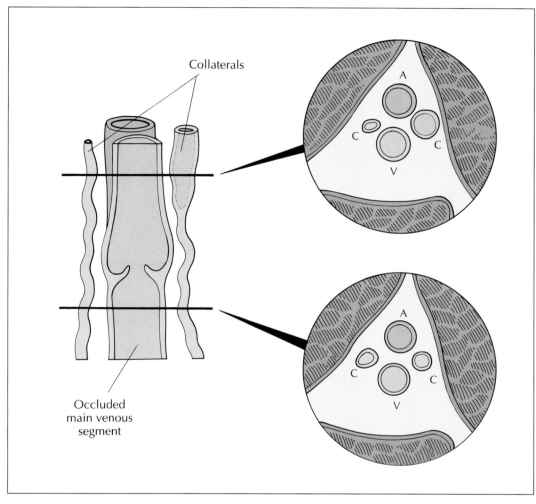

FIGURE 11-21. The typical appearance of acute venous thrombosis superimposed on chronic venous thrombosis. In this case, the native femoral vein is totally occluded because of a previous episode of venous thrombosis. The major collateral pathways that have developed can also become involved by acute venous thrombosis. Acute venous thrombosis within a collateral causes, on sonography, a loss of flow signals and of compressibility (*top inset*). There is also obvious distention of the involved venous channel. Displacement of the transducer to an uninvolved segment lower in the leg shows a decrease in vein diameter and a normal response to compression (*bottom inset*). The venographic findings include failure to visualize the obstructed venous segment of the true femoral vein. In this respect, sonography is superior to venography. The obstructed vein is seen on sonography whereas its presence is inferred on venography. Venography will show the patent collateral vein. A—artery; C—collaterals; V—vein.

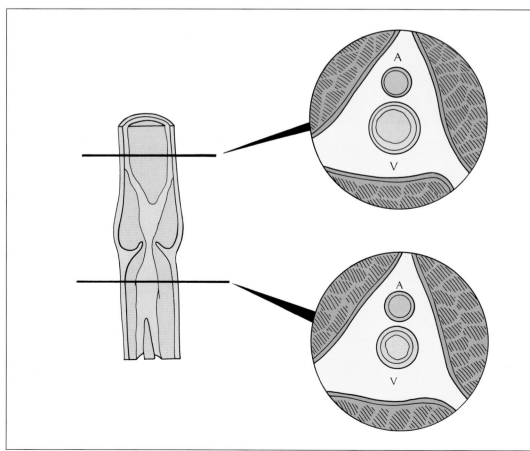

FIGURE 11-22. Acute venous thrombosis can also develop within a recanalized channel that was previously affected by venous thrombosis. Acute venous thrombosis superimposed on chronic venous thrombosis appears, on venography, as a transition from a small irregular channel with synechia (chronic deep vein thrombosis) to a channel that contains a large filling defect (acute deep vein thrombosis). Sonography depicts the more chronically affected portion of the vein (*bottom inset*). There is flow signal within the recanalized lumen. The wall typically has a thickened echogenic structure. The sonographic findings within the segment affected by acute venous thrombosis (*top inset*) include distention and loss of compressibility. Flow is elicited at the periphery of the thrombus located within the vein. A—artery; V—vein.

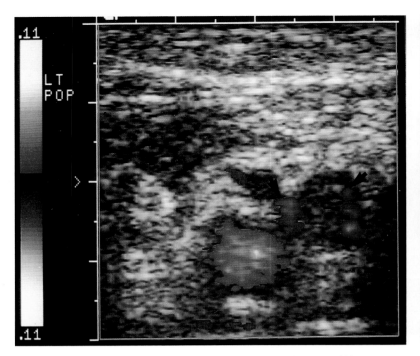

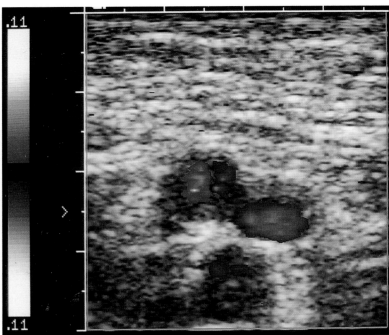

FIGURE 11-23. A rim of blue color surrounds a discrete filling defect. This defect is consistent with an acute thrombus. In acute venous thrombosis, flow signals are either absent in a distended segment or outline the contents of the vein.

FIGURE 11-24. An area where flow is in the central portion of the lumen lower in the leg (*blue area*). This is consistent with chronic venous thrombosis and corresponds to the scenario of recanalization with residual wall thickening.

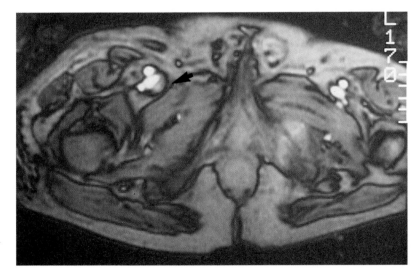

FIGURE 11-25. This magnetic resonance venogram shows a discrete filling defect at the periphery of the vein lumen (*arrow*), a finding that is consistent with chronic venous thrombosis. The thigh is markedly swollen because of the presence of chronic lymphatic obstruction.

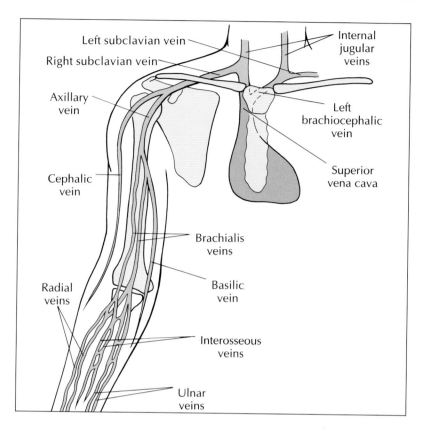

FIGURE 11-26. The two major superficial veins to the arm are the cephalic and basilic veins. The cephalic vein is situated more laterally and joins the subclavian vein at the distal one third of the clavicle. The proximal cephalic vein is often used as the site of insertion of chronic indwelling lines such as Hickman lines, port-a-cath catheters, and pacing wires. These can be the source of thrombi that extend into the subclavian vein. The basilic vein courses medially and joins one of the brachial veins at a variable level between the axilla proper and a point located midway up the humerus. This is a common location for superficial venous thrombosis, typically at the site of an intravenous line. The deep veins of the forearm and the brachial veins are duplicated. Duplications are less common at the level of the axillary vein and are absent at the level of the subclavian vein. The internal jugular veins drain the head and join the subclavian veins. They are often the site of thrombi associated with central line placements.

The subclavian vein joins the internal jugular vein to become the brachiocephalic vein. The right side of this venous segment is quite short. On the left, the brachiocephalic vein courses over a large distance behind the sternum. Its length may explain the higher prevalence of left-sided venous thrombi. Both brachiocephalic veins join into the superior vein cava in the upper mediastinum. The superior vena cava can have sites of venous thrombi, often caused by the presence of indwelling catheters. Mediastinal masses may also increase stasis in the superior vena cava and promote de novo thrombosis. Sonographic evaluation of the presence of upper extremity venous thrombosis relies on a combination of diagnostic criteria [17–19].

SONOGRAPHIC DIAGNOSTIC CHARACTERISTICS

CHARACTERISTIC	PRINCIPLE
Loss of vein compressibility	Thrombus occupies the lumen of the vein, which does not compress when external pressure is applied
Altered flow dynamics	The normal venous flow signals are blunted by obstructive thrombus; if color flow imaging is used, flow signals are absent or can be used to outline partly obstructive thrombus
Echogenic signals arising from thrombi in the vein	The thrombus has internal echoes due to the organizing fibrin; areas of decreased echoes can also be seen during thrombolytic therapy
Distention of the vein	Seen with obstructive thrombus
Venous collaterals	Develop parallel to an obstructed vein segment

FIGURE 11-27. Sonographic characteristics useful for diagnosing deep vein thrombosis. Distention of the vein and the presence of venous collaterals are considered secondary characteristics. The primary diagnostic criteria are loss of compressibility and loss of venous flow signals.

SONOGRAPHIC CRITERIA FOR DIAGNOSIS OF VENOUS THROMBOSIS IN THE ARM

VEIN	COMPRESSIBILITY	FLOW	ECHOGENICITY
Brachial veins	+++	±	±
Axillary	+++	±	±
Subclavian D1/3	+++	+	±
Subclavian M1/3	±	+	+
Subclavian P1/3	±	++	+
Jugular	+++	++	+

FIGURE 11-28. Sonographic criteria for the diagnosis of venous thrombosis in the arm. +++—always useful; ++—often useful; +—occasionally useful; ±—rarely useful; D1/3— distal third; M1/3— middle third; D1/3— proxomal third.

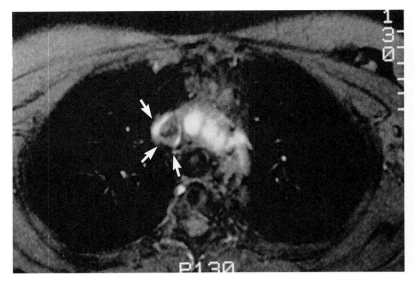

FIGURE 11-29. This magnetic resonance venogram shows a typical filling defect in the superior vena cava: an extension of thrombus from the right brachiocephalic vein (*arrows*). The thrombus is located centrally and is surrounded by flow signal, which is typical of an acute venous thrombosis.

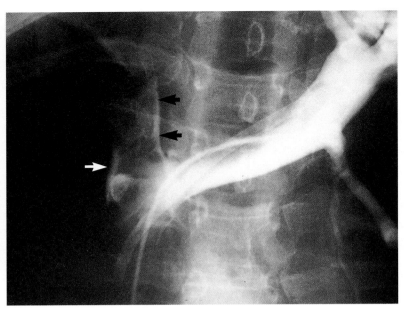

FIGURE 11-30. Acute venous thrombosis is seen as a filling defect (*arrows*) within the right innominate (brachiocephalic) vein on this patient's venogram.

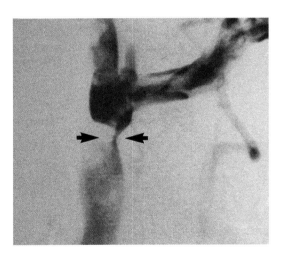

FIGURE 11-31. This venogram, taken following thrombolytic therapy, shows resolution of the filling defect. There is, however, a defect in the superior vein cava (*arrows*). This defect may represent acute thrombus or a more chronic process. Normally, thrombolytic therapy is more effective in situations in which a partly obstructive thrombus is present or when the agent is administered directly into the thrombus. The agent, once chosen, is commonly administered with a special catheter designed with side holes that help disperse the drug into the thrombus.

REFERENCES

1. Kakkar VV, Flanc C, Howe CT, *et al.*: Natural history of post-operative deep-vein thrombosis. *Lancet* 1969, 2:230–233.

2. Huisman MV, Buller HR, ten Cate JW, *et al.*: Serial impedance plethysmography for suspected deep venous thrombosis in outpatients: the Amsterdam general practitioner study. *N Engl J Med* 1986, 314:823–828.

3. Killewich LA, Bedford GR, Beach KW, *et al.*: Spontaneous lysis of deep venous thrombi: rate and outcome. *J Vasc Surg* 1989, 9:89–97.

4. Sevitt S, Gallagher N: Venous thrombosis and pulmonary embolism: a clinico-pathological study in injured and burned patients. *Br J Surg* 1961, 48:475–489.

5. Hull R, Hirsh J, Sackett DL: Combined use of leg scanning and impedance plethysmography in suspected venous thrombosis: an alternative to venography. *N Engl J Med* 1977, 296:1497–1500.

6. Baldridge ED, Martin MA, Welling RE: Clinical significance of free-floating venous thrombi. *J Vasc Surg* 1990, 11:62–69.

7. Liu G-C, Ferris EJ, Reifsteck JR, *et al.*: Effect of anatomic variations on deep venous thrombosis of the lower extremity. *AJR Am J Roentgenol* 1986, 146:845–848.

8. Polak JF: *Peripheral Vascular Sonography: A Practical Guide*. Baltimore: Williams and Wilkins; 1992.

9. Effeney DJ, Friedman MB, Gooding GA: Iliofemoral venous thrombosis: real-time ultrasound diagnosis, normal criteria, and clinical application. *Radiology* 1984, 150:787–792.

10. Hillner BE, Philbrick JT, Becker DM: Optimal management of suspected lower-extremity deep vein thrombosis: an evaluation with cost assessment of 24 management strategies. *Arch Intern Med* 1992, 152:165–175.

11. Heijboer H, Buller HP, Lensing AWA, *et al*.: A comparison of real-time compression ultrasonography with impedance plethysmography for the diagnosis of deep-vein thrombosis in symptomatic outpatients. *N Engl J Med* 1993, 329:1365–1369.

12. Patterson RB, Fowl RJ, Keller JD, *et al*.: The limitations of impedance plethysmography in the diagnosis of acute deep venous thrombosis. *J Vasc Surg* 1989, 9:725–730.

13. Cronan JJ, Dorfman GS, Scola FH, *et al*.: Deep venous thrombosis: US assessment using vein compression. *Radiology* 1987, 162:191–194.

14. Lensing AW, Prandoni P, Brandjes D, *et al*.: Detection of deep-vein thrombosis by real-time B-mode ultrasonography. *N Engl J Med* 1989, 320:342–345.

15. White RH, McGahan JP, Daschbach MM, *et al*.: Diagnosis of deep-vein thrombosis using duplex ultrasound. *Ann Intern Med* 1989, 111:297–304.

16. Alanen A, Kormano M: Correlation of the echogenicity and structure of clotted blood. *J Ultrasound Med* 1985, 4:421–425.

17. Grassi CJ, Polak JF: Axillary and subclavian venous thrombosis: follow-up evaluation with color Doppler flow US and venography. *Radiology* 1990, 175:651–654.

18. Haire WD, Lynch TG, Lieberman RP, *et al*.: Utility of duplex ultrasound in the diagnosis of asymptomatic catheter-induced subclavian vein thrombosis. *J Ultrasound Med* 1991, 10:493–496.

19. Burbridge SJ, Finlay DE, Letourneau JG, *et al*.: Effects of central venous catheter placement on upper extremity duplex US findings. *J Vasc Interv Radiol* 1993, 4:399–404.

TREATMENT OF VENOUS THROMBOSIS

12

CHAPTER

Samuel Z. Goldhaber

Venous thrombi differ markedly in anatomic location, burden, and clinical implication. Therefore, the severity and hazard of venous thrombi vary greatly among individual patients. Accordingly, treatment regimens must be tailored to the type of venous thrombus that is identified as well as to the patient's need for (or contraindications to) aggressive therapy.

The classic approach of providing about 1 week of continuous infusion of unfractionated heparin followed by 3 months of oral warfarin is appropriate only in a subset of patients. Our contemporary therapeutic armamentarium encompasses two extremes: from no treatment and serial noninvasive monitoring to thrombolytic therapy or placement of a filter into the inferior vena cava. Furthermore, the ideal duration of treatment of patients with venous thrombosis is uncertain, especially because the rate of recurrent thrombosis after completion of anticoagulation therapy has recently been shown to be surprisingly high.

Although unfractionated heparin has been the cornerstone of treatment of venous thrombosis, the availability of low molecular weight heparins will make outpatient treatment or abbreviated inpatient treatment feasible in some patients with venous thrombosis. Treatment with low molecular weight heparins will probably receive Food and Drug Administration (FDA) approval because of the prolonged half-life and excellent bioavailability of these agents, which make them suitable for once- or at most twice-daily subcutaneous administration. The lower mortality rate, particularly among cancer patients, associated with low molecular weight heparins compared with unfractionated heparins is particularly deserving of clinical attention.

Innovations in bolus thrombolysis regimens hold promise for streamlining administration of this potent type of therapy as well as for maximizing efficacy and safety. Certain characteristics of the thrombus at baseline can help predict whether thrombolytic agents administered through a peripheral vein will succeed (more likely with nonobstructive thrombi) or whether local administration through a catheter will be necessary (more likely with totally occlusive thrombi). Finally, a new generation of smaller, technically improved vena cava filters has been developed. These new filters are easier to insert percutaneously, and the ferromagnetism of some is so low that high-quality magnetic resonance imaging can be obtained.

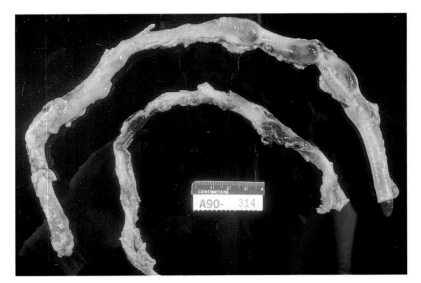

FIGURE 12-1. One of the rationales for treating deep venous thrombosis is to prevent propagation of thrombi, which might eventually embolize and cause death from pulmonary embolism. In this figure, an autopsy specimen is shown from a woman who died from adenocarcinoma and massive bilateral deep venous thrombosis associated with recurrent embolization to the lungs; however, the extensive venous thrombosis demonstrated in this illustration is uncommon. In most cases, the rationale for treatment is to alleviate the pain and discomfort from the phlebitis. For patients with thrombosis of the upper extremities, aggressive therapy may preserve an indwelling central venous catheter that may become obstructed by a clot and subsequently cease to function.

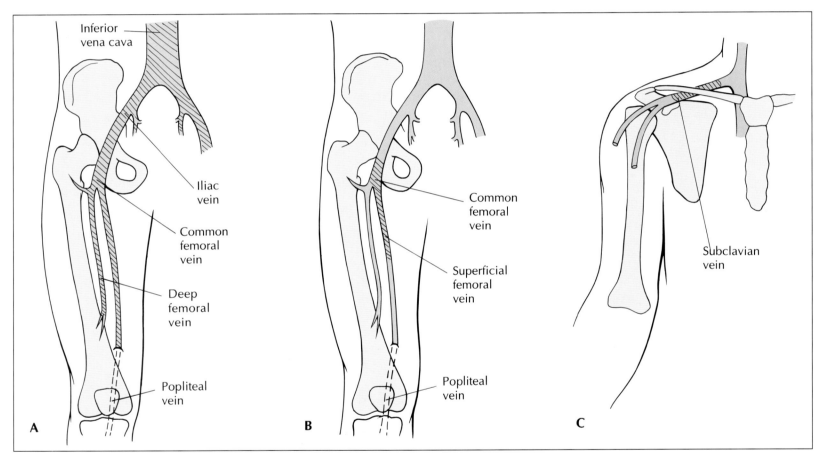

FIGURE 12-2. Syndromes of venous thrombosis. **A,** Massive venous thrombosis. Patients with massive venous thrombosis commonly have involvement of the inferior vena cava as well as the pelvic and deep leg veins. The clot may occur bilaterally. These patients may suffer pain and leg swelling. They are at high risk of clinically important pulmonary embolism. Extension of thrombosis may continue despite administration of therapeutic levels of heparin. Thrombolytic therapy is warranted to debulk the thrombus medically.

B, Moderate-size venous thrombosis. This is the most common syndrome of venous thrombosis. There usually is no involvement of pelvic veins and, of the three major proximal deep leg veins (*ie*, common femoral, superficial femoral [which is a deep vein despite being named *superficial*], and popliteal), thrombus is unilaterally present in only one or two of these types of veins. Patients with moderate-size venous thrombosis are treated with anticoagulants alone. Recent studies have shown that injections of low molecular weight heparin once or twice daily are effective, safe, and practical. About one fourth of patients may be eligible for either outpatient treatment of the thrombosis or for a short inpatient hospitalization, followed by self-injection at home.

C, Upper-extremity vein thrombosis. The most common causes are an indwelling central venous catheter, effort thrombosis in an otherwise healthy, athletic person, or thrombus caused by intravenous drug use. Patients with thrombosis of the upper extremities are often good candidates for thrombolytic therapy. **D,** Isolated calf vein thrombosis. Whether patients with thrombosis of isolated calf veins should be anticoagulated or followed up with serial imaging examinations is persistently debated, although the trend is to anticoagulate them. (*continued*)

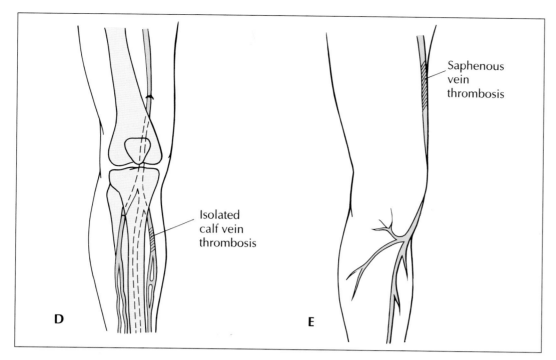

FIGURE 12-2. (*continued*) Without treatment, about one fourth of the thrombi will propagate in a proximal direction and may cause extensive deep vein thrombosis in the leg or even pulmonary embolism [1]. In patients with paradoxic embolism, occult isolated calf vein thrombosis is often present [2].

E, Superficial, or saphenous, vein thrombosis. This condition is often manifested by palpable cords and erythema. The risk of propagation to the deep venous system is low. Most patients respond to bedrest, leg elevation, hot packs, and nonsteroidal anti-inflammatory agents. Patients who are refractory to local treatment benefit from anticoagulation therapy, which also prevents extensive superficial vein thrombosis from propagating to the deep venous system. Occasionally, concomitant cellulitis necessitates antibiotic therapy.

ANTICOAGULATION

RECURRENCE FOLLOWING ORAL ANTICOAGULATION VS ORAL ANTICOAGULATION + HEPARIN

	SYMPTOMATIC RECURRENCE, %	ANY RECURRENCE, %
Oral anticoagulation only	20	40
Oral anticoagulation + heparin	7	8

FIGURE 12-3. The question often arises whether it is necessary to administer heparin concomitantly with initiation of oral anticoagulants to patients who are newly diagnosed with acute venous thrombosis. In this era of cost containment, it might be tempting to write a prescription for oral anticoagulation when patients are diagnosed with venous thrombosis. If no parenteral therapy were needed, most patients could be treated at home. A group of Dutch investigators randomly assigned venous thrombosis patients into two groups. One group was given oral anticoagulants alone, and the other was given heparin plus oral anticoagulants. The recurrence rate of symptoms was 20% in patients given oral anticoagulants alone versus 7% in those given heparin plus oral anticoagulants. Asymptomatic extension of venous thrombosis occurred in 40% of the patients who received oral anticoagulants alone versus 8% who received heparin plus oral anticoagulants [3]. Thus, it is clear that patients with acute venous thrombosis must receive heparin as well as oral anticoagulants.

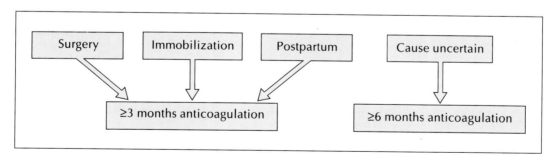

FIGURE 12-4. One of the most challenging aspects of treating venous thrombosis is to determine the optimum time to discontinue anticoagulation therapy. It is clear that not all patients with venous thrombi require the same length of treatment. Patients with venous thrombosis as a result of surgery, immobilization, or the postpartum state may do very well with as little as 3 months of anticoagulation; however, the length of treatment for patients with idiopathic venous thrombosis is not as well defined but should be continued for 6 months or more. When 145 patients with idiopathic venous thrombosis were treated with anticoagulants for 3 months and followed up for the next 1.5 years, 24% suffered recurrent venous thrombosis [4].

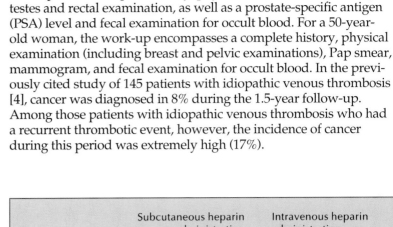

VENOUS THROMBOSIS AND OCCULT CANCER

WORK-UP

MEN

Complete history

Testicular exam

Rectal exam/test of stool for
occult blood

PSA test

WOMEN

Complete history

Pelvic exam/Pap smear

Breast exam/mammogram

Test of stool for occult blood

FIGURE 12-5. Relationship between venous thrombosis and occult cancer. All patients with recently diagnosed venous thrombosis should have, at a minimum, the work-up for cancer patients advised by the American Cancer Society. For a 50-year-old man, this work-up encompasses a complete history, physical examination including testes and rectal examination, as well as a prostate-specific antigen (PSA) level and fecal examination for occult blood. For a 50-year-old woman, the work-up encompasses a complete history, physical examination (including breast and pelvic examinations), Pap smear, mammogram, and fecal examination for occult blood. In the previously cited study of 145 patients with idiopathic venous thrombosis [4], cancer was diagnosed in 8% during the 1.5-year follow-up. Among those patients with idiopathic venous thrombosis who had a recurrent thrombotic event, however, the incidence of cancer during this period was extremely high (17%).

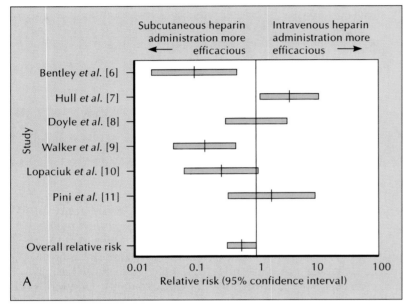

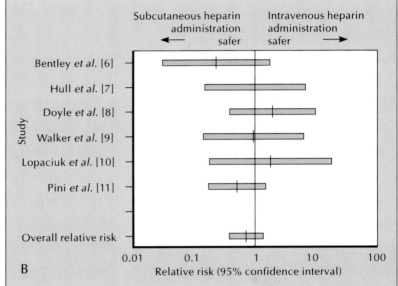

FIGURE 12-6. The administration of high-dose subcutaneous unfractionated heparin adjusted to a mid-interval partial thromboplastin time of 1.5 to 2.5 times the upper limit of normal would greatly simplify the treatment of patients with venous thrombus. With subcutaneous administration of heparin, no intravenous tubing or catheters would be necessary. Furthermore, there would be no need for automated infusion pumps to regulate continuous intravenous heparin administration. To determine whether such therapy would be worthwhile, Hommes *et al.* [5] undertook a meta-analysis of six studies that provided comparable efficacy (**A**) and safety (**B**) data. The results indicate that high-dose subcuta-neous unfractionated heparin compares favorably with continuous intravenous heparin. Efficacy meta-analysis (*A*) shows that overall efficacy of high-dose subcutaneous heparin was greater than that of intravenous heparin for prevention of the extension and recurrence of venous thrombosis. There were 38% fewer recurrences (95% confidence interval, 2% to 61%). Safety meta-analysis (*B*) shows that the occurrence of major hemorrhage associated with subcutaneous administration of high-dose heparin was the same as that of continuous intravenous administration. (*Adapted from* Hommes and coworkers [5]; with permission.)

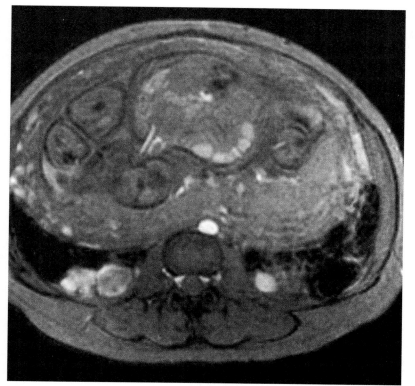

FIGURE 12-7. Ovarian vein thrombosis. A 23-year-old woman who was 35 weeks pregnant was transferred to Brigham and Women's Hospital with a chief complaint of severe right groin pain for 2 days. She had mild palpation tenderness in the right lower quadrant, just above her right groin. Ultrasonography of the leg, chest roentgenogram, and ventilation-perfusion lung scan were normal. However, magnetic resonance imaging demonstrated a dilated and thrombosed right ovarian vein. The patient was treated with continuous intravenous heparin for 1 week and was then discharged home on high-dose subcutaneous heparin every 8 hours, which she continued for the remainder of the pregnancy. Blood was obtained 4 hours after each injection so that the subcutaneous heparin dose could be adjusted to maintain a partial thromboplastin time of two to three times the control value. After delivery, heparin was overlapped with Coumadin (DuPont Pharmaceuticals, Wilmington, DE) until the patient achieved a stable and therapeutic level of Coumadin, based on an International Normalized Ratio of 2.0 to 3.0. The differential diagnosis of ovarian vein thrombosisis broad and is most often confused with acute appendicitis. The majority of cases are recognized postpartum. Although ovarian vein thrombosis was previously diagnosed clinically, contemporary imaging tests such as computed tomography and magnetic resonance imaging now are considered essential. When ovarian vein thrombosis is recognized, it can almost always be treated successfully [12]. (Courtesy of Ramin Khorsani, MD, Brigham and Women's Hospital, Boston, MA.)

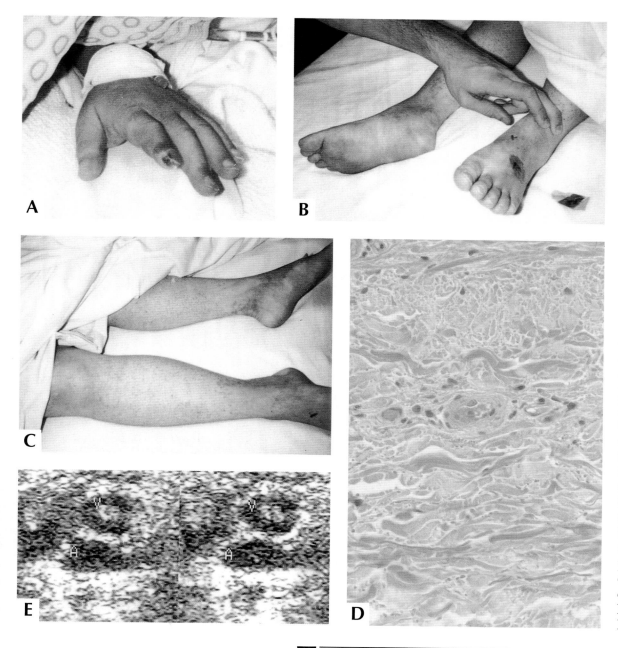

A

B

C

E

D

FIGURE 12-8. Disseminated intravascular coagulation with manifestations of proximal deep leg vein thrombosis. A 31-year-old woman with systemic lupus erythematosus presented with a chief complaint of a painful left index finger, which became necrotic despite antibiotic therapy (**A**). Her feet became mottled and ulcerated (**B**), and petechiae developed on her legs (**C**). Skin biopsy showed a microvessel in the reticular dermis that was occluded by pink amorphous material characteristic of fibrin thrombi (**D**). In addition to the patient's dermatologic abnormalities, physical examination revealed left medial thigh tenderness. Venous ultrasound of the legs demonstrated that the left common femoral vein was not compressible because of a partially obstructing thrombus (*labelled* V) (**E**). After being treated with continuous intravenous heparin and Coumadin (DuPont Pharmaceuticals, Wilmington, DE) therapy, the patient gradually recovered. This case indicates that venous thrombosis can be a manifestation of a systemic disease process. The association between disseminated intravascular coagulation and systemic lupus erythematosus has been described previously [13]. The cutaneous features of the antiphospholipid syndrome have also been extensively reviewed [14]. (Part D courtesy of Raymond L. Barnhill, MD, Brigham and Women's Hospital, Boston, MA.)

DIFFERENCES BETWEEN LMWH AND UNFRACTIONATED HEPARIN

VARIABLE	LMWH	UNFRACTIONATED HEPARIN
Molecular weight average	4000–6000 D	12,000–15,000 D
Bioavailability	Good at low doses due to minimal binding to plasma proteins	Unpredictable at low doses due to marked binding to plasma proteins
Frequency of administration	Can administer once or twice daily	Usually administer three times daily if given subcutaneously
Ratio of factor Xa to factor IIa inhibition	At least 2:1	1:1
Platelet effects	Minimal (resistant to inactivation by platelet factor 4)	May be proaggregatory (susceptible to platelet factor 4)

FIGURE 12-9. Differences between low molecular weight heparins (LMWHs) and unfractionated heparin. LMWHs are fragments of unfractionated heparin produced by either chemical or enzymatic depolymerization [15]. They have a mean molecular weight of about 4000 to 6000 D, whereas the average molecular weight of unfractionated heparin is 12,000 to 15,000 D. LMWHs have good bioavailability at low doses and have a longer half-life than unfractionated heparin because they are less avidly bound to plasma proteins. The clearance of LMWHs is predictable and not dose-dependent. LMWHs preferentially inhibit factor Xa more than factor IIa (thrombin), which could lead to an increased antithrombotic effect. As molecular weight decreases, LMWHs become progressively less likely to aggregate with platelets. For an equivalent antithrombotic activity, LMWHs appear to be associated with less bleeding than unfractionated heparin. Consequently, the efficacy, safety, and bioavailability of these agents will probably make them an attractive therapeutic option for management of patients with venous thrombosis in North America. Use of LMWHs in the treatment of venous thrombosis is increasing, especially in Europe. The possibility of once- or twice-daily subcutaneous injections leaves open the potential for treatment of low-risk individuals on an outpatient basis.

CANCER MORTALITY RESULTS OF SUBCUTANEOUS LMWH VS CONTINUOUS INTRAVENOUS INFUSION OF UNFRACTIONATED HEPARIN

STUDY, DURATION OF FOLLOW-UP	LMWH REGIMEN	LMWH CANCER DEATHS AND TOTAL NUMBER OF LMWH CANCER PATIENTS, n/n	UNFRACTIONATED HEPARIN CANCER DEATHS AND TOTAL NUMBER OF UNFRACTIONATED HEPARIN CANCER PATIENTS, n/n
Prandoni et al. [17], 6 mo	Fraxiparine (weight-adjusted)	1 (uterine)/15	8 (3 lung, 2 renal, 1 bladder, 1 gallbladder, 1 breast)/18
Hull et al. [18], 3 mo	Logiparin (175 U once daily)	7 (not specified; 2 abrupt, 5 insidious)/46	14 (not specified; 8 abrupt, 6 insidious)/49
Simonneau et al. [19], 3 mo	Enoxaparin (1 mg/kg twice daily)	2 (not specified)/7	1 (not specified)/2

FIGURE 12-10. The effect of low-molecular weight heparins (LMWHs) on mortality. An overview of randomized controlled trials indicates that patients who received LMWH for treatment of deep venous thrombosis had approximately a 50% lower mortality rate than patients who received unfractionated heparin (4% vs 8%, respectively). The mortality reduction could be attributed mostly to a decreased death rate in cancer patients, especially to fewer abrupt deaths in patients with adenocarcinoma (Lensing and coworkers, Personal communication). It is intriguing that, among subjects with cancer, there was a risk reduction of 68% (95% confidence interval, 28% to 86%; $P<0.006$). The decreased mortality associated with LMWH is not well understood. Perhaps occult pulmonary embolism precipitated the deaths in cancer patients and simply occurred less often among those who received LMWH. Alternatively, heparins may have antineoplastic effects, and LMWHs may enter tumor cells and inhibit tumor growth more readily than unfractionated heparins do. Heparin, with its low-molecular-weight fractions, inhibits thymidine uptake, endothelial cell growth, and the intimal thickening that follows endothelial injury. Heparin or heparin fragments have inhibited angiogenesis and have caused tumor regression in mice [20].

EFFICACY AND SAFETY OF SUBCUTANEOUS LMWH VS CONTINUOUS INTRAVENOUS INFUSION OF UNFRACTIONATED HEPARIN

STUDY	LMWH REGIMEN	EFFICACY	SAFETY
Bratt et al. [16]	Fragmin (120 U/kg twice daily)	Same	Same
Prandoni et al. [17]	Fraxiparine (weight-adjusted)	Same	Same
Hull et al. [18]	Logiparin (175 U once daily)	Trend toward fewer recurrences with LMWH	Trend toward less major bleeding with LMWH
Simonneau et al. [19]	Enoxaparin (1 mg/kg twice daily)	Fewer recurrences with LMWH	Same

FIGURE 12-11. Low molecular weight heparin (LMWH) versus unfractionated heparin in the treatment of venous thrombosis. In these four large, randomized, controlled trials, LMWH was at least as efficacious and safe as a continuous intravenous infusion of unfractionated heparin.

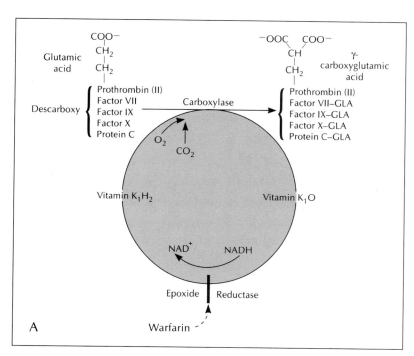

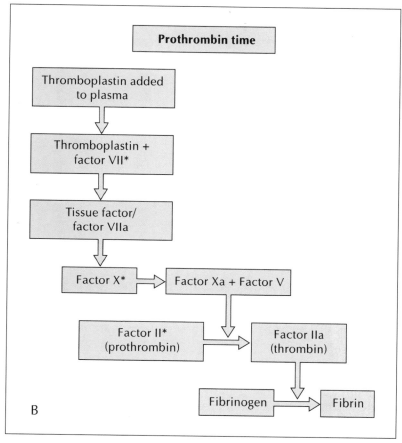

FIGURE 12-12. Management of oral anticoagulation. The only available form of warfarin in the United States is Coumadin (DuPont Pharmaceuticals, Wilmington, DE). The excellent bioavailability and consistency of this drug from lot to lot have not been matched by generic formulations, which have been voluntarily withdrawn by their manufacturers.

A, Mechanism of action of warfarin. Warfarin inhibits an important step in vitamin K metabolism, decreasing vitamin K_1H_2-dependent carboxylation of factors II, VII, IX, and X, and protein C. The gamma-carboxyglutamic acid (GLA) residues on the vitamin K–dependent factors are essential for participation of these factors in coagulation reactions.

B, Activation of coagulation produced by adding thromboplastin to plasma for the prothrombin time assay. *Asterisks* indicate factors that are vitamin K–dependent.

C, Formula for calculation of the International Normalized Ratio (INR). Although we used to monitor warfarin dosing based on prothrombin time (PT) expressed in seconds or in terms of the prothrombin time ratio (patient's prothrombin time divided by the laboratory control prothrombin time), the new standard of care requires that prothrombin time be expressed in terms of the INR. The reason is that, even within the United States and Canada, prothrombin time assays are carried out with thromboplastins that have markedly different sensitivities [21].

The INR is the prothrombin time ratio that would be obtained if the World Health Organization reference thromboplastin were always used to perform the prothrombin time test [22]. Most available thromboplastins are supplied with a calibration factor known as the International Sensitivity Index (ISI). By using the ISI, laboratories can express prothrombin time results in terms of the INR. For example, within North America, a prothrombin time of 18 seconds and a prothrombin time ratio of 1.5 at one laboratory may be equivalent to a prothrombin time of 22 seconds and a prothrombin time ratio of 1.8 at another laboratory. (*continued*)

$$INR= \left(\frac{PT \ patient}{PT \ normal}\right)^{ISI}$$

C

Figure 12-12. (*continued*) The same blood specimen in a European laboratory might yield a prothrombin time of 30 seconds and a prothrombin time ratio of 2.5. Nevertheless, the INR for this blood sample would be 3.0 at all laboratories, despite the three markedly different prothrombin times and ratios given in this example [23]. The target INR for oral anticoagulation of patients with venous thrombosis should be 2.0 to 3.0. The overlap of intravenous heparin and oral anticoagulants should generally be maintained for at least 5 days, even if the target INR is achieved more quickly. (Part A *adapted from* Stead [20a]; part B *adapted from* Hirsh [22]; with permission.)

THROMBOLYSIS

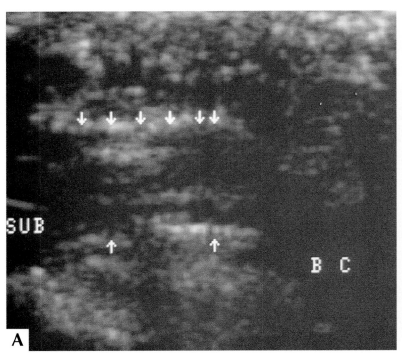

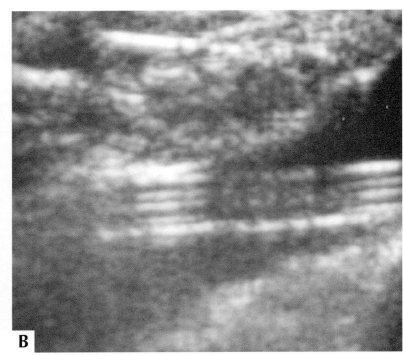

A **B**

Figure 12-13. Thrombolysis of venous thrombosis with an FDA–approved regimen. Streptokinase is the only thrombolytic agent approved by the FDA for the treatment of venous thrombosis. The dose is a bolus of 250,000 U given over approximately 20 minutes followed by a continuous infusion of 100,000 U/h for 24 to 72 hours. Thrombolytic therapy for venous thrombosis is recommended *without* concomitant heparin, although I have recently begun administering heparin simultaneously to help prevent the development of a new thrombus. The fibrinogen level should be checked periodically during prolonged infusion of streptokinase because resistance to this agent occurs frequently. If the fibrinogen level remains within the normal range, the dose of streptokinase should be doubled. Patients receiving prolonged infusions of streptokinase often develop fever, chills, and flushing during therapy. These side effects may be averted by premedication with high-dose acetaminophen (*eg*, 1500 mg orally), which may be repeated if symptoms or signs of a reaction to streptokinase begin to develop during treatment. If high-dose acetaminophen is not effective, then diphenhydramine (25 to 50 mg intravenously) and hydrocortisone (100 mg intravenously) may be administered.

A, Indwelling subclavian catheter surrounded by and occluded by a thrombus. **B,** The subclavian catheter is visible after a prolonged infusion of streptokinase successfully lysed the occluded catheter.

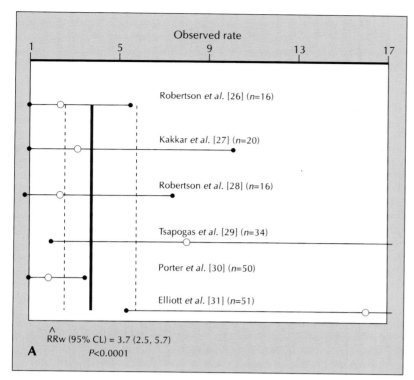

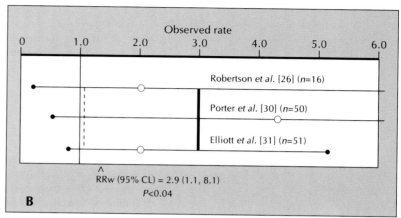

FIGURE 12-14. Pooled analysis of streptokinase (SK) efficacy and safety. About one in five patients with venous thrombosis of the legs may be eligible for thrombolytic therapy [24]. The major contraindications are recent trauma or surgery, recent gastrointestinal bleeding, or history of a serious bleeding disorder. In randomized trials comparing SK followed by heparin versus heparin alone, SK was more efficacious in lysing the clot, as evidenced by venography [25]. Major bleeding complications were, however, more common among patients treated with SK than among those who received heparin alone. **A,** Overview of six randomized trials of SK versus heparin for acute deep venous thrombosis indicates that the lysis rate is 3.7 times greater (*heavy vertical line*) for SK than for heparin. An observed rate greater than 1 indicates a beneficial effect of SK for clot lysis. The pooled risk ratio is statistically significant (P<0.001), with a 95% confidence limit (*dashed vertical lines*) of 2.5 to 5.7. In each

of the six trials, SK achieved superior lysis (*open circles*) than heparin alone. The lower 95% confidence limit (*closed circles, left side of each solid horizontal line*) was greater than 1, however, thereby indicating statistical significance in only two of six trials.

B, Overview of three trials of SK versus heparin (three of the trials discussed in *panel A* provided inadequate information on bleeding complications) for acute deep venous thrombosis. An overall 2.9-fold increase in the major bleeding rate (*heavy vertical line*) for SK compared with heparin is demonstrated. An observed rate greater than 1 indicates more major bleeding complications associated with SK than with heparin. The pooled observed rate is statistically significant (P<0.04), but the 95% confidence limit is wide, reflecting the small sample size among the trials. RRW—weighted (or adjusted) relative risk. (*Adapted from* Brown and Goldhaber [24]; with permission.)

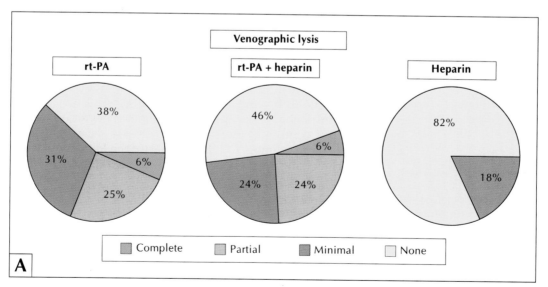

FIGURE 12-15. Recombinant tissue-type plasminogen activator (rt-PA) is the treatment of proximal venous thrombosis of the leg. In an attempt to improve the efficacy and safety of thrombolysis for deep venous thrombosis of the leg, we organized a randomized, controlled trial of rt-PA, rt-PA plus heparin, and heparin alone [32]. The patients assigned to rt-PA received a prolonged infusion of a low concentration: 0.05 mg/kg/h for 24 hours via a peripheral vein, with a maxi-

mum dose of 150 mg. Follow-up venography was performed 24 to 36 hours after initiation of therapy. **A,** Results of rt-PA versus heparin. Complete lysis or lysis of more than 50% occurred in 28% of patients treated with rt-PA and 29% of patients treated with rt-PA plus heparin; no lysis occurred in patients treated with heparin alone. There was one major bleeding complication—a nonfatal intracranial hemorrhage in a patient who received rt-PA alone. (*continued*)

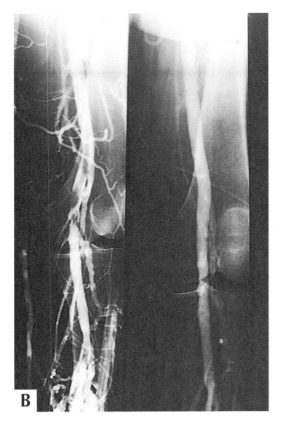

Figure 12-15. (*continued*) **B,** This 31-year-old woman with popliteal vein thrombosis was treated with rt-PA. Venogram (*left panel*) demonstrates nonobstructive popliteal vein thrombosis. Complete clot lysis is observed on venography after a 24-hour rt-PA infusion (*right panel*).

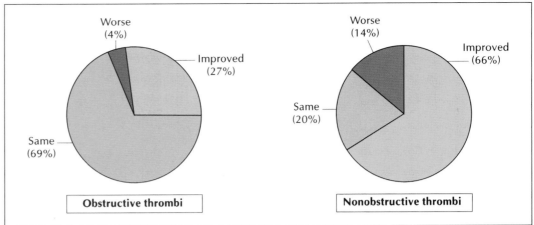

Figure 12-16. Nonobstructive thrombi are more likely to be lysed successfully than are totally obstructive thrombi. The venographic appearance of leg thrombuses may help to predict whether peripherally administered thrombolytic agents can successfully dissolve the clot [33]. In the study of deep venous thrombosis discussed in Fig. 12-15, the response to recombinant tissue-type plasminogen activator (rt-PA) plus heparin or rt-PA alone was significantly greater among venous segments showing nonobstructive thrombi than in those showing obstructive thrombi. Nonobstructive venous thrombi may respond more often to thrombolytic therapy simply because the lytic agent has more contact with the clot than in cases of totally obstructive thrombi. Therefore, catheter-directed thrombolytic therapy, with administration of the agent directly into the clot, should be considered for patients with completely obstructed venous segments.

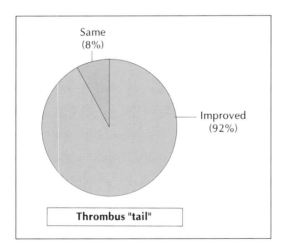

Figure 12-17. Free-floating venous thrombi. Although clots with "tails" look threatening, most free-floating thrombi do not embolize but instead become attached to the vein wall or resolve, as evidenced by noninvasive duplex scanning [34]. We have found that patients who have thrombi with tails respond especially well to peripherally administered thrombolytic agents, with no clinical evidence of clot embolization.

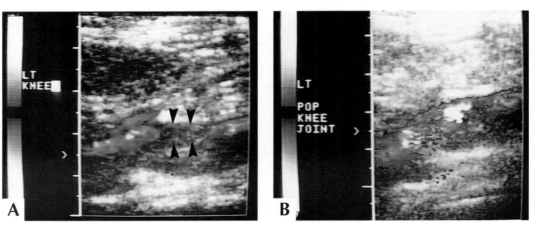

Figure 12-18. Bolus thrombolysis. The bleeding problems observed with streptokinase for venous thrombolysis may be ascribed, at least in part, to administration of the drug as a prolonged, continuous infusion rather than to the agent itself. Shorter periods of thrombolytic drug administration may reduce the frequency of bleeding complications while still conferring efficacy. Therefore, we tested the efficacy and safety of bolus thrombolysis among 27 cases of deep venous thrombosis [35]. During a 24-h period, patients received three doses of urokinase administered as 1 million-unit boluses over 10 minutes via a peripheral vein; patients also received heparin overnight between boluses. This regimen of boluses urokinase resulted in clot lysis in about one half of the cases.

A, A 37-year-old man was diagnosed with left popliteal deep venous thrombosis 19 days after surgery for left leg vein stripping. Baseline compression ultrasonography with color Doppler imaging demonstrates subtotal obstruction (*arrowheads*). On the day after this ultrasound examination, the patient began a course of bolus urokinase treatments.

B, Five days after initiation of urokinase, follow-up ultrasonography showed marked improvement, according to physicians on the vascular imaging panel, who were unaware of the sequence of the studies. The clinical treatment course for all patients studied was remarkable, however, because of no bleeding complications occurred. As a result, the safety record of the bolus regimen that we used appears superior to that of prolonged thrombolysis regimens reported in previous trials. (*continued*)

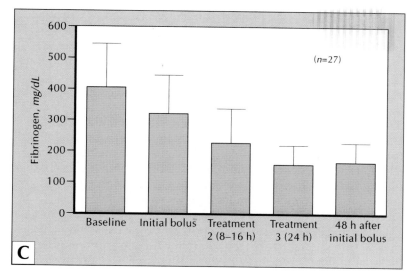

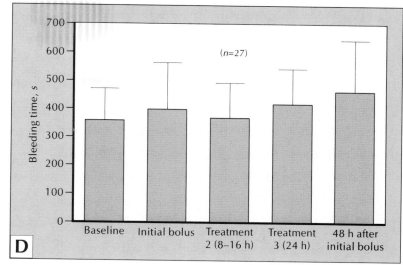

FIGURE 12-18. (*continued*) After therapy, the decrease in fibrinogen levels was more profound than the rise in bleeding times.

C, Baseline plasma fibrinogen (FBN) levels averaged 411±131 mg/dL. The levels were also assayed 2 hours after each administration of bolus thrombolysis and decreased after each additional bolus of urokinase. Two days after initiation of urokinase, the plasma fibrinogen levels were persistently low compared with baseline, averaging 161±67 mg/dL (*P*<0.0001).

D, Baseline bleeding time (BT) averaged 359±104 seconds. Additional bleeding times were obtained 10 to 60 minutes after administration of bolus thrombolysis. By 2 days after initiation of urokinase, BT increased to 458±-164 seconds (*P*=0.01), which is within the normal range (up to 570 seconds) and is only of borderline statistical significance after accounting for multiple comparisons. The sustained fibrinolytic state probably accounted for the clot lysis. The small rise in bleeding times, which did not exceed the normal range after thrombolytic therapy, suggests that qualitative platelet function remained intact. Therefore, normal platelet function may have contributed to the absence of bleeding, despite prolonged fibrinogenolysis.

MECHANICAL INTERVENTION

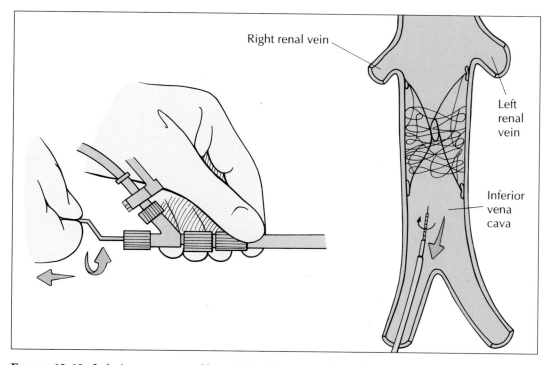

FIGURE 12-19. Inferior vena cava filters. Most filters are placed percutaneously via the right femoral vein. The three major indications are: 1) active major hemorrhage (*eg*, gastrointestinal or intracranial), 2) recurrent venous thrombosis despite adequate anticoagulation

therapy, and 3) prophylaxis against pulmonary embolism among patients at extremely high risk for embolism, especially when embolism might be fatal because of underlying cardiopulmonary disease. Long-term anticoagulation, if not contraindicated, should be used in conjunction with filters [36].

Our current preference is percutaneous placement of a Bird's Nest filter (Cook Incorporated, Bloomington, IN), which has low rate of failure, thrombogenicity, and occlusion. Its small sheath size may help minimize the risk of bleeding during and after the procedure. To insert the Bird's Nest filter, the right-angled handle of the wire guide pusher is rotated counterclockwise for 10 to 15 turns to disengage it from the filter. Then the wire guide pusher is removed first, followed by the empty filter catheter. The introducing sheath is left in place so that a post-procedure venacavogram can be obtained. Retrievable filters intended for temporary placement are widely available in Europe but have not received approval by the FDA.

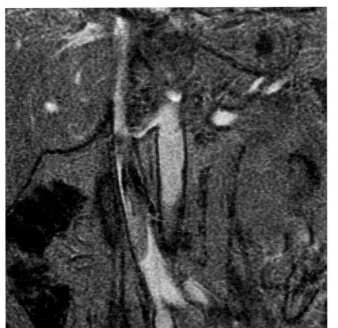

FIGURE 12-20. Lifesaving effect of a properly functioning titanium Greenfield filter. An 82-year-old man was admitted with a chief complaint of pain behind his right knee for 2 days. Three months previously, he had left leg proximal venous thrombosis that was managed with placement of a titanium Greenfield inferior vena caval filter (because of a subarachnoid hemorrhage 4 months earlier that precluded anticoagulation). Ultrasound examination of the legs showed a new right-leg deep vein thrombosis. To check the integrity of the vena caval filter, magnetic resonance imaging was obtained. With the GRASS (Gradient Recalled Acquisition at Steady State) images, flowing blood is bright and thrombus appears dark. A coronal magnetic resonance image showed that the filter was properly in place. An oblong thrombus could be visualized just inferior to it. The extensive thrombus, if not trapped by the filter, would probably have resulted in a fatal pulmonary embolism in this patient who had not received anticoagulation therapy because of prior subarachnoid hemorrhage. This case underscores that vena caval filters can prevent massive pulmonary embolism, but that they do not alter an underlying hypercoagulable state. (Courtesy of Ramin Khorsani, MD, Brigham and Women's Hospital, Boston, MA.)

TREATMENT PROTOCOLS

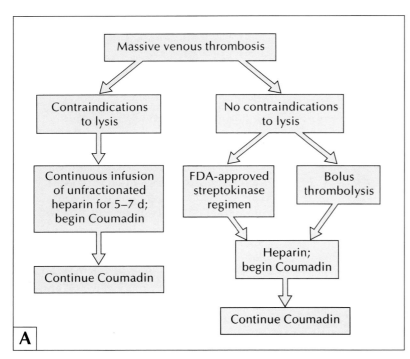

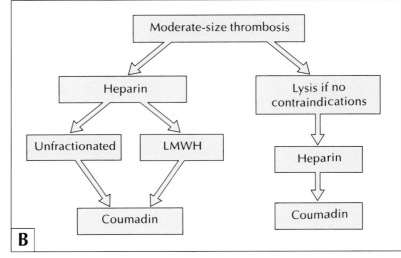

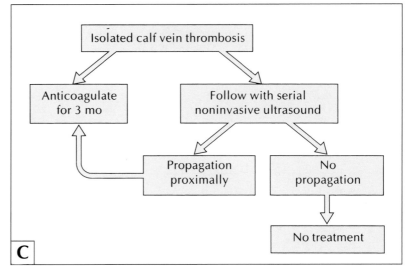

FIGURE 12-21. Protocols for treating different types of venous thrombosis. **A,** Massive venous thrombosis. Thrombolytic therapy is often warranted to debulk the thrombus medically and possibly to prevent chronic venous insufficiency. If the patient has underlying cardiopulmonary disease and a limited life expectancy, placement of a filter in the inferior vena cava should be considered. **B,** Moderate-size venous thrombosis. Whether such patients should undergo thrombolytic therapy, even if there are no contraindications, is currently undetermined. Theoretically, more complete clot dissolution would help minimize damage to venous valves and would thus decrease the likelihood of development of chronic venous insufficiency. **C,** Isolated calf vein thrombosis. Anticoagulation (*continued*)

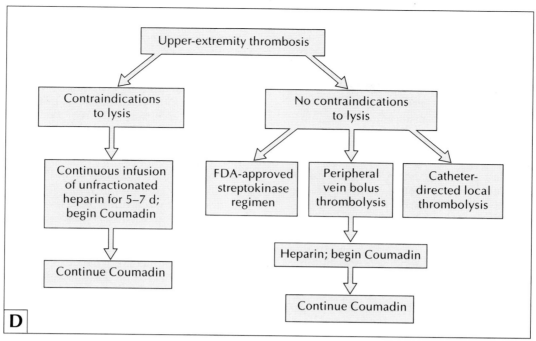

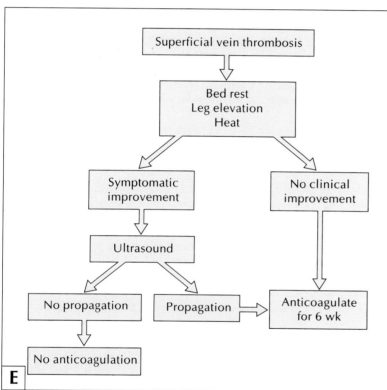

FIGURE 12-21. (*continued*) therapy is often indicated for patients with this type of thrombosis. However, if the physician chooses to follow such patients without anticoagulation therapy, it is important that they undergo several serial noninvasive tests within the ensuing 7 to 14 days to monitor potential propagation of thrombus to the proximal leg veins.

D, Upper-extremity (UE) vein thrombosis. Such patients are often good candidates for thrombolytic therapy, which may restore patency of a thrombosed, indwelling central venous catheter.

E, Superficial vein thrombosis. Most patients improve with bedrest, leg elevation, and heat to the affected veins. Nonsteroidal anti-inflammatory drugs (NSAIDs) may provide symptomatic relief. Ultrasonography of the legs usually will show no propagation to the deep venous system. Occasionally, however, patients do not improve merely with local treatment to the leg or demonstrate propagation of the thrombus. Such patients should receive anticoagulation therapy. LMWH—low molecular weight heparin.

REFERENCES

1. Lagerstedt CI, Olsson C-G, Fagher BO, *et al.*: Need for long-term anticoagulant treatment in symptomatic calf-vein thrombosis. *Lancet* 1985, 2:515–518.

2. Stöllberger C, Slany J, Schuster I, *et al.*: The prevalence of deep venous thrombosis in patients with suspected paradoxical embolism. *Ann Intern Med* 1993, 119:461–465.

3. Brandjes DPM, Heijboer H, Büller HR, *et al.*: Acenocoumarol and heparin compared with acenocoumarol alone in the initial treatment of proximal-vein thrombosis. *N Engl J Med* 1992, 327:1485–1489.

4. Prandoni P, Lensing AWA, Büller HR, *et al.*: Deep-vein thrombosis and the incidence of subsequent symptomatic cancer. *N Engl J Med* 1992, 327:1128–1133.

5. Hommes DW, Bura A, Mazzolai L, *et al.*: Subcutaneous heparin compared with continuous intravenous heparin administration in the initial treatment of deep vein thrombosis: a meta-analysis. *Ann Intern Med* 1992, 116:279–284.

6. Bentley PG, Kakkar VV, Scully MF, *et al.*: An objective study of alternative methods of heparin administration. *Thromb Res* 1980, 18:177–187.

7. Hall RD, Raskob GE, Hirsh J, *et al.*: Continuous intravenous heparin compared with intermittent subcutaneous heparin in the intimal treatment of proximal-vein thrombosis. *N Engl J Med* 1986, 315:1109–1114.

8. Doyle DJ, Turpie AG, Hirsh J, *et al.*: Adjusted subcutaneous heparin or continuous intravenous heparin in patients with acute deep vein thrombosis. *Ann Intern Med* 1987, 107:441–445.

9. Walker MG, Shaw JW, Thomson GJ, *et al.*: Subcutaneous calcium heparin versus intravenous sodium heparin in treatment of established acute deep vein thrombosis of the legs: a multicentre prospective randomised trial. *Br Med J [Clin Res]*, 1987, 294:1189–1192.

10. Lopaciuk S, Meissner AJ, Ciesielski L, Korzycki J: Subcutaneous sodium heparin versus intravenous sodium heparin in the treatment of deep vein thrombosis. Proceedings of the 6th International Meeting of the Danubian League Against Thrombosis and Haemorrhagic Disorders. Vienna, Austria, May 31 to June 3, 1989:389–393.

11. Pini M, Pattacini C, Quintavalla R, *et al.*: Subcutaneous vs intravenous heparin in the treatment of deep venous thrombosis. A randomized clinical trial. *Thromb Haemost* 1990, 64:222–226.

12. Simons GR, Piwnica-Worms DR, Goldhaber SZ: Ovarian vein thrombosis. *Am Heart J* 1993, 126:641–647.

13. Shimamoto Y, Ohta A, Sano M, *et al.*: Improved or fatal acute disseminated intravascular coagulation in systemic lupus erythematosus. *Am J Hematol* 1993, 42:191–195.

14. Stephens CJM: The antiphospholipid syndrome. Clinical correlations, cutaneous features, mechanism of thrombosis and treatment of patients with the lupus anticoagulant and anticardiolipin antibodies. *Br J Dermatol* 1991, 125:199–210.

15. Hirsh J, Levine MN: Low molecular weight heparin. *Blood* 1992, 79:1–17.

16. Bratt G, Åberg W, Johansson M, *et al.*: Two daily subcutaneous injections of Fragmin as compared with intravenous standard heparin in the treatment of deep venous thrombosis (DVT). *Thromb Haemost* 1990, 64:506–510.

17. Prandoni P, Lensing AWA, Büller HR, *et al.*: Comparison of subcutaneous low-molecular-weight heparin with intravenous standard heparin in proximal deep-vein thrombosis. *Lancet* 1992, 339:441–445.

18. Hull RD, Raskob GE, Pineo GF, *et al.*: Subcutaneous low-molecular-weight heparin compared with continuous intravenous heparin in the treatment of proximal-vein thrombosis. *N Engl J Med* 1992, 326:975–982.

19. Simonneau G, Charbonnier B, Decousus H, *et al.*: Subcutaneous low-molecular-weight heparin compared with continuous intravenous unfractionated heparin in the treatment of proximal deep vein thrombosis. *Arch Intern Med* 1993, 153:1541–1546.

20. Folkman J, Langer R, Linhardt RJ, *et al.*: Angiogenesis inhibition and tumor regression caused by heparin or a heparin fragment in the presence of cortisone. *Science* 1983, 221:719–725.

20a. Stead RB, Clinical pharmacology. In *Pulmonary Embolism and Deep Venous Thrombosis*. Philadelphia: WB Saunders Co.; 1985:107.

21. Bussey HI, Force RW, Bianco TM, *et al.*: Reliance on prothrombin time ratios causes significant errors in anticoagulation therapy. *Arch Intern Med* 1992, 152:278–282.

22. Hirsh J: Oral anticoagulant therapy. Urgent need for standardization. *Circulation* 1992, 86:1332–1335.

23. Goldhaber S, Morpurgo M, for the WHO/ISFC Task Force on Pulmonary Embolism: diagnosis, treatment, and prevention of pulmonary embolism. Report of the WHO/International Society and Federation of Cardiology Task Force. *JAMA* 1992, 268:1727–1733.

24. Brown WD, Goldhaber SZ: How to select patients with deep vein thrombosis for tPA therapy. *Chest* 1989, 95:276S–278S.

25. Goldhaber SZ, Buring JE, Lipnick RJ, *et al.*: Pooled analyses of randomized trials of streptokinase and heparin in phlebographically documented acute deep venous thrombosis. *Am J Med* 1984, 76:393–397.

26. Robertson BR, Nilsson IM, Nylander G: Value of streptokinase and heparin in treatment of acute deep venous thrombosis: a coded investigation. *Acta Chir Scand* 1968, 134:203–208.

27. Kakkar VV, Flanc C, Howe CT, *et al.*: Treatment of deep vein thrombosis: a trial of heparin, streptokinase, and arvin. *Br Med J* 1969, 1:806–810.

28. Robertson BR, Nilsson IM, Nylander G: Thrombolytic effect of streptokinase as evaluated by phlebography of deep venous thrombi of the leg. *Acta Chir Scand* 1970, 136:173–180.

29. Tsapogas MJ, Peabody RA, Wu KT, *et al.*: Controlled study of thrombolytic therapy in deep vein thrombosis. *Surgery* 1973, 74:973–984.

30. Porter JM, Seaman AJ, Common HH, *et al.*: Comparison of heparin and streptokinase in the treatment of venous thrombosis. *Am J Surg* 1975, 41:511–519.

31. Elliott MS, Immelman EJ, Jeffery P, *et al.*: A comparative randomized trial of heparin versus streptokinase in the treatment of acute proximal venous thrombosis: an interim report of a prospective trial. *Br J Surg* 1979, 66:838–843.

32. Goldhaber SZ, Meyerovitz MF, Green D, *et al.*: Randomized controlled trial of tissue plasminogen activator in proximal deep venous thrombosis. *Am J Med* 1990, 88:235–240.

33. Meyerovitz MF, Polak JF, Goldhaber SZ: Short-term response to thrombolytic therapy in deep venous thrombosis: predictive value of venographic appearance. *Radiology* 1992, 184:345–348.

34. Baldridge ED, Martin MA, Welling RE: Clinical significance of free-floating venous thrombi. *J Vasc Surg* 1990, 11:62–69.

35. Goldhaber SZ, Polak JF, Feldstein ML, *et al.*: Efficacy and safety of repeated boluses of urokinase in the treatment of deep venous thrombosis. *Am J Cardiol* 1994, 73:75–79.

36. Becker DM, Philbrick JT, Selby JB: Inferior vena cava filters: indications, safety, effectiveness. *Arch Intern Med* 1992, 152:1985–1994.

PREVENTION OF VENOUS THROMBOSIS

13

CHAPTER

Samuel Z. Goldhaber

Pulmonary embolism (PE) is easier and less expensive to prevent than to diagnose or treat [1]. Consensus conferences of the National Institutes of Health [2] and World Health Organization/International Society and Federation of Cardiology [3] as well as those held in Europe [4] and Great Britain [5] have declared that virtually all hospitalized patients should receive prophylaxis against venous thromboembolism. For every 1 million patients undergoing general, orthopedic, or urologic surgery, preventive measures both improve patient outcomes and reduce total health care costs by about $60 million [6].

Pulmonary embolism may occur among postoperative patients as late as 1 month *after discharge* from the hospital [7]. About 400,000 elective total hip or knee replacements as well as about 400,000 coronary artery bypass operations are performed per year in the United States. These types of surgery, in particular, continue to be associated with high rates of venous thrombosis. Acquired risk factors for PE include increasing age; immobilization; adenocarcinoma (which may be occult); oral contraceptives; and the postpartum period, particularly among women confined to bed after cesarean section. Some patients have a genetic predisposition to PE. Obtaining a careful history about family members with venous thrombosis may help identify persons who are at greater-than-average risk. Each patient's level of risk for PE should be assessed to determine whether mechanical, pharmacologic, or combined prevention modalities should be used. Because the risk of PE continues after discharge from the hospital, prophylaxis should be continued at home among patients who are at moderate to high risk for venous thromboembolism.

The paradox of PE prevention is that despite the availability of effective measures to curb venous thromboembolism, prophylaxis continues to be underused, even among high-risk hospitalized patients. In a survey of 16 short-stay hospitals in central Massachusetts [8], only 32% of patients at high risk for venous thrombosis received prophylaxis. The rates of prophylaxis varied widely, from 9% to 56% at the different hospitals. Patients received prophylaxis at teaching hospitals more often than they did at nonteaching hospitals. In this survey, fixed low-dose subcutaneous heparin was the most popular method of prophylaxis and was used in about four fifths of patients who received preventive measures. Prevention programs should be established at all hospitals to ensure that adequate measures are implemented. To achieve this objective, nurses and physicians must collaborate to institute protocols that are streamlined and standardized [9]. In addition, risk managers and quality-assurance personnel should encourage the development and oversee the monitoring of such programs.

EPIDEMIOLOGY

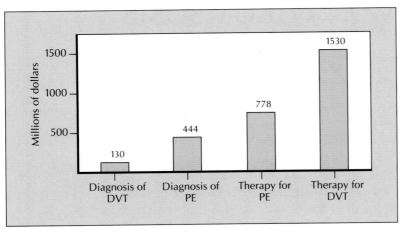

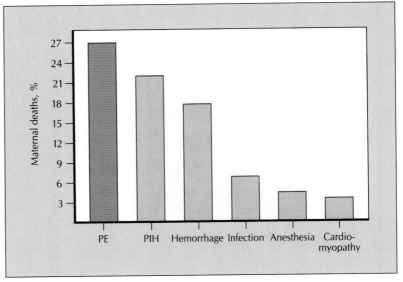

FIGURE 13-1. Annual direct costs of venous thrombosis. Pulmonary embolism (PE) and deep venous thrombosis (DVT) account for more than 250,000 hospitalizations per year in the United States and constitute one of the most common cardiovascular and cardiopulmonary illnesses. PE causes or contributes to as many as 50,000 deaths per year in the United States, a rate that has probably remained constant for the past three decades. Estimated annual charges for diagnosis and treatment of venous thrombosis in the United States are $2.9 billion [6]. This is merely the cost of medical care and excludes the cost of time lost from work, discomfort from chronic pulmonary hypertension caused by pulmonary embolism, and the value placed on the loss of life.

FIGURE 13-2. Pulmonary embolism (PE) and maternal mortality (a comparision of various causes of maternal mortality). PE is the most common medical cause of maternal mortality associated with live births in the United States [10]. The risk of PE is much greater during the first 6 weeks after parturition than during pregnancy [11]. PIH—pregnancy-induced hypertension.

PATHOPHYSIOLOGY

FIGURE 13-3. Common risk factors for venous thrombosis. Prophylaxis should be intensified when any of these risk factors are present. As the number of risk factors that are present increases, the likelihood of developing venous thrombosis increases.

COMMON RISK FACTORS FOR VENOUS THROMBOSIS

Genetic predisposition or family history

Surgery, trauma, immobilization

Obesity

Increasing age

Pregnancy, postpartum period, oral contraceptives

Cancer, especially adenocarcinoma

Spinal cord injury or stroke

Inflammatory bowel disease

Indwelling central venous catheter

Prior venous thrombosis

Anticardiolipin antibody or lupus anticoagulant

HYPERCOAGULABLE STATE	COMMENTS
Poor anticoagulant response to activated protein C	Detected in 21% of patients (aged <70 y) with venous thrombosis and among only 5% of controls [13]
Mutation in protein C gene	By age 45, 50% of heterozygotes and 10% of normal relatives develop venous thrombosis; about half of thrombotic events are associated with immobilization or surgery [12]
Protein S deficiency	In a cohort of 141 patients aged <45 y, 5% had this defect [14]
Presence of lupus anticoagulant	In a cohort of 141 patients with DVT aged <45 y, 3% had this defect [14]; in another cohort of 280 patients with acute DVT, 1% had this defect [15]
Presence of anticardiolipin antibodies	Acquired; usually not associated with lupus; often found in patients whose baseline PTT is elevated
	May be elevated in patients who also have lupus anticoagulant; associated with venous thrombosis and with recurrent first trimester miscarriages

FIGURE 13-4. Hypercoagulable states associated with venous thrombosis. Many patients with an inherited (*eg*, protein C deficiency) or acquired (*eg*, anticardiolipin antibody) hypercoagulable state do not manifest venous thrombosis unless they are stressed by immobilization, surgery, or other common acquired risk factors [12]. A poor anticoagulant response to activated protein C is the most exciting and far-reaching discovery in this field. Normally, adding a known amount of activated protein C to plasma will cause a twofold prolongation of the activated partial thromboplastin time (PTT). However, patients with a PTT prolongation less than twice control have a poor anticoagulant response. The abnormality appears to be due to a genetic mutation that causes a single amino acid substitution in the factor V molecule [16].

Work-up for possible hypercoagulable states is expensive and may be misleading. For example, obtaining levels of antithrombin III, protein C, or protein S should never substitute for carefully investigating a possible family history of venous thrombosis. Furthermore, a patient who has "consumption coagulopathy" or has recently begun heparin or warfarin therapy may be identified spuriously as having a genetic predisposition to venous thrombosis (*eg*, antithrombin III deficiency) when this is not really the case. Therefore, if a work-up is undertaken to diagnose a hypercoagulable state, it should typically be carried out after hospital discharge, at a time when the acute thrombotic process has been treated and the patient is clinically stable.

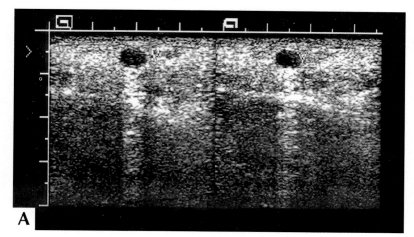

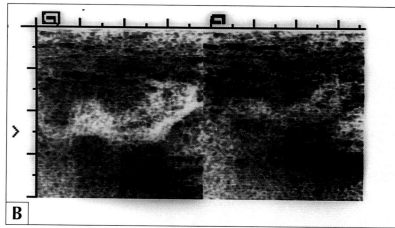

FIGURE 13-5. Although postoperative venous thrombosis is a well-known complication of orthopedic surgery, the disorder can be associated with virtually any type of surgery. **A,** A 70-year-old man underwent total nose reconstruction because of squamous cell carcinoma of the nose. Seventeen days after surgery, the patient complained of pain in the left calf. Noncompressible isolated thrombosis of the lesser saphenous vein was found on ultrasonography; this vein is superficial, not deep. Although in this case the thrombosis responded well to anti-inflammatory medication, warm soaks, and leg elevation, some patients have propagation of superficial vein thrombosis with conservative therapy and the thrombotic process eventually involves the deep venous system.

B, Ultrasound of a 55-year-old woman who had undergone cardiac transplantation 19 days before. Thrombosis of the greater saphenous vein was treated conservatively but progressed to involve the common femoral vein at the saphenovenous junction, shown at baseline in *A,* with compression of the ultrasound transducer shown in *B*. The patient required full-dose anticoagulation.

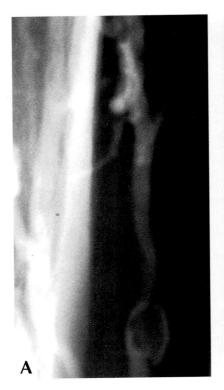
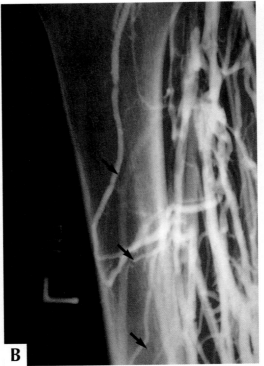
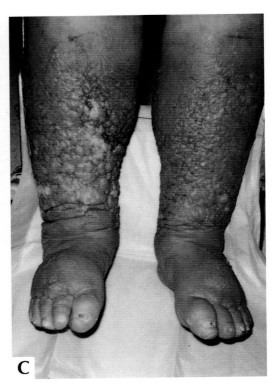

A

B

C

FIGURE 13-6. By preventing venous thrombosis, the eventual development of chronic venous insufficiency can also be prevented. **A,** A clot that has infiltrated a superficial venous valve. Chronic venous insufficiency almost always results from this situation. Often, however, clinically apparent venous insufficiency occurs several years after the initial venous thrombosis. **B,** Incompetent perforating veins in another patient with relatively severe chronic venous insufficiency. Perforating veins (*arrows*) provide channels that connect the superficial and deep venous systems.

C, The most severe case of chronic venous insufficiency that I have ever managed. Chronic venous insufficiency began to develop in this 82-year-old man about 3 years before. As a result, the patient was forced to retire from his job, which involved walking through each ward of a major hospital selling newspapers.

FIGURE 13-7. Prevention options for venous thrombosis are numerous and include mechanical or pharmacologic modalities (or a combination of both). Graduated compression stockings (GCS) and intermittent pneumatic compression (IPC) have complementary mechanisms. GCS provide continuous stimulation of blood flow and prevent dilation of the venous system in the legs. Intermittent pneumatic devices compress the veins more forcefully than do GCS, but compression only lasts for a relatively brief period. Low molecular weight heparins are the most recent innovation in the pharmacologic prophylaxis of venous thrombosis.

OPTIONS FOR PREVENTING VENOUS THROMBOSIS

Mechanical	GCS
	IPC
	Combined GCS and IPC
	Inferior vena caval filter
	Closure of patent foramen ovale
Pharmacologic	Unfractionated heparin
	Low molecular weight heparin
	Warfarin
	Dextran
	Aspirin
Combined mechanical + pharmacologic	GCS + heparin
	IPC + heparin
	IPC + warfarin
	Dextran + warfarin

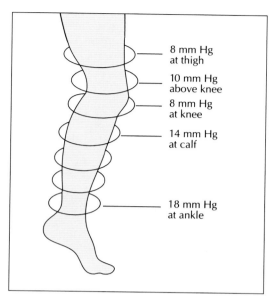

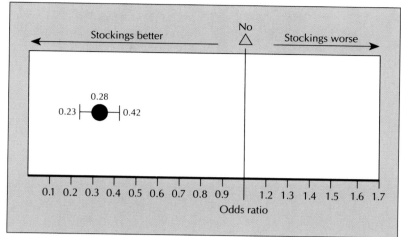

FIGURE 13-8. Graduated compression stockings (GCS) provide the greatest amount of pressure at the ankle, with decremental pressure at the calf and thigh. GCS prevent venous stasis, increase venous blood flow, and counter unopposed perioperative venodilatation. They are inexpensive, uncomplicated, and unlikely to cause serious complications, such as hemorrhage, which can occur with pharmacologic prophylaxis.

FIGURE 13-9. Efficacy of graduated compression stockings (GCS). In randomized trials studying the use of GCS for prevention of venous thrombosis after nonorthopedic procedures (*ie*, general surgery, gynecologic surgery, or neurosurgery), the likelihood of having deep venous thrombosis was reduced overall by 72% [17]. Thus, the odds ratio favoring GCS is 0.28, with very narrow confidence intervals (0.23 to 0.42). This meta-analysis of 1862 patients was derived from 12 trials that were properly randomized with objectively confirmed tests of venous thrombosis. The deep venous thrombosis rate was 6% in the GCS group compared with 18% among controls.

Therefore, GCS should be considered as first-line prophylaxis among all hospitalized patients, except for individuals with peripheral arterial disease whose condition may be exacerbated by vascular compression. Care should be taken to avoid a tourniquet effect at the proximal portion of the stockings. An analysis of general surgery patients indicates that use of GCS is the most cost-effective prophylaxis modality [18]. In this study, the cost of care averaged $34 less per admission for GCS patients than for those receiving no prophylaxis. Other prophylaxis methods further reduced thromboembolic risk but increased cost by $50 to $88 per patient relative to the cost of using GCS.

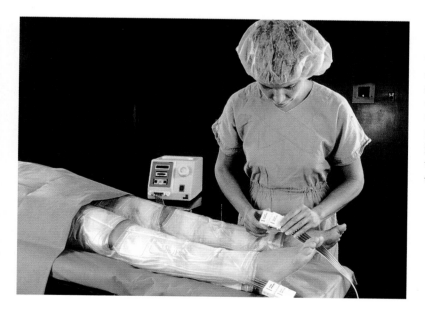

FIGURE 13-10. Intermittent pneumatic compression (IPC) devices ("boots") provide intermittent inflation of air-filled cuffs. These cuffs prevent venous stasis in the legs, accelerate venous return, and stimulate the endogenous fibrinolytic system. The IPC device shown in this illustration has four lower leg cuffs and two thigh cuffs that inflate sequentially from ankle to thigh. The pressure is usually adjusted so that it decreases from approximately 45 to 30 mm Hg. The inflation cycle is 11 seconds, and the deflation cycle is 60 seconds. The cuffs should be applied before surgery and worn after surgery, unless the patient is ambulating or being washed. (*Adapted from* Goldhaber [19]; with permission.)

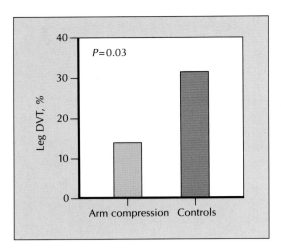

FIGURE 13-11. Intermittent pneumatic compression (IPC) devices cause systemic fibrinolysis in addition to their effects on venous blood flow. A trial of 121 general surgery patients tested specially constructed IPC devices of the arm to determine whether these *arm* devices might affect the rate of *leg* deep venous thrombosis (DVT) [20]. Patients either were assigned to arm compression (n=60) or served as controls (n=61). The frequency of postoperative leg DVT was assessed with serial ^{125}I fibrinogen leg scanning. The rate of leg DVT was markedly reduced among those patients who received arm compression. This indicates that IPC has systemic effects and causes endogenous fibrinolysis in addition to the local effects of accelerated venous blood flow. (*Adapted from* Knight and Dawson [20]; with permission.)

PHARMACOLOGIC PROPHYLAXIS

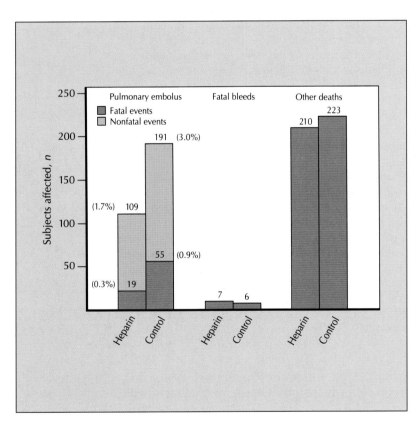

FIGURE 13-12. Fixed-dose unfractionated heparin trials. An International Multicenter Trial was organized by Kakkar [21]. The investigators recruited 4121 patients who were scheduled for major elective surgery. The patients were randomized to receive either low-dose unfractionated heparin (5000 U of subcutaneous calcium heparin 2 hours before surgery and every 8 hours thereafter for 7 days) or, alternatively, no prophylaxis. The principal endpoint was fatal postoperative pulmonary embolism (PE). Of the subjects on whom autopsy was done, PE was fatal in 16 controls, whereas only two patients in the heparin group died of PE. Although more wound hematomas occurred among heparin-treated patients, the number of deaths from hemorrhage was not increased among those who received heparin.

Collins *et al.* [22] pooled the data from 78 randomized controlled trials involving 15,598 patients on unfractionated heparin and confirmed the results of the International Multicenter Trial. Nonfatal PE was reduced by 40% and fatal PE was reduced by 64% among patients undergoing heparin prophylaxis. Patients given heparin had about one third as many deep venous thrombi as control patients, regardless of whether surgery was general, urologic, elective, orthopedic, or for trauma. In trials with an allocation ratio of 1:1, there were 6366 patients who received heparin versus 6426 controls. There was no significant difference in fatal hemorrhage between the heparin and control groups; however, an absolute excess in bleeding of about 2% was more likely to occur among patients assigned to heparin therapy—especially those who underwent urologic procedures. (*Adapted from* Collins and coworkers [22]; with permission.)

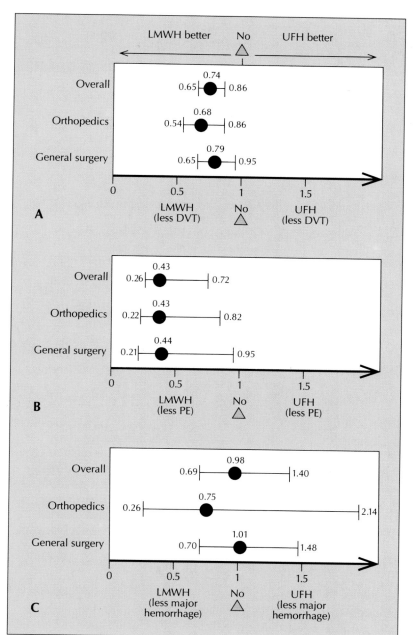

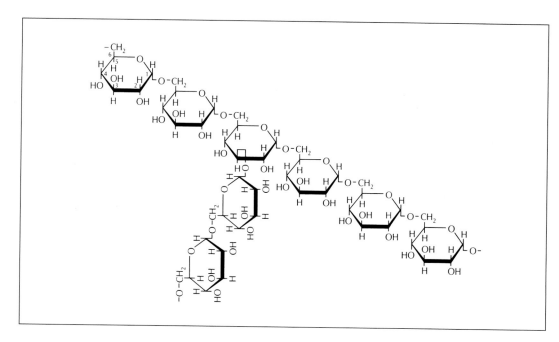

FIGURE 13-13. Low molecular weight heparins (LMWHs) versus unfractionated heparin (UFH). LMWHs exhibit less binding to plasma proteins and to endothelial cells than UFH. Therefore, LMWHs tend to have a more predictable dose response, a more dose-independent mechanism of clearance, and a longer plasma half-life than UFH. Theoretically, LMWHs can achieve higher plasma heparin levels with less protein binding than equivalent doses of UFH.

In most prophylaxis trials, LMWHs are administered as once- or twice-daily subcutaneous injections in fixed or weight-adjusted doses, without laboratory monitoring or dose adjustment.

This meta-analysis of LMWH versus standard UFH to prevent venous thrombosis in orthopedic and general surgery reveals that, overall, randomly selected patients given LMWH had 26% fewer leg thrombi (**A**) and 57% fewer pulmonary emboli (**B**) than patients who received UFH [23]. In trials of prophylaxis for orthopedic surgery, the decrease in deep venous thrombosis (DVT) rate was 32% (*A*) and the decrease in pulmonary embolism rate was 57% (*B*) with LMWH compared with UFH. There was, however, no difference in the rate of bleeding complications (**C**) between the two groups.

For prophylaxis in elective hip surgery, LMWHs have consistently performed well compared with other prevention modalities [24]. In 1993, the Food and Drug Administration approved the LMWH, enoxaparin, for prophylaxis against venous thrombosis among patients undergoing elective total hip replacement [25]. The approved dose is 30 mg subcutaneously twice daily for 10 to 14 days. No laboratory monitoring is needed.

FIGURE 13-14. Dextran was first used as a plasma substitute during World War II but subsequently has found limited application in preventing venous thromboembolism. It disaggregates erythrocytes, coats vessel wall endothelium, and decreases platelet adhesiveness [26]. We tend to use it in patients in whom heparin would pose an unacceptably high bleeding risk. After a 20-mL test dose of dextran 1, we usually administer 500 mL/24 hours of dextran 40 as a continuous intravenous infusion. The infusion is repeated daily for up to 1 week, depending on clinical necessity. (*Adapted from* Bergqvist [26]; with permission.)

PREVENTION OF DVT IN ELECTIVE TOTAL HIP REPLACEMENT

STRATEGY	ADVANTAGES	DISADVANTAGES
Adjusted-dose warfarin as inpatient only	Easy to obtain lab tests and target INR to 2.0–3.0 during inpatient hospitalization	Warfarin not effective for 3–5 d; if discontinued, does not provide protection after hospital discharge
Adjusted-dose warfarin as inpatient followed by predischarge ultrasound	If leg ultrasound is positive, treat with 6–12 wk of warfarin; negative ultrasound patients not given postdischarge warfarin	Leg ultrasound in patients after THR is notoriously insensitive; many patients are labeled as "normal" but really have DVT [27]
Adjusted-dose warfarin for 12 wk; no leg ultrasound [28]	Effective clinically in a series of 268 patients; saves cost of routine leg imaging	Silent DVT not identified by this, but all receive sufficient warfarin to treat most DVTs adequately
IPC device for 3–5 d plus adjusted-dose warfarin for 6 wk; no routine leg imaging	Provides protection before warfarin is fully effective	More expensive initially, but presumably minimizes DVT rate
Enoxaparin (30 mg SC) twice daily for 7–10 d	No laboratory monitoring needed; easy to administer to hospitalized patients	More expensive than warfarin; does not provide protection after discontinuation; requires injection
Fixed minidose (1 mg) warfarin	Inexpensive and easy to administer; no laboratory monitoring	Ineffective; failure rate of 40% in hip replacement and 70% in knee replacement [29]

FIGURE 13-15. Prevention of deep venous thrombosis (DVT) in elective total hip replacement (THR). Most North American strategies currently use warfarin, target International Normalized Ratio (INR) of 2.0 to 3.0, as part of the prevention of DVT associated with elective THR. Controversy centers on the duration of warfarin as well as on whether surveillance imaging of the legs is worthwhile. Low molecular weight heparin has gained more widespread use in Europe than in North America. Aspirin is inexpensive, easy to administer, and involves no laboratory monitoring. A meta-analysis from Oxford [31] (including studies using fibrinogen leg scanning as an endpoint) suggests it is effective. Conversely, a meta-analysis from the Mayo Clinic (including only studies using venographic assessment) shows that aspirin is no more effective than placebo [30]. IPC—intermittent pneumatic compression; SC—subcutaneous.

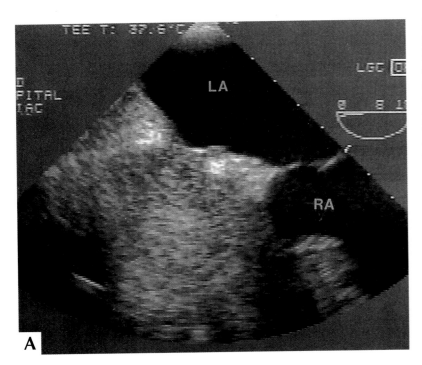

FIGURE 13-16. Case presentation: stroke after elective total knee replacement (TKR). A 65-year-old man was admitted for elective bilateral TKR as a staged procedure with a 1-week interval between operations. The right TKR lasted 4 hours and was performed under epidural anesthesia. Estimated blood loss was 600 mL. Tourniquet time was 124 minutes. Within 1 minute of tourniquet release, the patient developed acute confusion, dysarthria, and hypotension with a systolic arterial pressure of 80 mm Hg. His oxygen saturation decreased to 94% while receiving 3 L/min of oxygen. His blood pressure was restored to 120/60 mm Hg within 10 minutes of receiving intravenous fluids and ephedrine. There was no past history of hypertension, heart disease, or stroke. Cardiovascular consultation was requested to evaluate what clinical event had occurred and when the left TKR could be undertaken. Examination revealed elevation of the left hemipalate and deviation of the tongue to the right. Computed tomography of the brain and a cerebral angiogram were normal. Over the next 5 days, the dysarthria gradually improved and, upon discharge from the hospital, there were no residual neurologic deficits. **A,** The patient underwent transesophageal echocardiography (TEE) to look for a cardiac source of embolism. Initially, none was found. LA—left atrium; RA—right atrium. (*continued*)

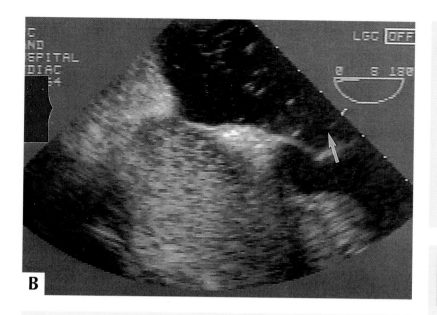

B

C. COINCIDENT THROMBOEMBOLISM WITH TKR TOURNIQUET DEFLATION

Population: 29 consecutive TKR patients

Methods: Intraoperative TEE (*n*=29) and PA monitoring (*n*=10)

Findings: All have showers of echogenic material, lasting 3–15 min, in RA and RV, within 15 s of tourniquet deflation; three patterns ("snow storm;" large, discrete particles >1 mm; and combinations).

E. ALTERNATIVE APPROACHES TO THE PREVENTION OF TKR EMBOLISM

Do not use a tourniquet (increases blood loss, wound hematoma, and subsequent wound infection)

Use a tourniquet just for cementing

Cementless TKRs (out of vogue because of poor 5-year results)

Operate with systemic anticoagulation (increases blood loss, wound hematoma, and subsequent infection; epidural anesthesia can be problematic)

D. TKR TOURNIQUET DEFLATION

HEMODYNAMICS	BASELINE	DEFLATION
MAP, *mm Hg*	94	78
PA saturation %	80	67
PA systolic pressure, *mm Hg*	36	43

FIGURE 13-16. (*continued*) **B**, Agitated saline was then injected into a peripheral vein, and microbubbles were observed crossing the atrial septum from right to left (*arrow*), thus demonstrating the presence of a patent foramen ovale. The decision was made to operate on the left knee after temporary transcatheter closure of the patent foramen ovale.

In a study of 406 patients with embolic stroke [32], 49 were found to have a patent foramen ovale. Although only five of the 49 had clinically suspected venous thrombosis, 42 of the 49 underwent bilateral contrast venography of the legs. Twenty-four of the 42 (57%) had DVT and 13 of the 24 DVTs were confined to the calf veins. This indicates that prevention of isolated calf vein thrombosis is important, not only to reduce the frequency of pulmonary embolism but also to reduce the rate of embolic stroke through a patent foramen ovale.

C, Every subject in a series of 29 patients undergoing elective TKR had intraoperative monitoring with TEE; 10 subjects also received intraoperative pulmonary arterial monitoring [33]. All 29 patients had showers of echogenic material in the right atrium (RA) and right ventricle (RV) that appeared within 15 seconds of tourniquet deflation and were 3 to 15 minutes in duration. These echogenic emboli could consist of bone marrow, bone cement, or thrombus. One embolus that was retrieved with suction through a pulmonary artery catheter was a fresh thrombus that was 6 mm in its longest dimension.

D, A decrease in systemic artery pressure and oxygen saturation with a concomitant increase in pulmonary artery systolic pressure occurred immediately after tourniquet deflation in subjects with pulmonary artery catheters. **E**, No simple, satisfactory prevention strategy currently exists. MAP—mean artery pressure.

STANDARD APPROACHES TO PREVENT TKR AND THR EMBOLISM HAVE HIGH FAILURE RATES

Randomized controlled trial of 1207 THR and TKR patients; warfarin (INR target 2.0–3.0) vs Logiparin 175 U/kg/d; endpoint was DVT (by venography)

37% warfarin DVT vs 31% LMWH DVT; 8% vs 6% proximal DVT; 1% vs 3% major bleeding

FIGURE 13-17. The standard preventive approaches in elective total hip (THR) and total knee replacement (TKR) have high failure rates. The ability of warfarin and low molecular weight heparin (LMWH) to prevent venous thrombosis was compared in a randomized trial [35] of 1207 patients undergoing elective THR or TKR. Both strategies resulted in surprisingly high rates of deep venous thrombosis (DVT) proven by venography. Although the rate of isolated venous thrombosis in the calf was slightly higher in the warfarin-treated patients, the rate of major bleeding complications was three times higher among those who received LMWH. INR—International Normalized Ratio.

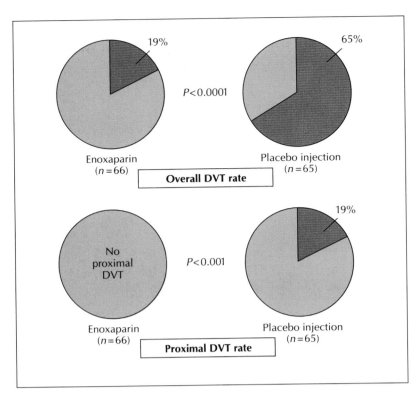

FIGURE 13-18. Use of low molecular weight heparin to prevent venous thrombosis after total knee replacement (TKR). One hundred thirty-one consecutive patients undergoing TKR or tibial osteotomy were randomly selected to receive either 30 mg of enoxaparin every 12 hours or a placebo injection, beginning on the first morning after surgery [34]. Bilateral contrast venography was performed on the legs at day 14 or at the time of hospital discharge, if sooner. Nineteen percent of the patients given enoxaparin had deep venous thrombosis (DVT) compared with 65% in the placebo group ($P<0.0001$). None of the patients given enoxaparin had venous thrombosis in the proximal leg, compared with 19% of the patients given placebo ($P<0.001$). There was no difference in clinical bleeding complications, estimated blood loss, nadir hemoglobin levels, or the number of blood transfusions between the two groups.

Enoxaparin appears to be effective and safe for reducing the frequency of DVT after major knee surgery; however, isolated calf vein thrombosis occurred at a rate of 19% among those who received low molecular weight heparin. This indicates that further effort must be directed toward improving efficacy rates within this area of prevention.

A. FAT EMBOLISM SYNDROME

PARADOXICAL EMBOLISM VIA PATENT FORAMEN OVALE	
GURD'S CRITERIA	Petechial rash, respiratory distress, and CNS dysfunction
Mechanical theory	Intramedullary vein trauma leads to intravasation and embolization of marrow fat
Findings	Complete opacification of RA and RV; many highly echogenic bodies (1-cm diameter; 1–7 cm in length), plus a mass of smaller echoes

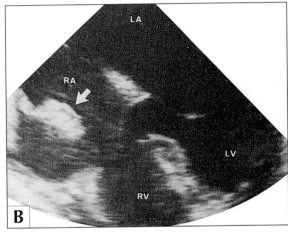

B

FIGURE 13-19. Posttraumatic fat embolism syndrome. Patients with long-bone fractures are susceptible to posttraumatic fat embolism syndrome, a multisystem disorder [36]. **A,** Trauma to intramedullary veins leads to extravasation and embolization of marrow fat, which can traverse a patent foramen ovale and cause neurologic dysfunction and a petechial rash. **B,** A trans-esophageal echocardiographic (TEE) four-chamber view of a large fat embolus (*arrow*) among smaller echogenic masses in the right atrium. CNS—central nervous system; LA—left atrium; LV—left ventricle; RA—right atrium; RV—right ventricle. (*Adapted from* Pell and coworkers [36]; with permission.)

LIMITATIONS OF STANDARD PREVENTIVE APPROACHES TO TKR AND THR EMBOLISM

Anticoagulation (LMWH or warfarin) is started postoperatively and, therefore, cannot possibly be effective during tourniquet deflation

IVC filters are probably ineffective for microthrombi or fat emboli

No known prophylactic agent will prevent emboli of cement

FIGURE 13-20. Problems with standard preventive approaches in total hip replacement (THR) and total knee replacement (TKR). Currently available modalities have surprisingly high failure rates. THR and TKR emboli may be caused by thrombus, fat, or cement, which are difficult to prevent. LMWH—low molecular weight heparin.

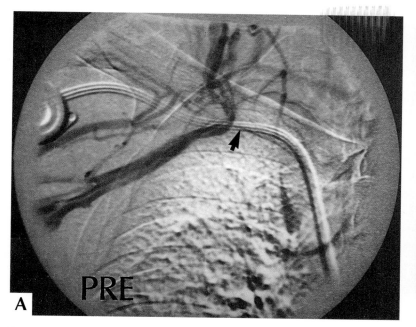

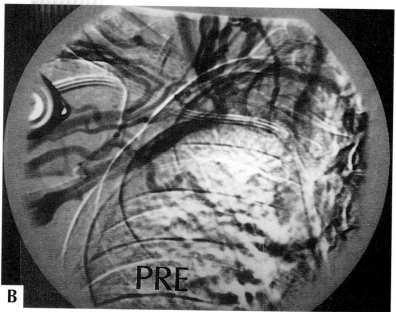

FIGURE 13-21. Case presentation: indwelling catheter–induced venous thrombosis of the upper extremities. A 29-year-old man had an indwelling catheter placed in the right subclavian vein so that repeated cycles of chemotherapy to treat Hodgkin's disease could be given.

A, Contrast venogram demonstrating thrombosis of the subclavian vein at the site of entry of the catheter (*arrow*). **B,** Flow of intravenous contrast medium into multiple collateral channels. The patient required 1 week of hospitalization and treatment with thrombolytic agents and anticoagulation.

Patients receiving indwelling central venous catheters should be considered for prophylaxis with fixed minidose warfarin (1 mg/d)

beginning at least several days before placement of the catheter. In a trial of 121 patients [37], 82 were randomly placed in a group given 1 mg of warfarin daily, beginning 3 days before catheter insertion and continuing for 90 days, or a control group that received no prophylaxis. Venograms of the subclavian vein, innominate vein, and superior vena cava were done at the onset of thrombotic symptoms or at the 90-day endpoint. Of the 42 subjects who completed the warfarin prophylaxis regimen, four had venogram-proven thrombosis. Of the 40 individuals who received no prophylaxis, 15 had venogram-proven thrombosis (*P*<0.001). Thus, this is the one particular population in which fixed minidose warfarin appears to be effective.

CASE SCENARIOS

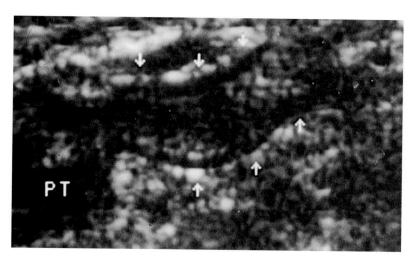

FIGURE 13-22. Venous thrombosis after coronary artery bypass grafting (CABG) surgery. *Arrows* outline the upper and lower borders of the vein wall.

Although pulmonary embolism has traditionally been considered a very rare complication of CABG, this belief is changing as new data are published. In a review of 819 consecutive patients undergoing CABG (without other concomitant cardiac surgery) at the Veterans Administration Medical Center

at Brockton/West Roxbury [38], 3.9% were found to have postoperative pulmonary embolism evidenced by autopsy, angiography, or high-probability lung scanning. Only one fourth of patients with postoperative pulmonary embolism were diagnosed within the first week after surgery—most were identified in the second week after surgery. Nineteen percent of patients with pulmonary embolism died, compared with an operative mortality of 3% of patients without pulmonary embolism.

In a series of 29 patients who had undergone uncomplicated CABG at Brigham and Women's Hospital, ultrasonography of the legs was done before hospital discharge [39]. None of the patients had postoperative signs or symptoms suggestive of deep venous thrombosis; however, 48% were found to have deep venous thrombosis on ultrasonography. In all but one case, the deep venous thrombosis was limited to the calf veins. Unexpectedly, half of the venous thrombi occurred in the leg contralateral to the harvest site of the saphenous vein. This ultrasonogram shows an early nonobstructive thrombus measuring 1.5 × 0.5 cm within a muscular vein sinusoid. This sinusoid communicates with the posterior tibial (PT) vein. All 29 patients in this report received prophylaxis with graduated compression stockings, thus suggesting that more intensive prevention strategies should be considered for CABG patients. (*Adapted from* Reis and coworkers [39]; with permission.)

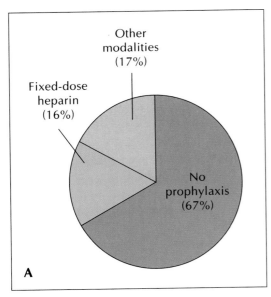

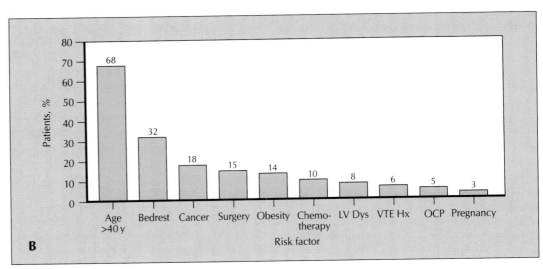

FIGURE 13-23. Low utilization rate of prophylaxis against venous thrombosis in medical intensive care unit (MICU) patients. To determine the prophylaxis rate in the MICU at Brigham and Women's Hospital, we undertook a prospective survey of 152 consecutive MICU patients [40].

A, Type of prophylaxis used. Overall, 67% of patients received no prophylaxis. This is unfortunate because MICU patients are at high risk for developing venous thrombosis. Of those who did receive some form of prophylaxis, there was an average delay of 2 days in the MICU before preventive measures were instituted.

B, Of the 152 patients, 88% had at least one risk factor for venous thrombosis and 53% had multiple risk factors. GCS—graduated compression stockings; IPC—intermittent pneumatic compression; LV Dys—left ventricular dysfunction; OCP—oral contraceptive pills; VTE Hx—history of venous thromboembolism.

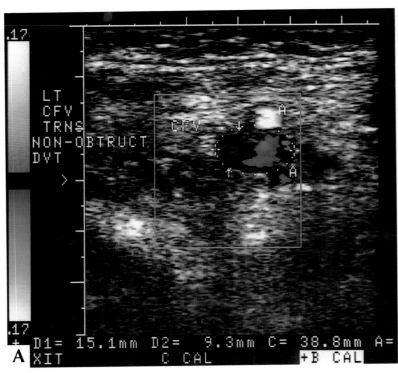

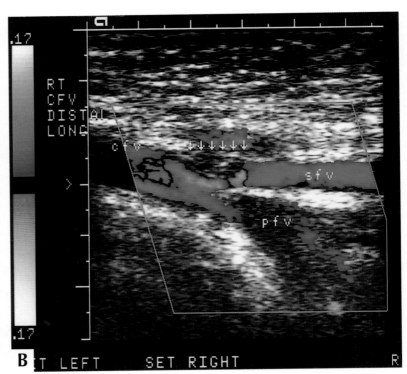

FIGURE 13-24. Case presentation of a medical intensive care unit (MICU) patient with venous thrombosis. As part of a survey of the frequency of venous thrombosis in MICU patients, this 63-year-old woman underwent venous ultrasonography of the leg and upper extremities. She presented 9 days previously with diffuse encephalopathy and necrotizing pneumonia and was immediately hospitalized in the MICU. **A,** Transverse view of nonobstructing deep venous thrombosis in the left common femoral vein (*arrows*). **B,** Thrombosis of the distal right common femoral vein in a longitudinal section (*arrows*). (*continued*)

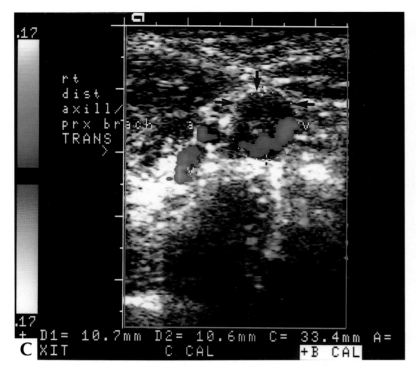

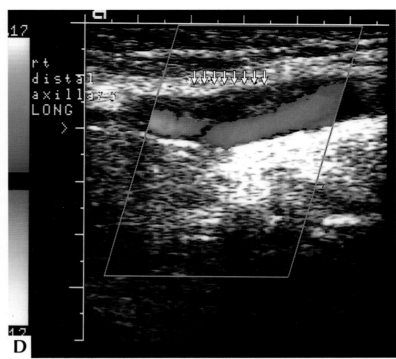

FIGURE 13-24. (*continued*) **C,** Transverse view of thrombosis of the right axillary vein (*arrows*). **D,** Longitudinal view of thrombus in the right distal axillary vein (*arrows*). After the results of the ultrasono-graphic examination were evaluated, a filter was inserted into the inferior vena cava. Nevertheless, the patient's condition deteriorated and she died 3 weeks later. Diffuse thrombi were confirmed at autopsy.

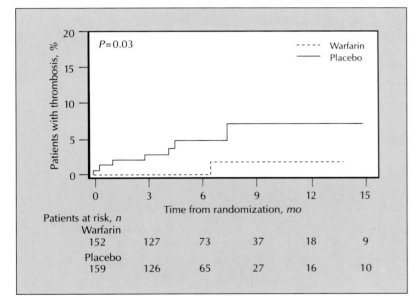

FIGURE 13-25. Very low dose warfarin prevents venous thrombosis in patients with stage IV breast cancer. Women receiving chemo-therapy for metastatic breast cancer were randomly assigned to receive either very low dose warfarin or placebo. The warfarin dose was 1 mg daily for 6 weeks and was then adjusted to a target International Normalized Ratio of 1.3 to 1.9. There were seven venous thromboembolic events in the placebo group compared with one in the warfarin group, a relative risk reduction of about 85% ($P=0.03$). Thus, very low dose warfarin is a safe and effective method for preventing thromboembolism in patients with metastatic breast cancer who are receiving chemotherapy. (*Adapted from* Levine and coworkers [41]; with permission.)

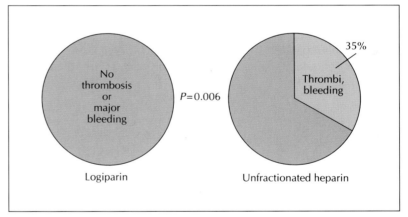

FIGURE 13-26. Prevention of venous thrombosis in patients with spinal cord injury. Venous thrombosis is a major problem in patients with complete motor paralysis after spinal cord injury. This randomized trial of 41 patients compared a once-daily fixed dose (3500 anti-Xa units) of low molecular weight heparin (Logiparin, Nordisk, Denmark) with standard unfractionated heparin (5000 U subcutaneously three times daily) [42]. The study lasted 8 weeks. None of the patients given Logiparin had throm-bosis or bleeding; however, five patients given unfractionated heparin had thrombosis, including two with fatal pulmonary embolism proven at autopsy. Two patients treated with unfraction-ated heparin had bleeding severe enough to necessitate withdrawal of the agent. This illustration shows the difference in adverse clin-ical outcomes between the two groups ($P=0.006$).

USE OF HORMONAL THERAPY IN WOMEN WITH A PRIOR HISTORY OF VENOUS THROMBOSIS

HORMONAL THERAPY	COMMENTS
Estrogen oral contraceptives	Should not be used in patients with prior DVT; however, no definitive evidence links progesterone contraceptive pills or implant with DVT; progesterone contraception can be considered if alternative methods are impractical or have failed
Estrogen replacement therapy	Consider transdermal rather than oral therapy in patients at very high risk of DVT
Progestins to treat dysfunctional uterine bleeding or endometriosis	.Although linked with hypertension, peripheral vascular disease, and cerebrovascular disease, they have not been associated with DVT
Tamoxifen to treat first relapse of breast cancer	Although slightly prothrombotic, the alternative (surgical oophorectomy) is more prothrombotic
Gonadotropin-releasing hormone agonists	Used to treat endometriosis, these produce a hypoestrogenic state and are not associated with hypercoagulability; can be used safely in women with prior venous thrombosis
Danazol (Sanofi Winthrop Pharmaceutical, New York) for endometriosis	Not prothrombotic; can be used safely in women with prior DVT
Pergonal (Serono Laboratories, Inc, Norwell, MA) for ovulation induction	Can be used safely in women with prior DVT

FIGURE 13-27. Women's health: use of hormonal therapy in women with a history of deep venous thrombosis (DVT). Oral contraceptives, which contain a much higher dose of estrogen than needed for postmenopausal estrogen replacement therapy, increase the risk of venous thrombosis. Estrogen replacement therapy decreases the risk of coronary heart disease, reduces the frequency and severity of osteoporosis, and reduces vaginal atrophy and hot flashes caused by menopause. However, physicians treating women with prior venous thrombosis are often confronted with dilemmas surrounding use of hormone therapy [43]. Should women with prior venous thrombosis not be given postmenopausal estrogen replacement therapy? Should an estrogen patch be used instead of oral therapy? The cardioprotective effects of estrogen diminish with transdermal therapy, which bypasses the liver (thereby failing to increase high-density lipoprotein cholesterol). Although no straightforward answers can be proffered, my recommendations are listed in this illustration.

REGIONAL ANESTHESIA IN PREVENTION OF VENOUS THROMBOSIS

VARIABLE	REGIONAL ANESTHESIA	GENERAL ANESTHESIA
Venodilatation	Mild (due to sympathetic blockade)	Marked (due to histamine release)
Blood loss	Less (decreased central venous pressure)	More (increased central venous pressure due to positive pressure ventilation)
Leg blood flow	Markedly increased	The same (with isoflurane) or slightly decreased
Volume administration	Patients are prehydrated (and hemodiluted) to minimize hypotensive response	Less volume administered; therefore, blood more viscous
Systemic effects of regional anesthetics (reduce coagulability and vessel damage)	Decreased platelet and erythrocyte aggregation; increased fibrinolysis; decreased neutrophil adherence, activation, and endothelial damage	NA

FIGURE 13-28. Utility of regional anesthesia for prevention of venous thrombosis. Regional anesthesia decreases the rate of venous thrombosis [44]; however, epidural hematoma can be a devastating complication. Therefore, if an agent used for pharmacologic prophylaxis, such as heparin, is combined with regional anesthesia, the prophylactic agent should either be withheld or coagulation studies should be obtained to ensure minimal anticoagulation at the time of epidural catheterization.

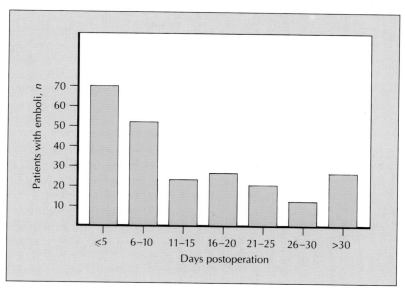

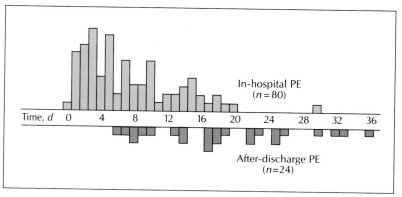

FIGURE 13-29. Autopsy study of the interval between surgery and pulmonary embolism. Although more pulmonary emboli occur during the first 5 days after surgery than during any other 5-day postoperative period, almost as many emboli occur during days 6 through 10. An important number of pulmonary emboli continue to occur during the first month after surgery. These data are based on a Swedish autopsy study [45] in which almost all of the city's deceased residents underwent routine postmortem examination.

These findings highlight one of the challenges involved in preventing venous thrombosis, because efforts must be directed toward continuing prophylactic measures after the patient has been discharged from the hospital. A follow-up study from the same investigators showed that the 13th day after surgery was the median time for postoperative pulmonary embolism [46]. (*Adapted from* Bergqvist and Lindblad [45]; with permission.)

FIGURE 13-30. Retrospective study of the frequency of postoperative pulmonary embolism (PE) after hospital discharge. Review of the general surgery experience at the University Hospital of Geneva [7] indicated that after accounting for patients readmitted to the hospital because of PE within 30 days of surgery, the overall rate of postoperative PE increased by 30%. Delayed embolic events occurred a median of 6 days after hospital discharge and 18 days after surgery. Delayed PEs were more common after low-risk surgery, such as hernia correction and appendectomy, than after higher-risk surgery on the colon, rectum, or stomach. This report, therefore, suggests that continuation of prophylactic measures should be considered for patients being discharged from the hospital after general surgery. (*Adapted from* Huber and coworkers [7]; with permission.)

SPECIFIC PREVENTION STRATEGIES

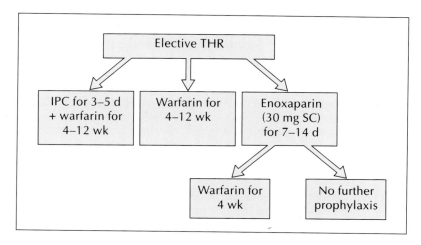

FIGURE 13-31. Elective total hip replacement (THR). The two principal choices are warfarin and low molecular weight heparin. If warfarin is used, consideration should be given to intermittent pneumatic compression (IPC) for the first 3 to 5 days after surgery, during which warfarin is not yet fully effective. The duration of prophylaxis must also be determined. Whereas some physicians use prophylaxis only for inpatients, others use as much as 12 weeks of warfarin therapy. At Brigham and Women's Hospital, we usually use IPC and about 4 to 6 weeks of warfarin. SC—subcutaneously.

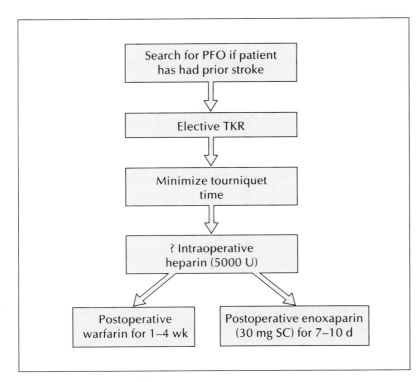

FIGURE 13-32. Elective total knee replacement (TKR). If the patient has had a stroke, preoperative echocardiographic assessment should be undertaken with agitated saline injection to search for a patent foramen ovale (PFO). If it is present, the patent foramen ovale should probably be closed before surgery. The likelihood of clinically significant pulmonary and paradoxical embolization should be taken into account during the period immediately after tourniquet deflation. To help prevent a shower of emboli, the surgeon should attempt to minimize tourniquet time or provide at least a modest level of intraoperative anticoagulation (bearing in mind that the patient probably has an epidural catheter). Warfarin is more effective after surgery than aspirin; however, low molecular weight heparins, although not approved by the Food and Drug Administration for this indication, may be more effective than warfarin. SC—subcutaneously.

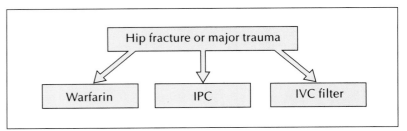

FIGURE 13-33. Hip fracture and major trauma. Posttraumatic fat embolism syndrome occurs especially after fracture of the pelvis or legs. To prevent thrombotic embolism, fracture patients should receive warfarin prophylaxis unless they are bleeding actively. If the legs are not fractured, intermittent pneumatic compression (IPC) can be used. If neither anticoagulation nor leg compression can be tolerated, however, placement of a filter in the inferior vena cava (IVC) should be considered.

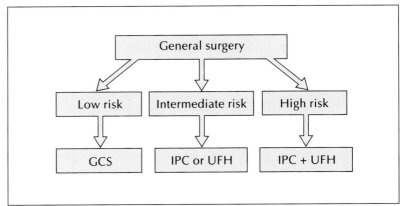

FIGURE 13-34. For low-risk patients, graduated compression stockings (GCS) should suffice. For intermediate-risk patients, either intermittent pneumatic compression (IPC) or fixed, low-dose unfractionated heparin (UFH) (*eg*, 5000 U twice or three times daily) should be adequate. The first dose of heparin should be administered 2 hours before the skin is incised. For high-risk patients, mechanical and pharmacologic prophylaxis can be combined.

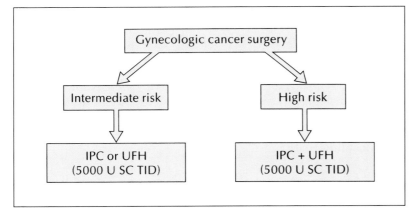

FIGURE 13-35. Gynecologic cancer surgery. Either intermittent pneumatic compression (IPC) or intensive fixed-dose unfractionated heparin (UFH) can be used. Subcutaneous (SC) heparin should be administered in a dosage of 5000 U three times daily because twice-daily administration has been associated with a high rate of venous thrombosis. For patients at very high risk, such as those with adenocarcinoma or a history of venous thrombosis, prophylaxis can be undertaken with both IPC and UFH.

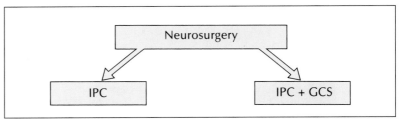

FIGURE 13-36. Neurosurgery. These patients are at very high risk of bleeding if pharmacologic prophylaxis is used. The bleeding risk appears to be higher with tumors that are metastatic to the brain (especially melanomas, germ cell tumors, and adenocarcinomas) than with primary brain tumors. Therefore, prevention of venous thrombosis ordinarily includes intermittent pneumatic compression (IPC) or a combination of IPC and graduated compression stockings (GCS).

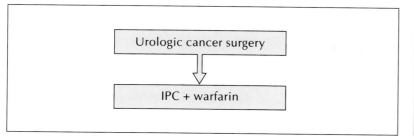

FIGURE 13-37. Urologic cancer surgery. This type of surgery results in a high rate of venous thrombosis unless prophylaxis is used. Open prostatectomy is associated with a higher risk of venous thrombosis than transurethral resection. Effective prophylaxis for these patients usually includes a combination of intermittent pneumatic compression (IPC) and warfarin.

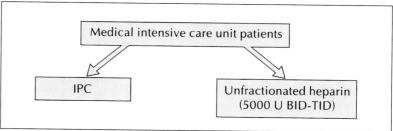

FIGURE 13-38. Medical intensive care unit patients. These patients are immobilized and are at substantial risk of venous thrombosis. Prophylaxis can be undertaken with either intermittent pneumatic compression (IPC) or fixed-dose unfractionated heparin.

REFERENCES

1. Goldhaber SZ: Practical aspects of venous thromboembolism prevention: an overview. In *Prevention of Venous Thromboembolism*. Edited by Goldhaber SZ. New York: Marcel Dekker; 1993:129–144.

2. National Institutes of Health Consensus Conference: Prevention of venous thrombosis and pulmonary embolism. *JAMA* 1986, 256:744–749.

3. Goldhaber SZ, Morpurgo M (for the WHO/ISFC Task Force on Pulmonary Embolism): Diagnosis, treatment, and prevention of pulmonary embolism: report of the WHO/International Society and Federation of Cardiology Task Force. *JAMA* 1992, 268:1727–1733.

4. European Consensus Statement: Prevention of venous thromboembolism. *Int Angiol* 1992, 11:151–159.

5. Thromboembolic Risk Factors (THRIFT) Consensus Group: Risk of and prophylaxis for venous thromboembolism in hospital patients. *BMJ* 1992, 305:567–574.

6. Landefeld CS, Hanus P: Economic burden of venous thromboembolism. In *Prevention of Venous Thromboembolism*. Edited by Goldhaber SZ. New York: Marcel Dekker; 1993:69–85.

7. Huber O, Bounameaux H, Borst F, *et al.*: Postoperative pulmonary embolism after hospital discharge: an underestimated risk. *Arch Surg* 1992, 127:310–313.

8. Anderson FA Jr, Wheeler HB, Goldberg RJ, *et al.*: Physician practices in the prevention of venous thromboembolism. *Ann Intern Med* 1991, 115:591–595.

9. Morrison RB: Nurse and physician collaborative responsibility. In *Prevention of Venous Thromboembolism*. Edited by Goldhaber SZ. New York: Marcel Dekker; 1993:577–582.

10. Koonin LM, Atrash HK, Lawson HW, *et al.*: Maternal mortality surveillance, United States, 1979–1986: CDC Surveillance Summaries. *MMWR* 1991, 40:1–13.

11. Morrison RB: Obstetrics. In *Prevention of Venous Thromboembolism*. Edited by Goldhaber SZ. New York: Marcel Dekker; 1993:445–462.

12. Allaart CF, Poort SR, Rosendaal FR, *et al.*: Increased risk of venous thrombosis in carriers of hereditary protein C deficiency defect. *Lancet* 1993, 341:134–138.

13. Koster T, Rosendaal FR, de Ronde H, *et al.*: Venous thrombosis due to poor anticoagulant response to activated protein C: Leiden Thrombophilia Study. *Lancet* 1993, 342:1503–1506.

14. Gladson CL, Scharrer I, Hach V, *et al.*: The frequency of type I heterozygous protein S and protein C deficiency in 141 unrelated young patients with venous thrombosis. *Thromb Haemost* 1988, 59:18–22.

15. Heijboer H, Brandjes DPM, Büller HR, *et al.*: Deficiencies of coagulation-inhibiting and fibrinolytic proteins in outpatients with deep-vein thrombosis. *N Engl J Med* 1990, 323:1512–1516.

16. Tuddenham EGD: Thrombophilia: the new factor is old factor V. *Lancet* 1994, 343:1515–1516.

17. Wells PS, Lensing AWA, Hirsh J: Graduated compression stockings in the prevention of postoperative venous thromboembolism: a meta-analysis. *Arch Intern Med* 1994, 154:67–72.

18. Oster G, Tuden RL, Colditz GA: Prevention of venous thromboembolism after general surgery: cost-effectiveness analysis of alternative approaches to prophylaxis. *Am J Med* 1987, 82:889–899.

19. Goldhaber SZ: Deep venous thrombosis. In *Current Management of Hypertensive and Vascular Diseases*. Edited by Frohlich E, Cook J. St. Louis: Mosby Yearbook; 1992:291.

20. Knight MTN, Dawson R: Effect of intermittent compression of the arms on deep venous thrombosis in the legs. *Lancet* 1976, 2:1265–1268.

21. International Multicenter Trial: Prevention of fatal postoperative pulmonary embolism by low doses of heparin. *Lancet* 1975, 2:45–51.

22. Collins R, Scrimgeour A, Yusuf S, *et al.*: Reduction in fatal pulmonary embolism and venous thrombosis by perioperative administration of subcutaneous heparin: overview of results of randomized trials in general, orthopedic, and urologic surgery. *N Engl J Med* 1988, 318:1162–1173.

23. Nurmohamed MT, Rosendaal FR, Büller HR, *et al.*: Low-molecular-weight heparin versus standard heparin in general and orthopaedic surgery: a meta-analysis. *Lancet* 1992, 340:152–156.

24. Mohr DN, Silverstein MD, Murtaugh PA, *et al.*: Prophylactic agents for venous thrombosis in elective hip surgery: meta-analysis of studies using venographic assessment. *Arch Intern Med* 1993, 153:2221–2228.

25. Enoxaparin—a low-molecular-weight heparin. *Med Lett Drugs Ther* 1993, 35:75–78.

26. Bergqvist D: Dextran. In: *Prevention of Venous Thromboembolism*. Edited by Goldhaber SZ. New York: Marcel Dekker; 1993:167–215.

27. Davidson BL, Elliott CG, Lensing AWA (for the RD Heparin Arthroplasty Group): Low accuracy of color Doppler ultrasound in the detection of proximal leg vein thrombosis in asymptomatic high-risk patients. *Arch Intern Med* 1992, 117:735–738.

28. Paiement GD, Wessinger SJ, Hughes R, *et al.*: Routine use of adjusted low-dose warfarin to prevent venous thromboembolism after total hip replacement. *J Bone Joint Surg [Am]* 1993, 75:893–898.

29. Dale C, Gallus A, Wycherley A, *et al.*: Prevention of venous thrombosis with minidose warfarin after joint replacement. *BMJ* 1991, 303:224.

30. Antiplatelet Trialists' Collaboration: Collaborative overview of randomised trials of antiplatelet treatment: Part III: Reduction in venous thrombosis and pulmonary embolism by antiplatelet prophylaxis among surgical and medical patients. *BMJ* 1994, 308:235–246.

31. Mohr DN, Silverstein MD, Murtaugh PA, *et al.*: Prophylactic agents for venous thrombosis in elective hip surgery: meta-analysis of studies using venographic assessment. *Arch Intern Med* 1993, 153:2221–2228.

32. Stöllberger C, Slany J, Schuster I, *et al.*: The prevalence of deep venous thrombosis in patients with suspected paradoxical embolism. *Ann Intern Med* 1993, 119:461–465.

33. Parmet JL, Berman AT, Horrow JC, *et al.*: Thromboembolism coincident with tourniquet deflation during total knee arthroplasty. *Lancet* 1993, 341:1057–1058.

34. Leclerc JR, Geerts WH, Desjardins L, *et al.*: Prevention of deep vein thrombosis after major knee surgery: a randomized, double-blind trial comparing a low molecular weight heparin fragment (enoxaparin) to placebo. *Thromb Haemost* 1992, 67:417–423.

35. Hull R, Raskob G, Pineo G, *et al.*: A comparison of subcutaneous low-molecular-weight heparin with warfarin sodium for prophylaxis against deep-vein thrombosis after hip or knee implantation. *N Engl J Med* 1993, 329:1370–1376.

36. Pell ACH, Hughes D, Keating J, *et al.*: Brief report: fulminating fat embolism syndrome caused by paradoxical embolism through a patent foramen ovale. *N Engl J Med* 1993, 329:926–929.

37. Bern MM, Lokich JJ, Wallach SR, *et al.*: Very low doses of warfarin can prevent thrombosis in central venous catheters: a randomized prospective trial. *Ann Intern Med* 1990, 112:423–428.

38. Josa M, Siouffi SY, Silverman AB, *et al.*: Pulmonary embolism after cardiac surgery. *J Am Coll Cardiol* 1993, 21:990–996.

39. Reis SE, Polak JF, Hirsch DR, *et al.*: Frequency of deep venous thrombosis in asymptomatic patients with coronary artery bypass grafts. *Am Heart J* 1991, 122:478–482.

40. Keane MG, Ingenito EP, Goldhaber SZ: Utilization of venous thromboembolism prophylaxis in the Medical Intensive Care Unit. *Chest* 1994, 106:13–14.

41. Levine M, Hirsh J, Gent M, *et al.*: Double-blind randomised trial of very-low-dose warfarin for prevention of thromboembolism in stage IV breast cancer. *Lancet* 1994, 343:886–889.

42. Green D, Lee MY, Lim AC, *et al.*: Prevention of thromboembolism after spinal cord injury using low-molecular-weight heparin. *Ann Intern Med* 1990, 113:571–574.

43. Zelop CM: Gynecology. In *Prevention of Venous Thromboembolism*. Edited by Goldhaber SZ. New York: Marcel Dekker; 1993:405–424.

44. Dehring DJ: Anesthesia. In *Prevention of Venous Thromboembolism*. Edited by Goldhaber SZ. New York: Marcel Dekker; 1993:345–371.

45. Bergqvist D, Lindblad B: A 30-year survey of pulmonary embolism verified at autopsy: an analysis of 1274 surgical patients. *Br J Surg* 1985, 72:105–108.

46. Lindblad B, Sternby NH, Bergqvist D: Incidence of venous thromboembolism verified by necropsy after 30 years. *BMJ* 1991, 302:709–711.

CHRONIC VENOUS INSUFFICIENCY

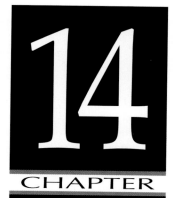

CHAPTER

C. Vaughan Ruckley

Chronic venous insufficiency (CVI) is a disorder of the lower limbs caused by unremitting high pressure in the venous system when the subject is standing erect, and also when mobile, giving rise to the term "chronic ambulatory venous hypertension." The manifestations—pigmentation, eczema, induration, and ulceration—collectively termed lipodermatosclerosis, occur in approximately 5% of the adult population in developed countries. They are more common in women (2:1) and rise in prevalence with increasing age [1,2]. The key pathophysiologic derangement in CVI is valve failure, giving rise to reflux when the patient is in the erect position and when the calf muscle pump is in diastole. Incompetence of valves in the superficial veins alone can give rise to lipodermatosclerosis and venous ulceration, but more often, and parti0cularly in the more intractable cases, there is also reflux in the deep venous system.

The causes of CVI are those diseases that impair function of venous valves or obstruct the venous channels of the limb. Primary valvular insufficiency is believed to result from a congenital or acquired connective tissue disorder in the vein wall. Secondary insufficiency results from direct valve impairment and follows either venous thrombosis or trauma. Aggravating factors are those that interfere with the mechanical function of the muscular pumps of the legs. These factors, which raise the venous pressure centrally or cause the limb to be chronically dependent, include locomotor disorders, arthropathies, neurologic disorders, obesity, pregnancy, cardiac failure, tricuspid incompetence, standing occupations, and senility. Associated diseases commonly found in patients with chronic leg ulceration, which may play a role in compounding the diagnosis, impairing healing, or complicating therapy, include arterial insufficiency, rheumatoid disease, hematologic disorders, diabetes, and the vasculitides. Approximately one third of CVI patients have a history of deep vein thrombosis, in which case it is termed *postthrombotic syndrome.* Swelling is usually more marked than in nonthrombotic CVI and there is sometimes enough outflow obstruction for the patient to experience venous claudication. More often, however, the crucial finding in the postthrombotic syndrome is the same as in nonthrombotic CVI, *ie*, valve reflux.

A thorough patient history is essential, with particular attention given to etiologic factors, aggravating factors, and associated diseases. In assessing primary varicose veins, simple physical examination may suffice, but additional investigation is required in CVI, beginning with Doppler measurement of arterial ankle-brachial pressure ratios and ultrasound imaging of potential sites of reflux. Assessment in the vascular laboratory is classified into tests of function, such as the various forms of plethysmography, or imaging, by means of the color-coded duplex scanner. Phlebography is not required unless there is doubt as to the patency of deep veins or valvular reconstruction is being contemplated.

The vast majority of patients with CVI are treated conservatively by simple physical measures, of which the most important are graduated compression therapy, high elevation of the leg when resting, and weight control. Most ulcers can be healed with ambulatory regimens, but extensive ulcers should be skin-grafted followed by surgical correction of the venous hypertension. Superficial venous incompetence is handled by conventional varicose vein surgery, and is supplemented if necessary by sclerotherapy. In any population of patients with CVI, the proportion suitable for reconstruction of the deep valves is very small.

PATHOPHYSIOLOGY

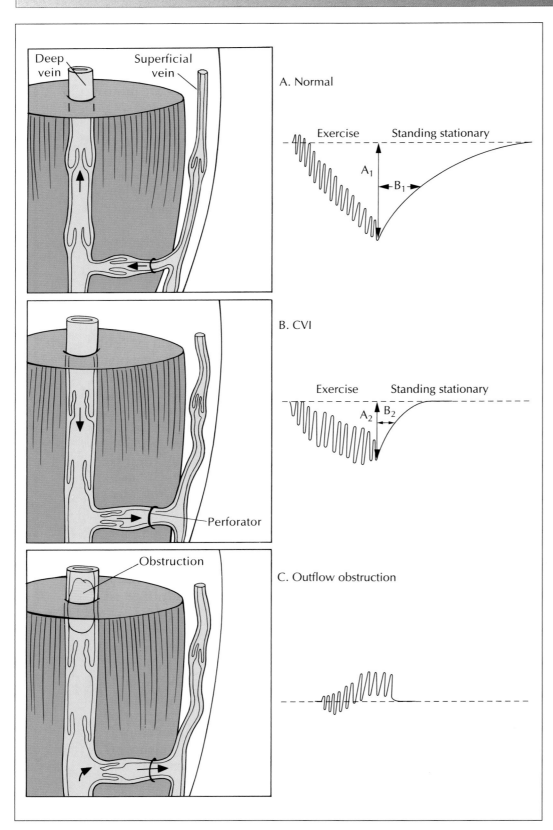

FIGURE 14-1. The pathologic changes in the skin and subcutaneous tissues are caused by ambulatory venous hypertension, *ie*, high pressure not only when standing stationary (which is normal) but also when walking.

A, The normal centripetal direction of venous flow in a perforating vein and the corresponding pressure tracing as obtained following puncture of a foot vein. During exercise the pressure falls (A_1) as a result of the action of the calf muscle pump in the presence of competent valves. Thus the fall in pressure is a measure of calf pump performance. When standing stationary, the pressure returns to its high baseline level. The slope of the refilling curve and the half refilling time (B_1) reflect venous filling by arterial inflow.

B, In chronic venous insufficiency (CVI), there is outward perforator flow during calf pump contraction and inward flow on relaxation, with little or no fall in pressure (A_2), *ie*, defective pump function. When exercise stops there is an immediate return to high baseline pressure caused by reflux through incompetent superficial or deep valves. Thus the slope of the curve and the refilling time (B_2) are a measure of the severity of venous insufficiency. **C,** When outflow is obstructed, the pressure does not fall with calf muscle contraction; it may even rise, as is shown in the tracing, which leads to the symptom of venous claudication.

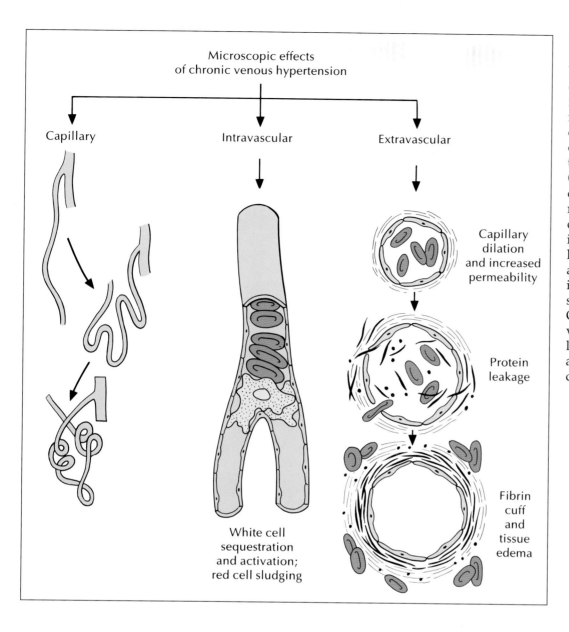

Microscopic effects
of chronic venous hypertension

Capillary   Intravascular   Extravascular

Capillary
dilation
and increased
permeability

Protein
leakage

White cell
sequestration
and activation;
red cell sludging

Fibrin
cuff
and
tissue
edema

FIGURE 14-2. Sustained hypertension impacts at the venous end of the capillary bed, upsetting the balance between hemodynamic and osmotic pressures (Starling forces). Increased capillary permeability results in the leaking out of proteins, white cells, and red cells, resulting in fibrin pericapillary cuffing, inflammatory infiltration, tissue edema, and pigmentation (hemosiderin) [3]. There is increased capillary tortuosity or "tufting." Sequestration of white cells has been shown to occur in association with chronic venous insufficiency, especially in the dependent limb [4]. Activation of these cells may play an important part in the severe chronic inflammatory change, tissue damage, and scarring that characterize the condition [5]. Observation of these events at the microvascular level has led to a search, with limited success as yet, for pharmacologic agents that may favorably influence chronic venous insufficiency.

CLINICAL PRESENTATION

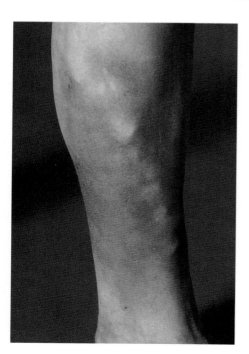

FIGURE 14-3. As with all of the skin changes involved in chronic venous insufficiency, pigmentation is usually maximal on the posteromedial aspect of the calf, where incompetent perforators connect to the long saphenous system. When there is short saphenous incompetence the skin changes are maximal on the posterolateral aspect of the lower calf.

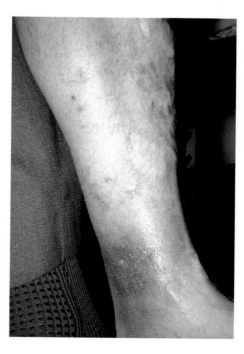

FIGURE 14-4. Acute lipodermatosclerosis should be distinguished from other common causes of acute inflammation in chronic venous insufficiency such as phlebitis and bacterial cellulitis. Lipodermatosclerosis relates to sites of perforator incompetence. Superficial phlebitis follows the course of a varicose vein. Cellulitis is more diffuse and usually relates to an infected open ulcer or the ingress of infection through a break in the skin of the foot, such as athlete's foot.

LABORATORY ASSESSMENT

TESTS OF THE VENOUS SYSTEM

	TRAINING PERIOD	COST	TYPE
Venous insufficiency			
Doppler	Long	Low	Functional
Duplex	Long	High	Anatomic and functional
Air plethysmography	Short	Medium	Functional
Photoplethysmography	Short	Medium	Functional
Foot volumetry	Short	Medium	Functional
Phlebography	Long	High	Anatomic
Outflow obstruction			
Duplex	Long	High	Anatomic and functional
Air plethysmography	Short	Medium	Functional
Strain-gauge plethysmography	Short	Medium	Functional
Impedance plethysmography	Short	Medium	Functional
Phlebography	Long	High	Anatomic

FIGURE 14-7. Tests of function are based on the response to exercise and the rate of refilling (*see* Fig. 14-1). Such tests enable quantification of the efficacy of the muscle pump, the degree of outflow obstruction, and the severity of valvular insufficiency; and, when combined with a venous tourniquet, can distinguish between superficial and deep valvular incompetence. The reference standard is direct ambulatory venous pressure measurement, but commonly used noninvasive methods include photoplethysmography, foot volumetry, and air plethysmography.

IMAGING

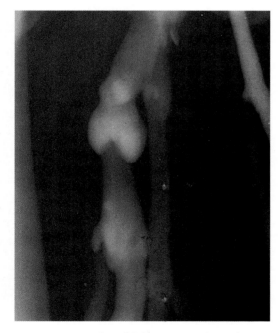

FIGURE 14-8. The phlebogram is the reference standard for imaging venous disease. For an overall display of the venous pattern of the limbs, phlebography is performed by the ascending route. For assessment of reflux, the descending route is employed. Note the superficial femoral vein, well outlined by contrast injected into the common femoral vein (descending phlebogram), with the patient standing erect. Some leakage of contrast medium through valves into the upper thigh is normal, but reflux down to the knee or beyond is pathologic and may be used as a criterion for valve reconstruction. As a result of the introduction of duplex scanning, it is now recognized that segments of deep vein, such as the popliteal segment, can sometimes be incompetent below competent proximal valves. (*Adapted from* Callam and Ruckley [6]; with permission.)

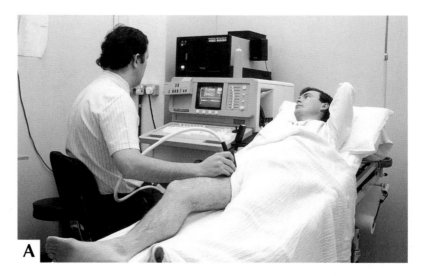

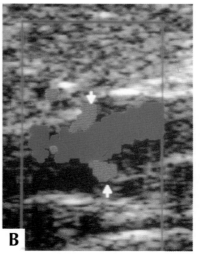

FIGURE 14-9. A, Because it is noninvasive, color-coded duplex ultrasound scanning represents the major advance in recent years in the investigation of venous disease. As well as enabling mapping of the venous system, it provides information on directions and flow velocities. Valve reflux can be directly visualized. However, we still lack a reliable formula for quantifying reflux on duplex scanning. **B,** This duplex scan shows flow through an open valve. The *red areas* indicate reversal of flow in the eddies behind the cusps.

CONSERVATIVE THERAPIES

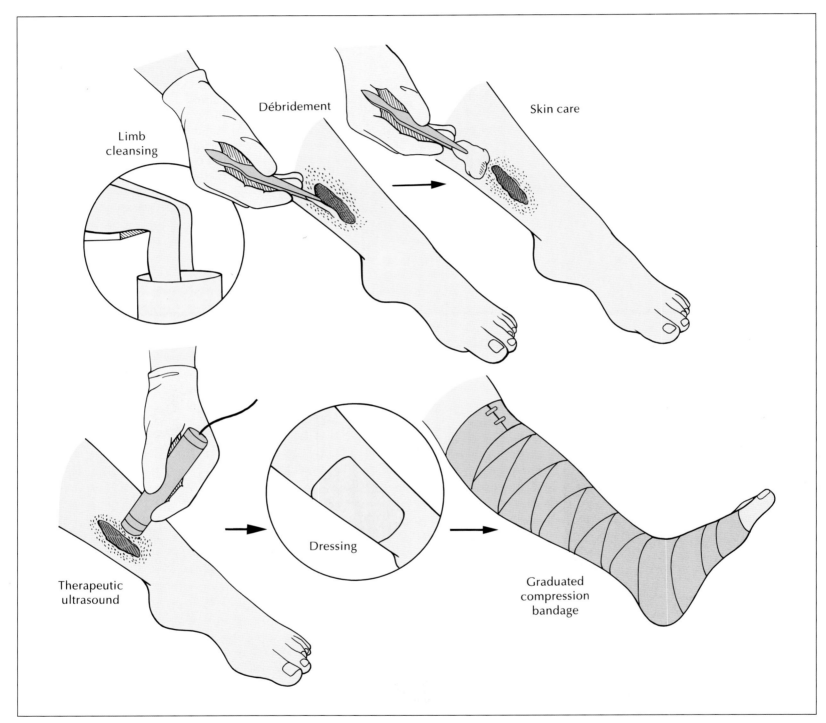

FIGURE 14-10. Because chronic leg ulcers invariably are colonized with bacteria the technique of ulcer dressing requires cleanliness rather than strict sterility. Ulcer care involves treatment of the whole patient, the limb, and the surrounding skin—as well as the ulcer itself—and is best provided by a trained wound care nurse. A simple regimen applicable to most cases would be as follows. The ulcer and the surrounding skin are washed with plain lukewarm water in a foot bath. Crusts, sloughs, and scaly skin are physically débrided. Dessicated skin is moisturized with arachis oil or 1% ichthammol. Weeping exfoliative eczema is dried with 2% eosin. Itchy eczema is treated sparingly with diluted steroid cream. Therapeutic ultrasound to the ulcer edge and surrounding skin has been shown to accelerate healing [7]. The ulcer itself is dressed with a hydrocolloid if it needs desloughing or with tulle once it has entered the clean, healing stage. The most important guiding principle is to avoid agents that may set up skin sensitivity reactions, *eg*, neomycin. Dressings should be bland, but their nature is of minor consequence compared with the crucial importance of dispelling edema and controlling the venous hypertension by physical means. Simple physical measures can effect dramatic improvement in chronic venous insufficiency. These include high elevation of the limb, graduated elastic compression, and weight control.

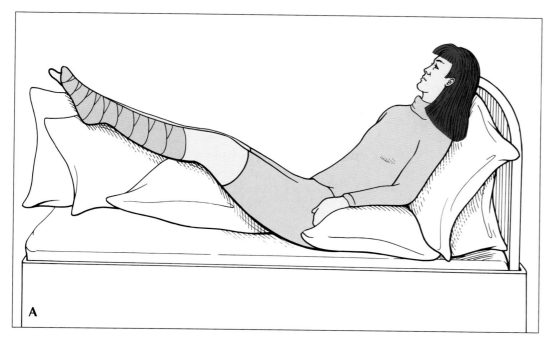

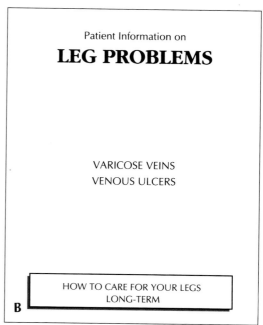

Patient Information on

LEG PROBLEMS

VARICOSE VEINS
VENOUS ULCERS

HOW TO CARE FOR YOUR LEGS
LONG-TERM

FIGURE 14-11. When advised to elevate the legs at rest, few patients will do so properly (**A**), unless given clear and precise instructions, preferably reinforced by an information sheet (**B**) and diagram. When sitting the feet should be higher than the hip and when lying down the feet should be higher than the heart. Elevation should be combined with active exercise of calf muscles, consisting of flexion, extension, and rotatory movements at the ankle. The exercises can be reinforced by providing the patient with a latex rubber band, which is held in the hands and looped around the foot so that the patient performs the exercises against elastic resistance.

PHYSIOLOGIC EFFECTS OF COMPRESSION	
INCREASE	DECREASE
Local interstitial pressure	Edema
Venous femoral flow velocity	Superficial venous pressure
Plasminogen activator release	Ambulatory venous pressure
Compression of superficial veins	Superficial vein distention
Expelled calf volume on exercise	
Venous refilling time	
Local capillary clearance	
Capillary refilling time	

FIGURE 14-12. The physiologic effects of compression therapy are beneficial in every type of venous disease ranging from simple primary varicose veins to advanced chronic venous insufficiency. Whether the therapy is bandaging or tailored hosiery the principles are the same: 1) the pressure exerted must be appropriate to the severity of disease and the build of the patient; 2) the pressure must be maximal at the ankle and in a diminishing gradient as it ascends the leg; 3) the bandage or stocking must be correctly measured and accurately and expertly applied; and 4) in chronic venous insufficiency, unlike extensive postthrombotic edema or lymphedema, compression should only be applied from the base of the toes to the tibial tuberosity.

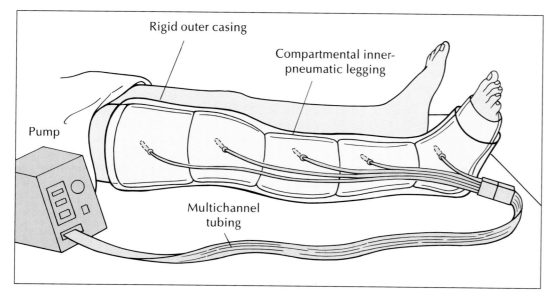

FIGURE 14-13. Sequential pneumatic compression may be employed to control edema and hasten ulcer healing. This consists of a plastic sleeve divided into compartments that are inflated in sequence, from distal to proximal, thus enhancing venous return and lymphatic clearance. The patient can use the device at home as required.

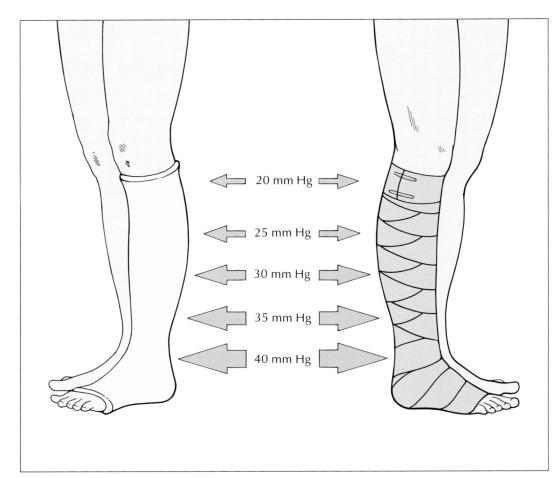

FIGURE 14-14. To control venous hypertension and heal a venous ulcer, the average patient requires a pressure of approximately 35 to 40 mm Hg at the ankle. A tall, heavily built individual will require higher pressures and a frail, elderly patient will require lower pressures. The pressures illustrated are not absolute but rather are intended to convey approximate levels and the need for a gradient. Bandaging is the preferred form of compression when there is open ulceration with exudation and when dressings require changing at regular intervals. Effective bandaging requires experience and skill. The bandage characteristics are vitally important, notably elasticity, handling qualities, conformity, and cohesiveness. Elastic bandaging has been shown to heal ulcers faster than minimal stretch bandaging [8]. Figure-of-eight application gives better and more sustained compression than simple spiral. Multilayer elastic bandaging is generally more effective than single-layer bandaging because it results in a more even distribution of pressure and is more likely to stay in place, especially if a cohesive bandage is used as the outer layer [9]. In the late stages of ulcer healing and in the long-term treatment of chronic venous insufficiency, bandaging is replaced by below-knee elastic stockings.

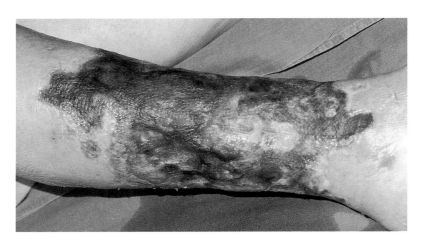

FIGURE 14-15. Although graduated compression is beneficial for the majority of patients with chronic venous insufficiency, approximately 20% of the population over 60 years of age has some degree of arterial impairment, as demonstrated by Doppler pressure measurements [10]. Compression therapy can be dangerous in these patients, and especially in diabetics [11]. Severe tissue damage can result from the application of tight elastic compression to an ischemic limb. However, a venous ulcer, if it is to be managed on an ambulatory basis, will not heal without effective compression. Therefore, coexisting arterial insufficiency should first be corrected by reconstruction or angioplasty.

OPERATIVE TREATMENT

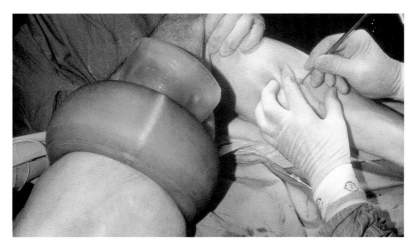

FIGURE 14-16. Depending on the sites of incompetence, superficial varicose veins are dealt with by conventional techniques including saphenofemoral and saphenopopliteal ligation, stripping of the thigh portion of the long saphenous vein, and multiple avulsions of varices. After saphenofemoral incompetence has been corrected, my preference is to carry out all subsequent surgery under roll-on pneumatic tourniquet. The sterile pneumatic cuff is inflated to approximately 160 Hg mm, rolled on from the toes to exsanguinate the limb, and then secured in place at thigh level by a latex wedge.

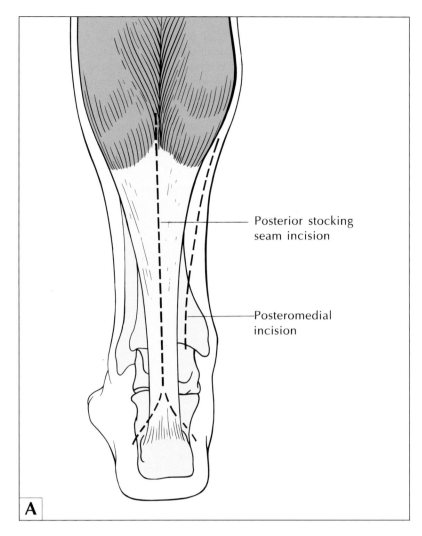

Posterior stocking
seam incision

Posteromedial
incision

A

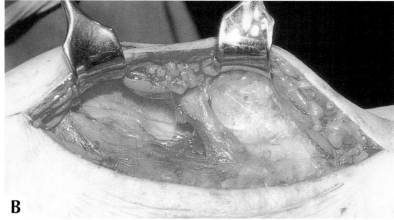

B

FIGURE 14-17. When the lower leg is heavily inflamed or scarred, a direct extrafascial approach to perforators is difficult and is associated with healing problems. **A,** The subfascial approach is therefore preferred, and can be achieved through a posteromedial approach or, better still, a posterior "stocking seam" incision, which is carried straight through the deep fascia to access to perforators as they enter the posterior compartment. **B,** To avoid healing problems, the posterior stocking seam incision should veer off the Achilles tendon at its lower end to the medial or lateral aspects. The side chosen depends on which perforators are sought.

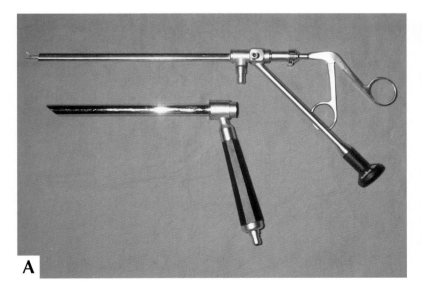

A

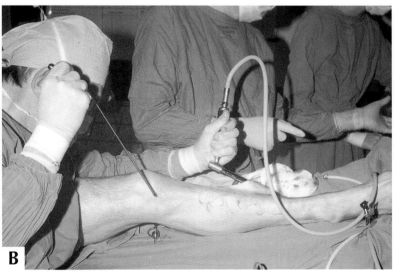

B

FIGURE 14-18. Endoscopic perforator division. The incisions described in Fig. 14-17 tend to heal poorly and commonly require prolonged postoperative bedrest. Other methods of dealing with perforators have therefore been described, including endoscopic perforator interruption. **A,** The Wolf cannula, the endoscope, and scissors. **B,** The cannula, with connected fiberoptic cable, is inserted under the deep fascia of the calf to give access to the perforator, which can then be clipped or cauterized.

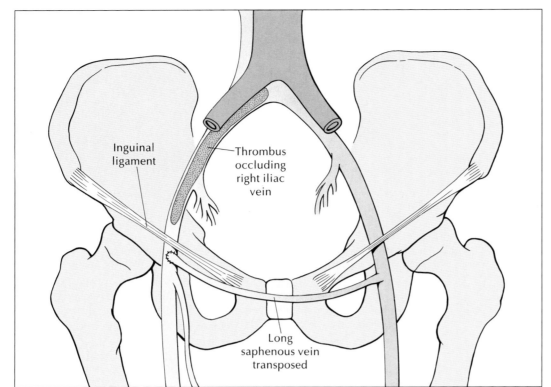

Inguinal
ligament

Thrombus
occluding
right iliac
vein

Long
saphenous vein
transposed

FIGURE 14-19. When chronic venous insufficiency is associated with proximal venous outflow occlusion, venous claudication tends to be the most disabling symptom. If direct venous pressure measurement shows a substantial rise in pressure with exercise, then a Palma crossover femorofemoral venous bypass may be indicated. Some authors advocate the simultaneous construction of an arteriovenous fistula, which is closed a few weeks later. My preference is rather to rely on the pressure gradient, simple physical measures, and anticoagulation to maintain venous flow through the graft.

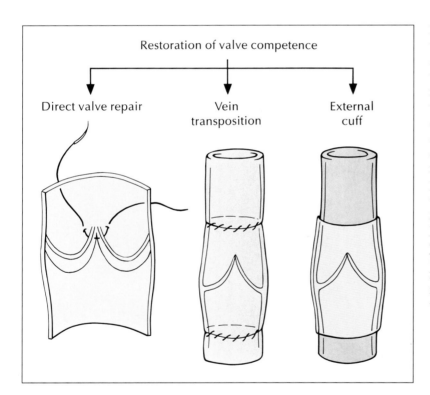

Restoration of valve competence

Direct valve repair   Vein
transposition   External
cuff

FIGURE 14-20. In approximately one third of patients with chronic venous insufficiency, valvular insufficiency is limited to the superficial veins and perforators. In this group, accurate surgery to the saphenous systems and perforators will be sufficient to relieve symptoms and ameliorate the skin changes. In another third, postthrombotic damage will be observed in the deep veins, and will render valve reconstruction impracticable. Thus in only about a third of patients with chronic venous insufficiency is it appropriate to consider deep valve reconstruction. This number is further reduced by the general frailty of the chronic leg ulcer population and because a substantial proportion of these patients can be kept ulcer-free by means of properly fitted and supervised graduated compression therapy. There remains a small group of patients whose ulceration proves intractable, despite effective correction of superficial venous incompetence. Such patients may be considered for valve repair, valve transposition, or an externally positioned valve cuff [12–14]. Until larger series and longer follow-up studies and preferably randomized trials are available, this type of surgery should be considered investigational.

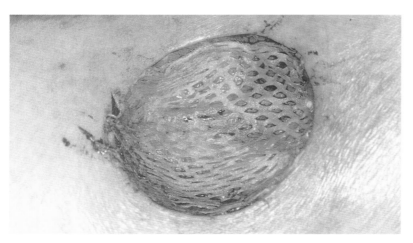

FIGURE 14-21. An excised ulcer that has been covered with a mesh graft. The majority of ulcers (<10 cm^2) can be healed within 3 months by an ambulatory regimen of dressings and graduated compression therapy. Larger ulcers and those proving intractable to ambulatory care should be skin-grafted. Recurrence is likely unless the underlying vascular abnormality is also corrected.

REFERENCES

1. Bobek K, Cajzl L, Cepelak V, *et al.*: Etudes de la frequence des maladies phlebologiques et de l'influence de quelques facteurs etiologiques. *Phlebologie* 1966, 19:217–230.

2. Borshberg E: The prevalence of varicose veins in the lower extremities. Basel: S. Karger; 1967:85–97.

3. Browse NL, Gray L, Jarrett PEM, *et al.*: Blood and vein-wall fibrinolytic activity in health and vascular disease. *BMJ* 1977, 1:478–481.

4. Thomas PRS, Nash GB, Dormandy JA: White cell accumulation in the dependent legs of patients with venous hypertension: a possible mechanism for trophic changes in the skin. *BMJ* 1988, 296:1693–1695.

5. Coleridge Smith PD, Thomas P, Scurr JH, *et al.*: Causes of venous ulceration: a new hypothesis. *BMJ* 296:1726–1727.

6. Callam MJ, Ruckley CV: Chronic venous insufficiency and leg ulcer. In *Surgical Management of Vascular Disease.* Edited by Bell PRF, Jamieson CW, Ruckley CV. London: Saunders; 1992:1267–1303.

7. Callam MJ, Harper DR, Dale JJ, *et al.*: A controlled trial of weekly ultrasound therapy in chronic leg ulceration. *Lancet* 1987, II:204–206.

8. Callam MJ, Harper DR, Dale JJ, *et al.*: Lothian and Forth Valley Leg Ulcer Healing Trial. Part 1: elastic versus nonelastic bandaging in the treatment of chronic leg ulceration. *Phlebology* 1992, 7:136–141.

9. Blair SD, Wright DDI, Backhouse CM, *et al.*: Sustained healing and compression of chronic venous ulcers. *BMJ* 1988, 297–230.

10. Callam MJ, Harper DR, Dale JJ, *et al.*: Arterial disease in chronic leg ulceration: an underestimated hazard. *BMJ* 1987, 294:929–930.

11. Callam MJ, Ruckley CV, Dale JJ: Hazards of compression treatment of the leg: an estimate from Scottish surgeons. *BMJ* 1987, 295:1382–1383.

12. Ferris EB, Kirstner RL: Femoral vein reconstruction in the management of chronic venous insufficiency. *Arch Surg* 117:1571–1579.

13. Raju S: Venous insufficiency in the lower limb and stasis ulceration. *Ann Surg* 1983, 197:688–697.

14. Eriksson I: Vein valve surgery for deep valvular incompetence. In *Controversies in the Management of Venous Disorders.* Edited by Eklof B, Gjores JE, Thulesius O, *et al.* London: Butterworths; 1989:267–290.

Cardiac Tumors

PRIMARY CARDIAC TUMORS

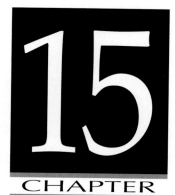

15

CHAPTER

Michael F. Allard, Glenn P. Taylor, Janet E. Wilson, and Bruce M. McManus

Neoplasms that arise in the heart are relatively rare. Even the most common primary tumors (*ie*, myxomas) have been estimated to occur in fewer than two or three people per 10,000 population. When primary cardiac tumors occur, however, the chances of morbid or fatal consequences are considerable because of the crucial nature of the various cardiac structures involved. The complications attributed to such tumors are as protean as the tumors themselves and depend on the tumor's location, size, mobility, friability, and invasiveness. Primary tumors of the heart and pericardium are important more for their local effects than for their potential metastatic behavior. Cardiac tumors present primarily as rhythm disturbances, contractility abnormalities, obstructions, valvular regurgitations, embolic events, or pericardial effusions with tamponade. In addition, presentations may resemble conventional ischemia, cardiomyopathy, systemic or local infection, or intrinsic valvular disease. Mimicry of noninfectious inflammatory diseases, pulmonary vascular diseases, endocrinopathies, and intrinsic shunts is uncommon but should be considered. Both primary and secondary tumors may thus present in varied and unpredictable ways, and the manner in which they present may not necessarily reflect their pathologic nature or histogenetic origin.

The availability of numerous imaging modalities has enhanced the likelihood that the presence and nature of a tumor can be established during life. Surgical resection and, on occasion, intravascular endomyocardial biopsy may allow a tumor's pathobiologic features to be characterized. With these advances, the chances for definitive or adjunctive therapy are increased, and appropriate recommendations can be offered to patients and their families. To date, however, the natural history of many primary cardiac tumors remains ill defined.

The frequency of certain primary tumors of the heart and pericardium is distinct for particular age groups. Indeed, outcomes depend on the patient's age. The early occurrence of tumors with a subsequently rapid growth is a poor prognostic sign. For example, the growth of primary neoplasms in newborns or infants may outpace the normal growth rate of the heart and thus present as terminal disease. A more protracted course with a later clinical presentation is more likely when tumors that arise in the adult heart are similar in histology to those in children. Occasionally, transplantation is a therapeutic option.

Although the cell of origin is well established for such tumors as rhabdomyomas, the apparently pluripotential "reserve cells" of myxomas, for example, are much less clearly understood. Similarly, mesotheliomas of the atrioventricular node are now believed to reflect neoplastic endothelial proliferations, yet the reason for such localized growth abnormalities is not known. Cardiac tumors diagnosed during life can be excised and studied not only for a definitive histologic diagnosis but also to discern phenotypic and genotypic features using immunohistochemical, molecular, biochemical, and other biological studies. Such diagnostic studies may distinguish tissue damage due to interventional procedures from true proliferative (neoplastic) lesions [1,2].

In this chapter, we present the key epidemiologic findings, clinical presentations, morphologic features, natural history, results of imaging, and pathologic characteristics of common benign and malignant primary tumors of the heart and pericardial tissues, as well as current modes of therapy. Benign and malignant primary tumors of large and small veins, arteries, and lymphatic vessels may cause a spectrum of obstructive syndromes beyond the scope of this work. Readers should consult several major papers [3–11] that describe the features of cardiac tumors for details not provided here.

EPIDEMIOLOGY

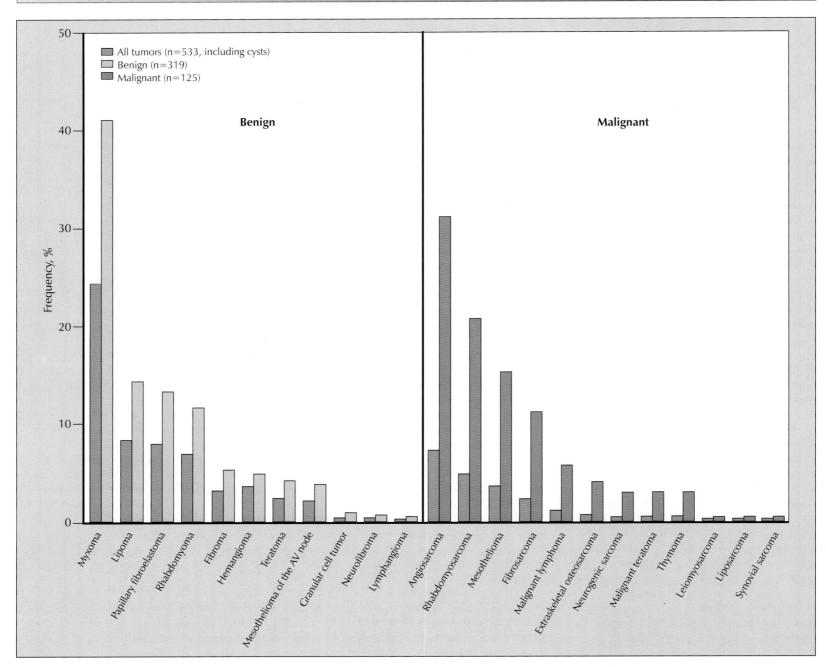

FIGURE 15-1. In 1978, the Armed Forces Institute of Pathology reported more than 500 cases of primary benign tumors and cysts and malignant tumors of the heart and pericardium [3]. The frequency of certain reported tumors is similar to that observed in other series [12–14]. Myxomas are by far the most common benign tumor, while lipomas, papillary fibroelastomas, and rhabdomyomas occur with almost equal frequency. Malignant tumors are primarily sarcomatous, including those that originate from the vasculature, cardiac muscle, and fibrous tissue. As a percentage of malignant tumors, angiosarcomas and rhabdomyosarcomas are by far the most common. In essence, any number of primary malignancies that represent the cells and tissues of the different germ layers may occur.

RESULTS OF AUTOPSY SERIES

STUDY	YEARS REPRESENTED	TOTAL AUTOPSIES, n	TOTAL PRIMARY TUMORS, n	BENIGN, %	INCIDENCE, %
Nadas and Ellison [12]	1914–1966	11,000	9	89	0.08
Fine [13]	1916–1962	12,600	10	100	0.08
	1957–1964	5764	7	100	0.12
Lam et al. [14]	1972–1991	12,485	7	100	0.06
Total	1914–1991	41,849	33	96	0.08

FIGURE 15-2. Three autopsy series emphasizing the number of primary benign and malignant cardiac tumors have been reported [12–14]. These series represent nearly 75 years of research and more than 41,000 autopsies. The rate of primary cardiac neoplasms found at autopsy has not changed during this period. Of 33 tumors, 96% were benign. The average rate of tumors in the series was 0.08%, which is similar to that in other reports. In a work by Chan et al. [15] that included 790 autopsies on children with malignant tumors, 16 primary cardiac tumors were found; of these, 94% were benign.

OPERATIVE EXPERIENCE

STUDY	YEARS REPRESENTED	TUMORS REPORTED, n	BENIGN, %
Simcha et al. [7]	1950–1970	8	100
Fine [13]	1957–1964	12	92
Cooley [16]	1957–1987	127	—
Tazelaar et al. [17]	1957–1991	106	100
Molina et al. [18]	1959–1989	124	83
Moosdorf et al. [19]	1960–1990	54	78
Dein et al. [20]	1961–1986	42	81
Guang-ying [21]	1962–1988	656	97
Tschirkov et al. [22]	1970–1988	66	98
Sezai [23]	1986–1987	317	—
	1984–1989	89	93
Blondeau [24]	25 years	533	90

FIGURE 15-3. Operative experience from institutions in seven countries gathered over a period of approximately 40 years illustrate that most of the cardiac tumors identified are likely to be benign [7,13,16–24]. Two of the tumors reported by Simcha et al. [7] were found at autopsy; the precise years of the Blondeau study [24] were not provided.

AUTOPSY RESULTS BY AGE: BENIGN TUMORS

BENIGN TUMOR	% OF GROUP		
	ADULTS	CHILDREN	INFANTS
Myxoma	46	15	0
Lipoma	21	0	0
Papillary fibroelastoma	16	0	0
Rhabdomyoma	2	46	65
Fibroma	3	15	12
Hemangioma	5	5	4
Teratoma	1	13	18
Mesothelioma of the AV node	3	4	2
Granular cell tumor	1	0	0
Neurofibroma	1	1	0
Lymphangioma	1	0	0
Hamartoma	0	1	0

FIGURE 15-4. Data representing the extensive investigations of the Armed Forces Institute of Pathology [3] as well as the cumulative experience of other researchers [12–14] (see also Fig. 15-5). A total of 265, 82, and 49 benign tumors were found in adults (aged >16 years), children (aged 1 to 16 years), and infants (aged <1 year), respectively. Myxomas were the most commonly reported benign tumors in adults, whereas rhabdomyomas were the most common benign tumors in both children and infants; benign teratomas also occurred frequently in children and infants. When no specific age group was reported (24 tumors), the data were included in the adult category. AV—atrioventricular.

AUTOPSY RESULTS BY AGE: MALIGNANT TUMORS

	% OF GROUP		
TUMOR TYPE	ADULTS	CHILDREN	INFANTS
Angiosarcoma	33	0	0
Rhabdomyosarcoma	21	33	66
Mesothelioma	16	0	0
Fibrosarcoma	11	11	33
Malignant lymphoma	6	0	0
Extraskeletal osteosarcoma	4	0	0
Thymoma	3	0	0
Neurogenic sarcoma	3	11	0
Leiomyosarcoma	1	0	0
Liposarcoma	1	0	0
Synovial sarcoma	1	0	0
Malignant teratoma	0	44	0

FIGURE 15-5. A total of 117, nine, and three malignant tumors were found in adults (aged >16 years), children (aged 1 to 16 years), and infants (aged <1 year), respectively. Angiosarcomas were the most commonly reported malignant tumors in adults, but rhabdomyosarcomas and mesotheliomas were also relatively common. Malignant teratomas were the most common tumors in children. Rhabdomyosarcomas were the most frequently reported malignant tumors in infants, with fibrosarcomas the second most common. When no specific age group was reported (24 tumors), the data were included in the adult category.

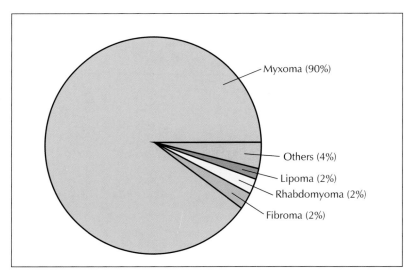

FIGURE 15-6. Relative frequency of various operatively removed benign cardiac tumors among 1619 gathered by researchers from more than 21 institutions in seven countries over approximately 40 years. The vast majority of benign tumors are myxomas. The category "others" includes papillary fibroelastomas, hemangiomas, mesotheliomas, lymphangiomas, teratomas, granular cell tumors, neurofibromas, hamartomas, angiomas, and papillomas.

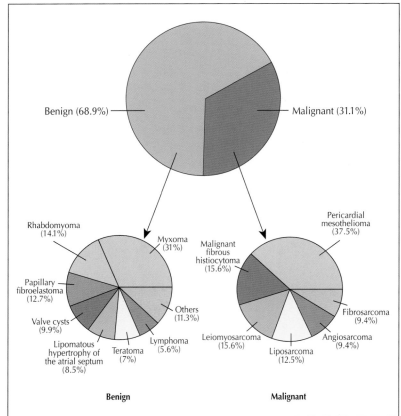

FIGURE 15-7. Since 1990, numerous individual cases and small series of primary and secondary tumor involvement of the heart and pericardium have been reported based on autopsy results. In these studies, 71 benign and 32 malignant tumors were reported. Valve cysts, angiomatous and lipomatous lesions, and mesotheliomas were emphasized. In addition, numerous examples of cardiac myxomas, papillary fibroelastomas, and rhabdomyomas were reported, and the occurrence of leiomyosarcoma in the heart and great vessels was highlighted. The category "others" includes lipomas, mesotheliomas of the atrioventricular (AV) node, fibromas, hemangiomas, granular cell tumors, and neurofibromas.

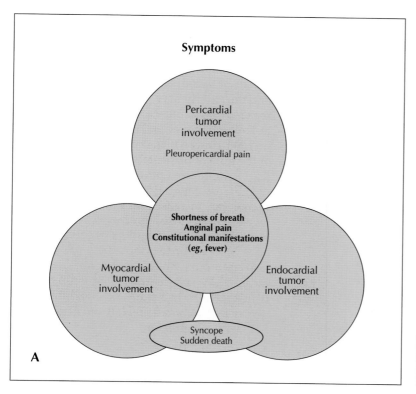

Symptoms

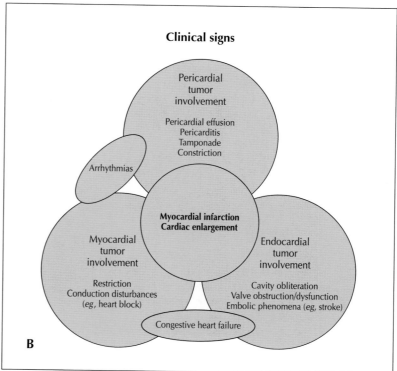

Clinical signs

FIGURE 15-8. Cardiac tumors can have protean effects depending on their location. Clinical manifestations are directly related to the site of tumor involvement, *ie*, the particular chamber as well as the distribution of the tumor within the pericardium, myocardium, and/or endocardium. The Venn diagrams show the general correspondence of symptoms (**A**) and clinical signs (**B**) to tumor site. Almost any cardiologic syndrome may result from tumors involving the heart and pericardium. Angina and myocardial infarction may occur secondary to extrinsic (*ie*, compressive, invasive) or intrinsic (*ie*, embolic) involvement of a coronary artery.

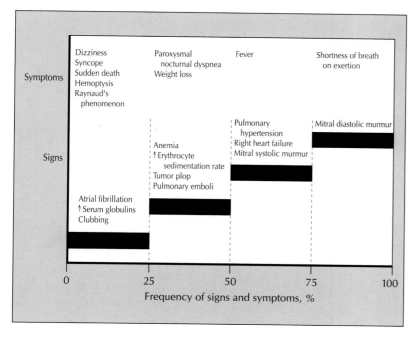

FIGURE 15-9. Patients with myxoma typically present with a clinical triad that includes systemic symptoms, embolic phenomena, and manifestations related to valvular or intracavitary disease [25]. Physical findings reflect the obstructive nature of the myxoma. The intensity of valve-related murmurs often varies with changes in body position or respiratory movements. A *tumor plop* is an auscultatory finding that follows the second heart sound; it is often confused with a third heart sound or the opening snap of the mitral valve. Tumor plop is believed to be caused by sudden tension on the stalk as the tumor prolapses into the left ventricle during diastole or by tumor striking the myocardium [26].

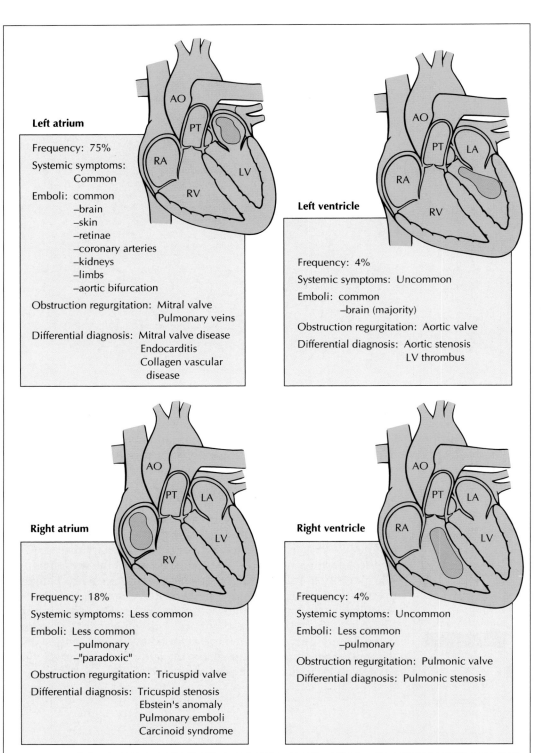

Left atrium

Frequency: 75%

Systemic symptoms:
    Common

Emboli: common
    –brain
    –skin
    –retinae
    –coronary arteries
    –kidneys
    –limbs
    –aortic bifurcation

Obstruction regurgitation: Mitral valve
                         Pulmonary veins

Differential diagnosis: Mitral valve disease
                      Endocarditis
                      Collagen vascular
                         disease

Left ventricle

Frequency: 4%

Systemic symptoms: Uncommon

Emboli: common
           –brain (majority)

Obstruction regurgitation: Aortic valve

Differential diagnosis: Aortic stenosis
                      LV thrombus

Right atrium

Frequency: 18%

Systemic symptoms: Less common

Emboli: Less common
        –pulmonary
        –"paradoxic"

Obstruction regurgitation: Tricuspid valve

Differential diagnosis: Tricuspid stenosis
                      Ebstein's anomaly
                      Pulmonary emboli
                      Carcinoid syndrome

Right ventricle

Frequency: 4%

Systemic symptoms: Uncommon

Emboli: Less common
        –pulmonary

Obstruction regurgitation: Pulmonic valve

Differential diagnosis: Pulmonic stenosis

FIGURE 15-10. Clinical manifestations of cardiac myxomas according to chamber involvement. Most myxomas occur sporadically [27]. Patients are predominantly female and middle-aged, although children and the elderly may also be affected. Myxomas may be familial, occurring more often in young patients, and are often multiple, involving more than one cardiac chamber at the time of presentation (*ie*, synchronous) [27]. Systemic symptoms may include fever, weight loss, fatigue, anemia (possibly hemolytic), increased immunoglobulin levels, leukocytosis, thrombocytopenia, erythrocytosis, Raynaud's phenomenon, and clubbing; breast fibroadenomas may also be found [28]. Ao—aorta; LA—left atrium; LV—left ventricle; PT—pulmonary trunk; RA—right atrium; RV—right ventricle. (*Adapted from* Hall and Cooley [29]; with permission.)

CASE 1: LEFT ATRIAL MYXOMA

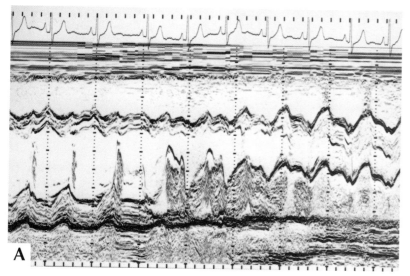

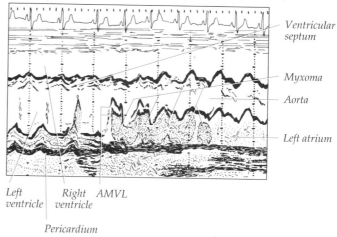

Ventricular
septum

Myxoma

Aorta

Left atrium

Left
ventricle   Right   AMVL
ventricle

Pericardium

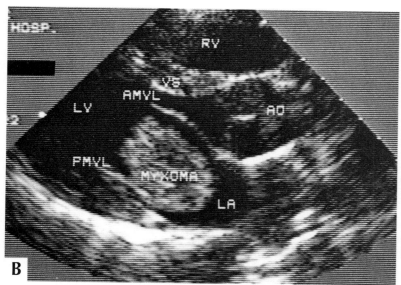

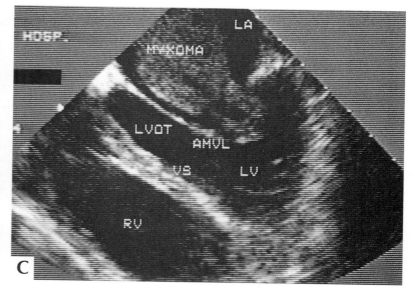

FIGURE 15-11. A, M-mode echocardiogram showing a collection of echoes behind the anterior leaflet of the mitral valve (AMVL). Transthoracic two-dimensional echocardiogram (**B**) and transesophageal two-dimensional echocardiogram (**C**) showing a left atrial (LA) mass prolapsing into and obstructing the mitral valve orifice. Note the superior resolution of the transesophageal echocardiogram. Although not visible here, the myxoma was attached to the mid-portion of the atrial septum.

Typically, LA myxomas attach to the fossa ovalis; although myxomas are rarely located posteriorly, a mass in this location should arouse suspicion of malignancy. During diastole, an atrial myxoma is visualized on M-mode echocardiography as multiple echoes behind the AMVL on the left and the tricuspid valve on the right. M-mode echocardiography is most useful for intracavitary,

pedunculated masses of the LA; however, it is less effective for visualizing tumors during systole and immobile tumors. Although ventricular myxomas can be seen as multiple intracavitary echoes, they are less frequently detected by this method. Two-dimensional echocardiography provides sufficient information (ie, size, attachment, and mobility) for surgical treatment. This imaging modality reveals intracavitary masses with alternating areas of echodensity and lucency and is useful for visualizing small, ventricular, and nonprolapsed tumors. Two-dimensional echocardiography also allows recognition of multiple masses. LV—left ventricle; LVOT—left ventricular outflow tract; PMVL—posterior leaflet of mitral valve; RV—right ventricle; VS—ventricular septum. (Courtesy of C.R. Thompson, MD, St. Paul's Hospital, Vancouver, BC.)

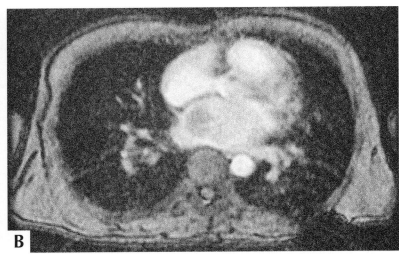

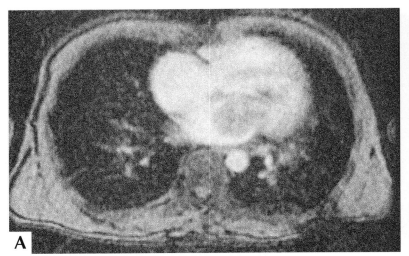

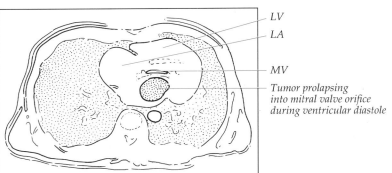

LV
LA
MV
Tumor prolapsing
into mitral valve orifice
during ventricular diastole

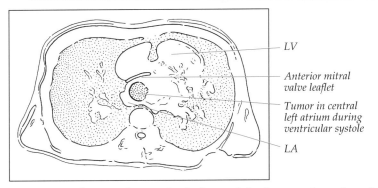

LV
Anterior mitral
valve leaflet
Tumor in central
left atrium during
ventricular systole
LA

FIGURE 15-12. Axial magnetic resonance images during diastole (**A**) and systole (**B**). In *A*, the left atrial (LA) mass has prolapsed into the mitral valve orifice during diastole, whereas in *B*, the mass has moved cephalad during systole into the body of the LA. Magnetic resonance imaging typically allows a large field of view with increased definition of prolapse, valvular obstruction, and chamber size.

Various other invasive and noninvasive diagnostic modalities can be used to evaluate intracavitary masses. Computed tomography can provide high resolution and a degree of tissue discrimination and is also useful for evaluating the extent of myocardial, pericardial, or extracardiac tumor involvement. Radionuclide imaging using isotopically labeled erythrocytes can identify myxomas, which appear as areas of diminished activity with altered myocardial uptake or, using ventriculography, can reveal an intracavitary filling defect. This technique is less sensitive than echocardiography or angiography, however.

Angiography may be particularly useful when noninvasive visualization of the mass is inadequate, when not all chambers can be visualized, or when other cardiac disease is suspected. Angiography may identify LA myxomas when opaque medium is injected into the left ventricular (LV) cavity and if sufficient regurgitation is present. Injection into the superior or inferior vena cava can be used to identify myxomas in the right atrium; however, embolization may occur during angiography, particularly if myxoma is not suspected. To reduce this risk, echocardiographic studies can be performed prior to angiography.

Coronary angiography may demonstrate a vascular blush in the myxoma, although vascularization of a LA thrombus may also be demonstrated. Cardiac catheterization typically reveals elevation in intracavitary pressures upstream from the tumor. In particular, increases in pulmonary wedge pressure and right atrial pressure as well as pulmonary hypertension may be observed with LA myxomas. (Courtesy of P. Cooperberg, MD, St. Paul's Hospital, Vancouver, BC.)

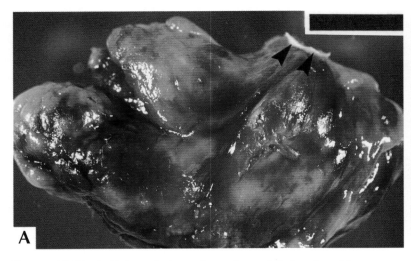

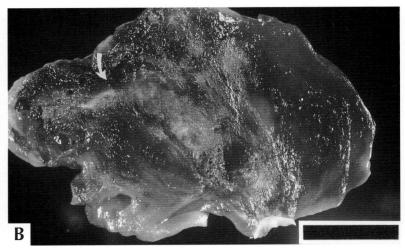

FIGURE 15-13. A, External view of a pedunculated polypoid myxoma with an irregular and glistening surface. The cut surface contains a short stalk with an accompanying rim of tissue from the atrial sep-

tum (*arrowheads*). **B,** The surface appears gelatinous with focal areas of hemorrhage (*curved arrow*). These findings are typical for pedunculated myxomas; sessile myxomas are uncommon. Bar = 2 cm.

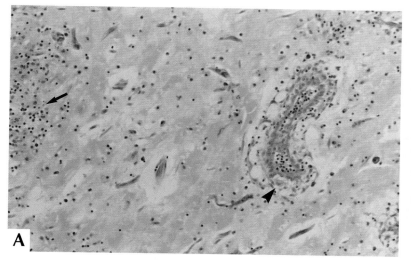

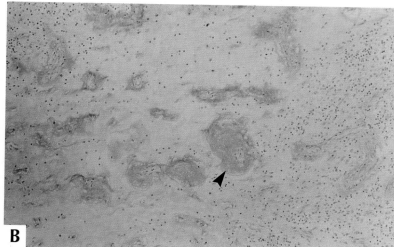

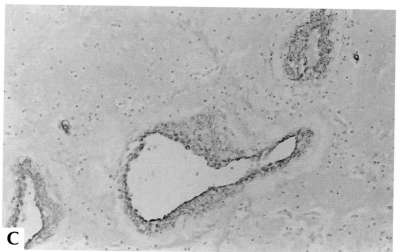

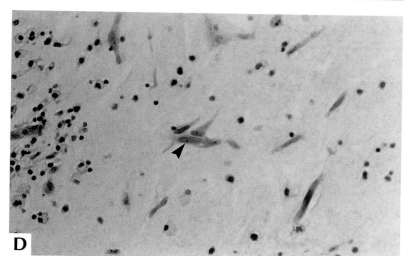

FIGURE 15-14. **A,** Abundant eosinophilic myxoid matrix containing polygonal to stellate myxoma cells distributed singly, in small groups, and around thin-walled vascular channels (*arrowhead*). Focal collections of mononuclear cells (macrophages, lymphocytes, plasma cells) are also seen (*arrow*). Myxomas may also contain areas of recent and old hemorrhage as well as calcification and metaplastic bone formation (hematoxylin and eosin, × 200).

B, Large quantities of acid mucopolysaccharide are present in the myxoma matrix, primarily in the vicinity of vascular channels (*arrowhead*) (Alcian blue, × 100).

C, Cells forming the vascular channels show endothelial differentiation and are positive for factor VIII. Myxomas contain a diverse population of cells that are positive for such differentiation markers as S-100, a protein present in Schwann cells and melanocytes, and neuron-specific enolase, a cytoplasmic protein in axons [30]. Ultrastructurally, myxoma cells resemble multipotential mesenchymal cells. The exact nature of the differentiation and histogenesis of myxo-mas remains unknown (immunoperoxidase, factor VIII, × 200). **D,** The myxoma cells embedded within the matrix are polygonal to stellate, so-called *lepidic cells* (*arrowhead*) (Movat pentachrome stain, × 400).

CASE 2: CALCIFIED MYXOMA

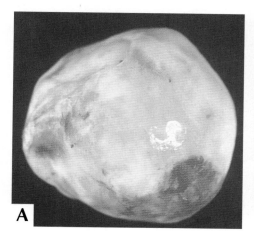

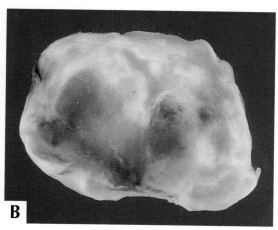

FIGURE 15-15. Gross photograph of an operatively excised myxoma from a 71-year-old woman. **A,** Myxoma with typical irregular and glistening surface. **B,** The cut surface reveals focal hemorrhage (*see also* Fig. 15-13). (*continued*)

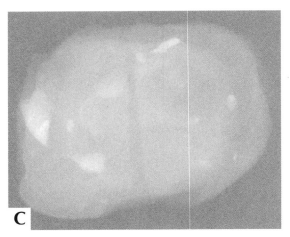

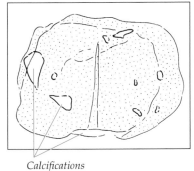

FIGURE 15-15. (*continued*) **C,** The myxoma contains areas of calcification, which should lead one to suspect a cardiac neoplasm, especially in children. (Courtesy of J. Radio, MD, University of Nebraska Medical Center, Omaha, NE.)

C

Calcifications

CASE 3: RHABDOMYOMA

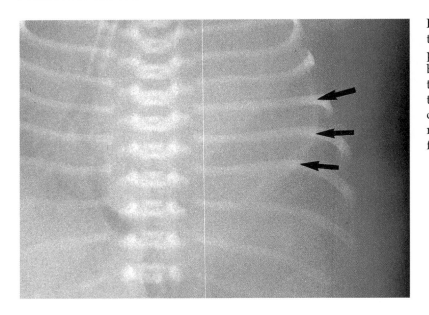

FIGURE 15-16. Radiograph in a neonate showing marked soft tissue edema with a thin, partial rim of calcification at the left lateral periphery of the cardiac shadow (*arrows*). A large cardiac mass had been identified in a female fetus at 29 weeks of gestation. Connection of the flow circuits of the fetal heart at the atrial level increases the possibility that alterations in blood flow to any chamber will cause congestion in the right atrium. The resultant heart failure is manifest by gross fetal edema [31]. The presence or suspicion of fetal hydrops suggest cardiac rhabdomyoma.

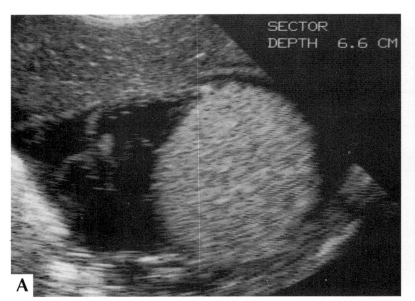

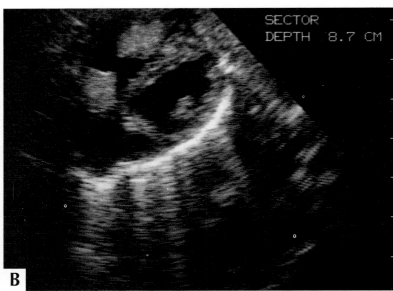

A

B

FIGURE 15-17. **A,** Two-dimensional echocardiogram obtained shortly after birth showing a large cardiac mass with several smaller echogenic foci. **B,** An echocardiogram from a different patient depicts the multiple nodules typical of rhabdomyoma. Clinically, rhabdomyo-mas may also be suggested by electrocardiographic evidence of ectopic atrial rhythm with retrograde atrial depolarization or ventricular preexcitation syndrome [31,32].

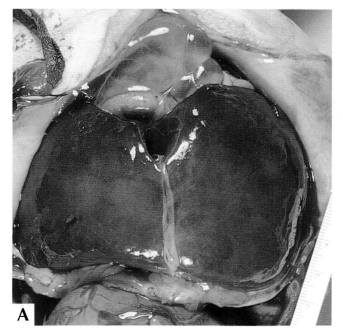

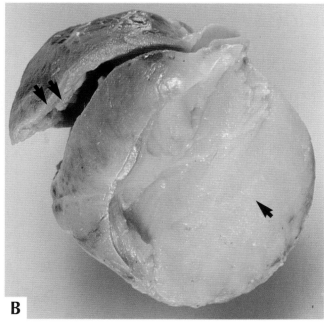

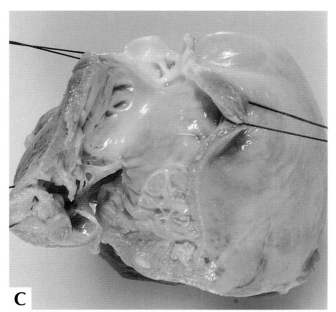

FIGURE 15-18. The infant died 5 hours after birth from a combination of respiratory failure caused by pulmonary hypoplasia (related to pleural effusion and cardiomegaly) as well as cardiac failure caused by left ventricular outflow obstruction. **A**, The exposed body cavity demonstrates marked cardiomegaly and congesting hepatomegaly. **B**, The right ventricular outflow tract is compressed by a large septal tumor (*arrow*), and smaller rhabdomyomas (*double arrows*) are present in the apex of the right ventricle. **C**, The septal rhabdomyoma has a homogeneous, slightly soft cut surface. There is no hemorrhage or necrosis; however, there is a thin rim of peripheral dystrophic calcification.

  Rhabdomyomas may vary in diameter from millimeters to several centimeters and are multiple in more than 90% of patients [3]. Smaller rhabdomyomas are often intramural in position, whereas a larger one may extend into the ventricular cavity [33]. Although most rhabdomyomas are intramyocardial, some may cover the epicardial or endocardial surface of the heart [3].

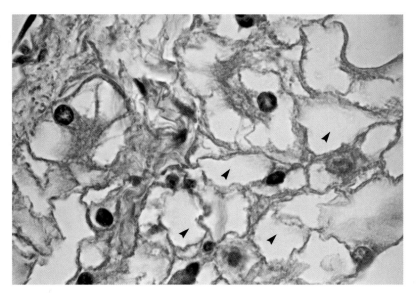

FIGURE 15-19. Photomicrograph showing the large, vacuolated spider cells of rhabdomyomas (*arrowheads*). Loss of glycogen during routine histologic processing results in the vacuolated appearance. A typical spider cell has a central nucleus and cytoplasmic mass, with cytoplasmic strands extending to the periphery of the cell. Spider cells are always present and are the hallmark of rhabdomyomas. Other features of these tumors include bundles of myofilaments and a cytoplasm rich in mitochondria and glycogen, which have been demonstrated by electron microscopy [26].

CASE 4: FIBROMA

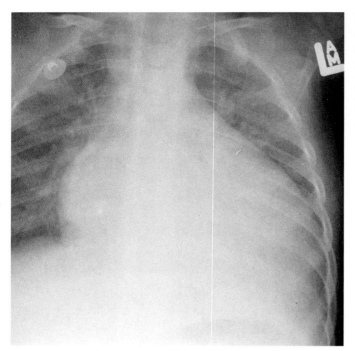

FIGURE 15-20. Chest radiograph of a 2 1/2-year-old boy showing marked cardiomegaly—a common finding in patients with fibroma. Because of the clinically obscure nature of the presenting symptoms, fibromas are usually not diagnosed before surgery or postmortem examination [34]. This patient presented with respiratory distress and heart failure. Fibromas are usually located in the ventricular myocardium, particularly the anterior free wall of the left ventricle or the ventricular septum, and can be readily defined on cardiac catheterization.

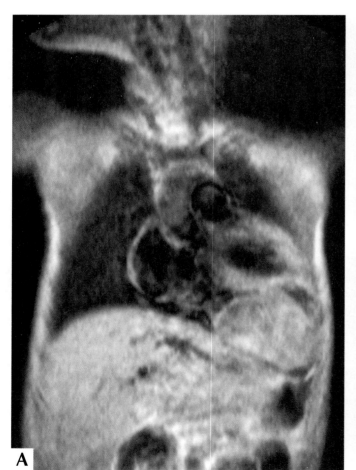

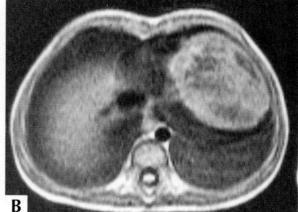

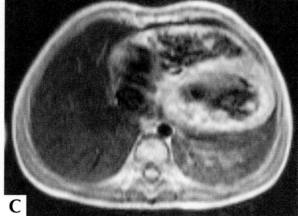

FIGURE 15-21. Magnetic resonance images illustrating a large tumor in the right ventricular apex, impinging on the apical septum. In the coronal view, the prominent mass indents the septum (**A**). In the axial views, the tumor shows areas of tissue inhomogeneity (**B**) and indents the ventricular septum (**C**).

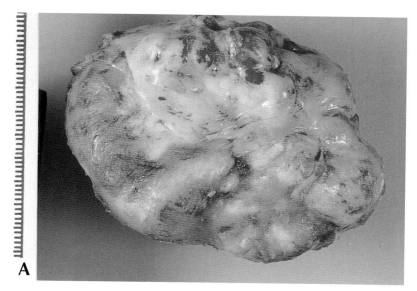

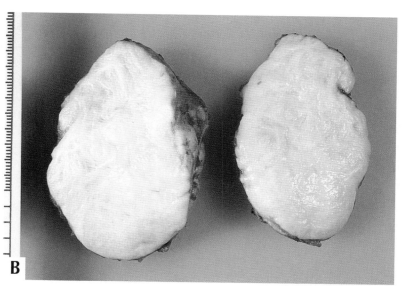

FIGURE 15-22. The tumor shown in Fig. 15-21 was excised, and the patient remained tumor-free at 4-year follow-up. **A**, On gross examination, the excised tumor was found to be solid and fibrous, without necrosis or hemorrhage. **B**, The cut surface was bosselated and firm. Fibromas are not encapsulated and extend into the surrounding myocardium [3]. When discovered, they typically range from 3 to 10 cm in diameter. They are composed of hyalinized fibrous tissues, and areas of dystrophic calcification and cystic degeneration may be seen in the central portion (probably owing to an inadequate blood supply).

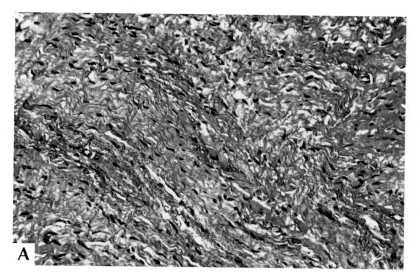

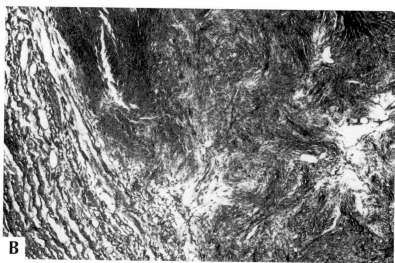

FIGURE 15-23. Photomicrographs of the fibroma discussed above showing fascicles of spindle cells (fibroblasts) with abundant extracellular collagen (**A**; Masson's trichrome, × 50). The degree of cellularity varies, and mitotic figures are rare. Fibrous tissue at the tumor periphery may contain prominent elastic and collagen tissue. The tumor may infiltrate adjacent myocardium (**B**; Masson's trichrome, × 10). A fibroma typically contains few myocytes and has limited vascularity.

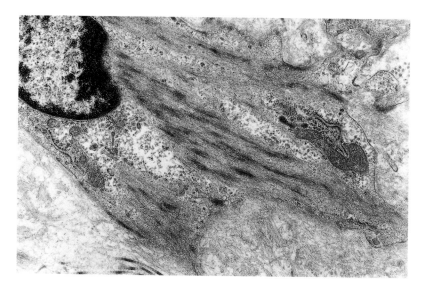

FIGURE 15-24. Electron micrograph of the fibroma discussed above showing typical myofibroblast tumor cells. Smooth muscle cell features include bundles of thin (actin) filaments with dense bodies, pinocytotic vesicles, and rough endoplasmic reticulum.

Rough endoplasmic reticulum

Pinocytotic vesicles

Filament bundle

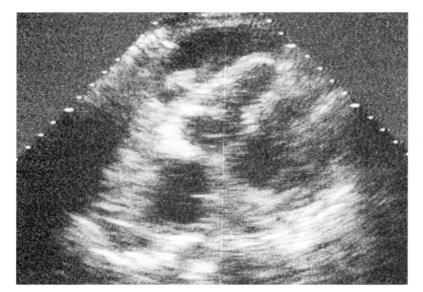

FIGURE 15-25. Echocardiogram from an 11-year-old girl showing an irregularly thickened pericardium. Physical findings included cardiac tamponade and pericardial effusion. The effusion was drained twice via pericardiocentesis. Open pericardial drainage was performed subsequently, revealing a diffusely thickened and hemorrhagic pericardium. Angiosarcomas may cause electrocardiographic disturbances, with sinus tachycardia and ST-T wave changes [35]. Chest roentgenograms generally show cardiomegaly in patients with angiosarcomas [3].

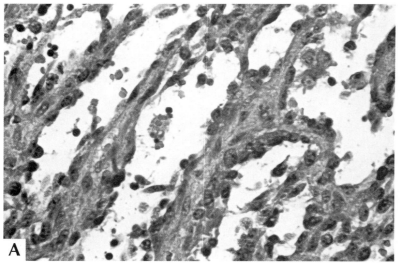

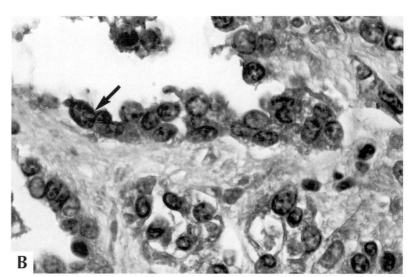

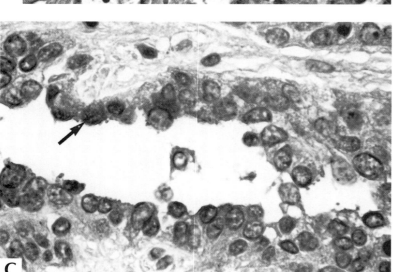

FIGURE 15-26. Biopsy revealed a tumor composed of anastomosing vascular channels lined with rounded, spindled endothelial cells having hyperchromatic, prominent nuclei (**A**; hematoxylin and eosin, × 100). Focally, more cellular areas with trabeculae of rounded cells were found. With immunohistochemical staining, the tumor cells were positive for the endothelial markers *Ulex europaeus* (*arrow*) (**B**; × 200) and factor VIII–related antigen (*arrow*) (**C**; × 200).

CASE 6: PAPILLARY FIBROELASTOMA

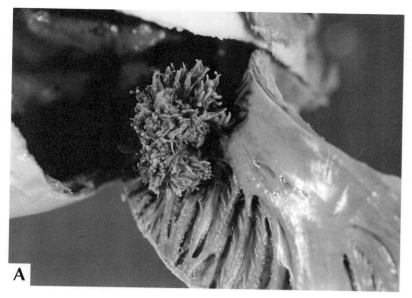

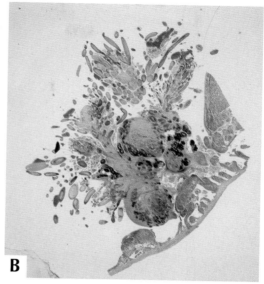

FIGURE 15-27. **A,** A papillary fibroelastoma is present on the atrial endocardial surface, with multiple papillary structures giving it a sea anemone–like appearance.

B, Photomicrograph showing typical findings that include numerous papillary structures containing a core of dense connective tissue (collagen), an overlying elastic tissue layer, and surrounding acid mucopolysaccharide–rich tissue, all of which are covered by endothelium (Masson's trichrome and Verhoeff–van Gieson elastin, × 6). Papillary fibroelastomas, which typically occur in older adults, are located most commonly on the aortic valve cusps but may be found anywhere in the heart and may be multiple. Although usually an incidental finding, they may cause valvular dysfunction, embolic phenomena, or direct obstruction of a coronary ostium. Operative excision is curative.

CASE 7: MESOTHELIOMA OF THE ATRIOVENTRICULAR (AV) NODE

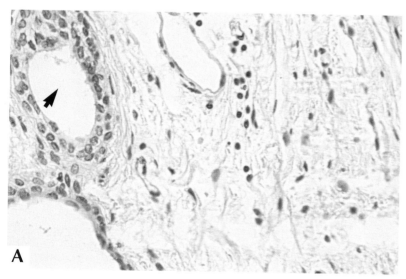

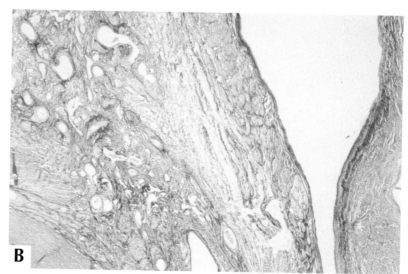

FIGURE 15-28. Photomicrographs showing the loose fibrous stroma with scattered mononuclear cells and numerous variably sized channels typical of a mesothelioma of the AV node (*arrow*). **A,** Cells that line the channels of the tumor are flat to cuboidal and either single or multilayered (hematoxylin and eosin, × 125).

B, Widespread disruption of the normal architecture can be seen in the region of the AV node owing to the accumulation of vascular channels (Verhoeff–van Gieson elastic, × 33).

Immunohistochemical staining [36–38] and ultrastructural analysis have shown the cells lining the channels of the tumor to be endothelial in origin. Therefore, the tumors are actually endotheliomas rather than mesotheliomas. A recent report by Balasundaram *et al.* [39] has detailed the successful operative excision of a mesothelioma of the AV node during repair of an ostium secundum atrial septal defect.

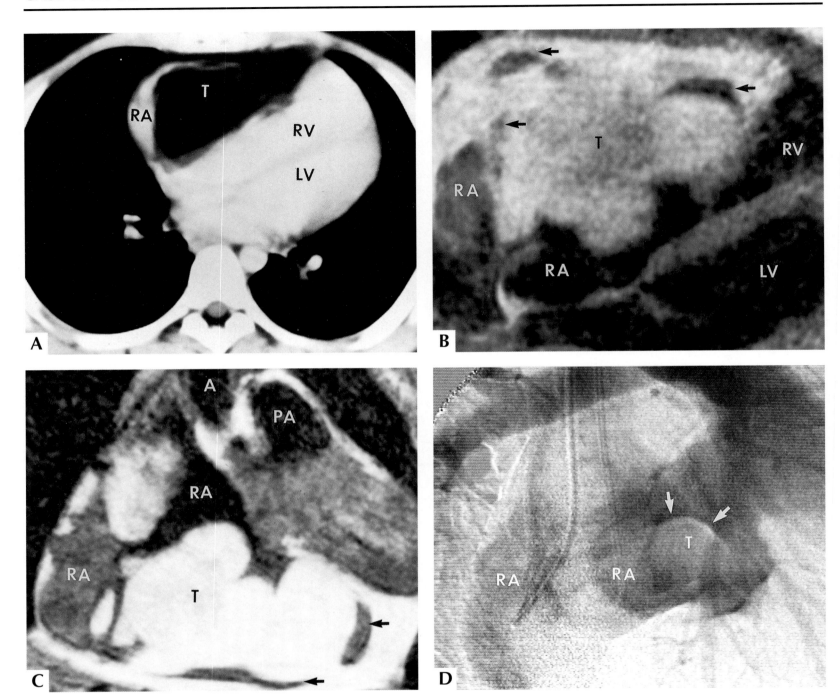

FIGURE 15-29. Images of an epicardial lipoma. **A,** Contrast-enhanced computed tomographic scan revealing a low-attenuation tumor (T). **B,** Axial magnetic image illustrating a tumor deforming the right ventricle (RV) (*arrows*). **C,** Coronal magnetic resonance image showing the lobular nature of the tumor, which is impinging on the right atrium (RA). **D,** Angiogram showing contrast medium flowing around the tumor, which is protruding into the RA (*arrows*). A—aorta; LV—left ventricle; PA—pulmonary artery. (*Adapted from* King and coworkers [40]; with permission.)

KEY MORPHOLOGIC FEATURES

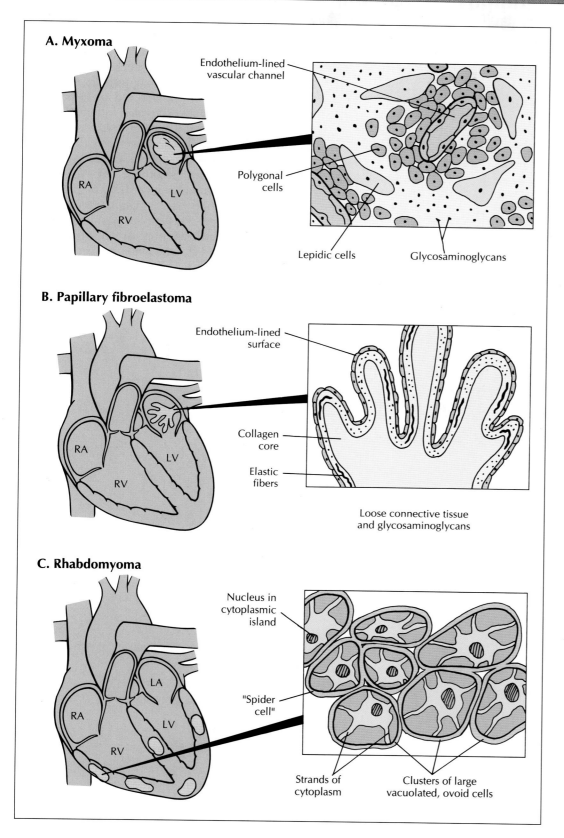

A. Myxoma

Endothelium-lined vascular channel

Polygonal cells

RA
LV
RV

Lepidic cells

Glycosaminoglycans

B. Papillary fibroelastoma

Endothelium-lined surface

Collagen core

Elastic fibers

RA
LV
RV

Loose connective tissue and glycosaminoglycans

C. Rhabdomyoma

Nucleus in cytoplasmic island

"Spider cell"

LA
RA
LV
RV

Strands of cytoplasm

Clusters of large vacuolated, ovoid cells

FIGURE 15-30. The five most common benign primary cardiac tumors—myxoma (**A**), papillary fibroelastoma (**B**), rhabdomyoma (**C**), (*continued*)

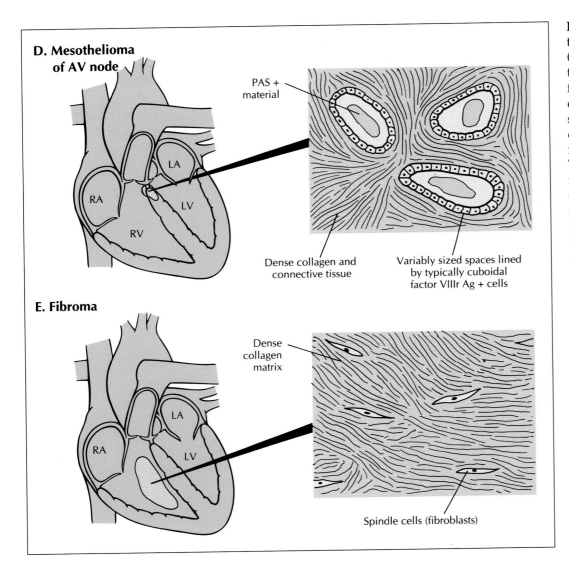

D. Mesothelioma of AV node

PAS + material

Dense collagen and connective tissue

Variably sized spaces lined by typically cuboidal factor VIIIr Ag + cells

E. Fibroma

Dense collagen matrix

Spindle cells (fibroblasts)

FIGURE 15-30. (*continued*) mesothelioma of the atrioventricular node (**D**), and fibroma (**E**)—are generally distinctive in their most typical location and gross and microscopic features. Myxomas have several features in common with "ball" thrombi, including small blood vessels, iron pigment, mononuclear cells, calcific areas, bone metaplasia, myxoid stroma, and mesenchymal cells. The main differential diagnosis for myxoma includes "ball" thrombus and aneurysm of the fossa ovalis. The main differential diagnosis for papillary fibroelastoma includes thrombus and Lambl's excrescence; for rhabdomyoma, it includes fibroma and myofibroma; for mesothelioma of the atrioventricular node, it includes other masses in the AV node region, malignant mesothelioma, and angiomatous tumors; and for fibroma, it includes fibrosarcoma, fibrous myxoma, and fibrous rhabdomyoma. LA—left atrium; LV—left ventricle; RA—right atrium; RV—right ventricle.

TUMOR TYPES

RHABDOMYOMA	RHABDOMYOSARCOMA	FIBROMA	FIBROSARCOMA
Most often in ventricular myocardium	Found in any chamber	Intracavitary	Often intracavitary, nodular, or infiltrative
Firm, grey-white	Pale, soft, nodular	Typically solitary	Single or multiple
Single or multiple	Multiple	Collagenous matrix	Cells lack basement membrane
Spider cells	Rhabdomyoblasts and giant cells	Numerous fibroblasts	Spindle cells
Vacuolation of cardiocytes due to glycogen	Common necrosis	Rare myocytes	Frequent mitosis
		Limited vascularity	Variably arrayed sheaths of tumor cells

FIGURE 15-31. In the differential diagnosis of primary cardiac tumors, it is essential to distinguish between benign and malignant tumors. The characteristics listed here can be used as a guide in differentiating benign and malignant forms of two common types of tumors, *ie*, rhabdomyoma from rhabdomyosarcoma and fibroma from fibrosarcoma.

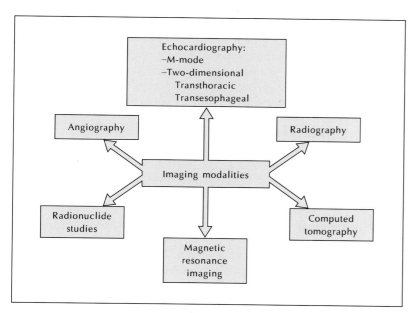

FIGURE 15-32. Imaging modalities in the diagnosis of primary cardiac tumors. On chest roentgenogram, myxoma may mimic mitral stenosis or there may be nonspecific cardiomegaly; however, when calcification can be seen in the mass, a tumor should be suspected. Echocardiography, magnetic resonance imaging, and computed tomography provide similar information but with varying degrees of resolution. Echocardiography is often sufficient to plan operative treatment of intracavitary neoplasms, which are readily visualized by this imaging modality. Other tumors that arise or extend outside the heart may not be visualized well with echocardiography, in which case magnetic resonance imaging or computed tomography is useful. All these modalities can be employed to determine the extent of cardiac and extracardiac involvement by neoplasm as well as operability and are helpful in planning the operative procedure [41]. Many centers proceed to surgery based on information obtained from echocardiography, magnetic resonance imaging, or computed tomography alone. Because more than one chamber may be involved, all four chambers should be visualized prior to operative intervention.

IMAGING MODALITIES

MODALITY	INTRACAVITARY	MYOCARDIAL	PERICARDIAL/EXTRACARDIAC
		SITE OF NEOPLASM	
Noninvasive			
Radiology			
Chest roentgenogram	Calcification in mass mimics mitral stenosis	Cardiomegaly	Cardiomegaly
Echocardiography	Intracavitary mass	Abnormal wall motion	Pericardial thickening
Computed tomography and magnetic resonance imaging	Intracavitary mass	Myocardial mass	Pericardial/extracardiac mass
Radionuclide imaging	Intracavitary filling defect	Altered myocardial uptake	
Invasive			
Angiography	Intracavitary filling defect	Compression or displacement of cardiac chamber; chamber deformity; variable myocardial thickness; abnormal wall motion	Pericardial effusion

FIGURE 15-33. Echocardiography is often sufficient for the operative treatment of intracavitary neoplasms. Cross-sectional images of cardiac, pulmonary, and mediastinal structures can be obtained with computed tomography or magnetic resonance imaging. Using these technologies, the extent of cardiac and extracardiac involvement by the neoplasm can be assessed. (*Adapted from* Colucci and Braunwald [26]; with permission.)

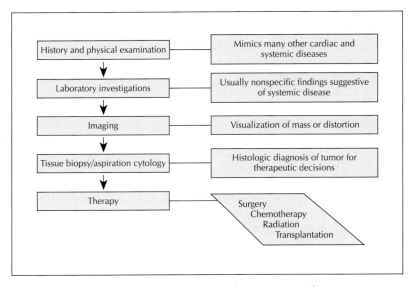

FIGURE 15-34. Approach to diagnosis of primary cardiac tumors. The history and physical examination may reveal signs and symptoms that mimic various cardiac or systemic diseases [4]. Laboratory investigations, including hematologic studies, blood chemistry, and the electrocardiogram, usually result in nonspecific findings that may suggest systemic disease. Both noninvasive and invasive imaging techniques may be used; however, echocardiography, magnetic resonance imaging, and computed tomography provide optimal visualization and tissue discrimination. Endomyocardial or pericardial biopsy may be useful in selected cases for histologic diagnosis.

No randomized clinical trials have been carried out to determine the optimal therapy for primary cardiac neoplasms [42]. The prognosis for survival of patients with primary malignant cardiac neoplasms is poor, with high rates of recurrence and metastases; survival seldom exceeds 1 year [43–45]. Surgery is the treatment of choice for small neoplasms localized to the heart. Partial resection of large neoplasms to relieve mechanical effects should be considered, especially in children [46]. It is not known whether adjuvant chemotherapy is beneficial in patients who have undergone curative surgery. Chemotherapy is the treatment of choice for cardiac neoplasms that have metastasized; in these cases, combination therapy is often more effective than single-agent therapy. The role of radiation in the treatment of cardiac neoplasms is not well defined. Although radiation is the therapy of choice for malignant lymphoma when combined with chemotherapy, it significantly increases the risk for myocardial and pericardial damage. When complete excision of benign neoplasms is not possible, heart transplantation may be considered.

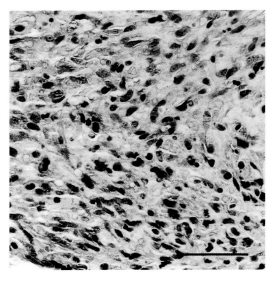

FIGURE 15-35. Endomyocardial biopsy has been used in the histopathologic diagnosis of neoplastic disease involving the heart and can be employed in conjunction with noninvasive imaging modalities [47]. This photomicrograph shows a tumor biopsy specimen with features typical of an angiosarcoma. The highly cellular tumor contains many pleomorphic malignant endothelial cells, and mitotic figures are apparent (hematoxylin and eosin; scale = 10 μm). (*Adapted from* Adachi and coworkers [48]; with permission.)

THERAPY AND OUTCOME

TREATMENT	RECURRENCE, %	COMMENTS
Operative excision		Mechanisms of recurrence
Removal of fossa ovalis and repair [49]	Sporadic: 1–5	Incomplete excision
Laser photocoagulation of attachment site and adjacent endocardium [50]		Operative implantation
		Metasynchronous ("new") focus
Removal of small rim of endocardium at base [51]	Familial: 12–22	More extensive excision recommended for familial myxomas
		Careful echocardiographic follow-up recommended, especially when familial or synchronous tumors are present initially
		Tumor emboli are the major operative risk

FIGURE 15-36. Therapeutic options and outcomes for patients with cardiac myxomas [49–51]. Operative excision may be most effective if careful attention is given to the point at which the tumor is attached to normal cardiac structures. Of note, myxomas occurring in a familial pattern are more likely to recur and warrant an even more extensive surgical approach and scrupulous follow-up.

FUTURE DIRECTIONS

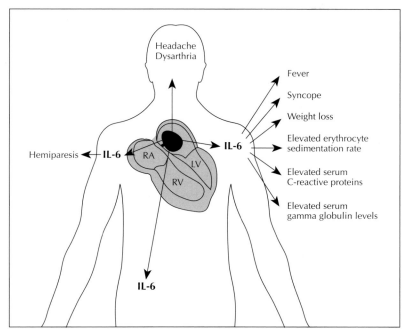

FIGURE 15-37. High serum concentrations of interleukin-6 (IL-6) have been demonstrated in patients with cardiac myxomas [52–56], and this circulating cytokine produces systemic symptoms. Elevated serum IL-6 subsides to normal levels after resection of the myxoma and after the systemic inflammatory or autoimmune manifestations have abated. Complaints pertaining to the central nervous system include headache, syncope, dysarthria, and hemiparesis, while fever, weight loss, elevation of erythrocyte sedimentation rate, serum C-reactive protein, and serum gamma globulin levels have also been demonstrated [52]. Thus, evidence to date suggests that IL-6 may play a key role in the immunologic alterations associated with cardiac myxomas.

REFERENCES

1. Courtice RW, Stinson WA, Walley VM: Tissue fragments recovered at cardiac surgery masquerading as tumoral proliferations: evidence suggesting iatrogenic or artefactual origin and common occurrence. *Am J Surg Pathol* 1994, 18:167–174.

2. Luthringer DJ, Virmani R, Weiss SW, *et al.*: A distinctive cardio-vascular lesion resembling histiocytoid (epithelioid) hemangioma: evidence suggesting mesothelial participation. *Am J Surg Pathol* 1990, 14:993–1000.

3. McAllister HA, Fenoglio JJ: Tumors of the cardiovascular system. In *Atlas of Tumor Pathology*, ed 2. Washington, DC: Armed Forces Institute of Pathology; 1978:111–119.

4. Tillmanns H: Clinical aspects of cardiac tumors. *J Thorac Cardiovasc Surg* 1990, 38:152–156.

5. Bloor CM, O'Rourke R: Cardiac tumors: clinical presentation and pathologic correlations. *Curr Prob Cardiol* 1984, 9:7–48.

6. Becker RC, Loeffler JS, Leopold KA, *et al.*: Primary tumors of the heart: a review with emphasis on diagnosis and potential treatment modalities. *Semin Surg Oncol* 1985, 1:161–170.

7. Simcha A, Wells BG, Tynan MJ, *et al.*: Primary cardiac tumors in childhood. *Arch Dis Child* 1971, 46:508–514.

8. Bini RM, Westaby S, Bargeron LM, *et al.*: Investigation and management of primary cardiac tumors in infants and children. *J Am Coll Cardiol* 1983, 2:351–357.

9. Wold LE, Lie JT: Cardiac myxomas: a clinicopathologic profile. *Am J Pathol* 1980, 101:219–230.

10. Goodwin JF: Symposium on cardiac tumors: the spectrum of cardiac tumors. *Am J Cardiol* 1968, 21:307–314.

11. Hehrlein FW, Dapper F: Tumors of the heart. *Thorac Cardiovasc Surg* 1990, 38:151.

12. Nadas AS, Ellison RC: Cardiac tumors in infancy. *Am J Cardiol* 1968, 21:363–366.

13. Fine G: Neoplasms of the pericardium and heart. In *Pathology of the Heart and Blood Vessels*, ed 3. Edited by Gould SE. Springfield, IL: Charles C. Thomas Publishers; 1968:851–883.

14. Lam KYL, Dickens P, Chan ACL: Tumors of the heart. *Arch Pathol Lab Med* 1993, 117:1027–1031.

15. Chan HSL, Sonley MJ, Moes CAF, *et al.*: Primary and secondary tumors of childhood involving the heart, pericardium, and great vessels. *Cancer* 1985, 56:825–836.

16. Cooley DA: Surgical treatment of cardiac neoplasms: 32-year experience. *J Thorac Cardiovasc Surg* 1990, 38:176–182.

17. Tazelaar HD, Locke TJ, McGregor CGA: Pathology of surgically excised primary cardiac tumors. *Mayo Clin Proc* 1992, 67:957–965.

18. Molina JE, Edwards JE, Ward HB: Primary cardiac tumors: experience at the University of Minnesota. *J Thorac Cardiovasc Surg* 1990, 38:183–191.

19. Moosdorf R, Scheld HH, Hehrlein FW: Tumors of the heart: experiences at the Giessen University Clinic. *J Thorac Cardiovasc Surg* 1990, 38:208–210.

20. Dein JR, Frist WH, Stinson EB, *et al.*: Primary cardiac neoplasms. *Thorac Cardiovasc Surg* 1987, 93:502–511.

21. Guang-ying L: Incidence and clinical importance of cardiac tumors in China: review of the literature. *J Thorac Cardiovasc Surg* 1990, 38:205–207.

22. Tschirkov A, Michev B, Topalov V, *et al.*: Incidences and surgical aspects of cardiac myxomas in Bulgaria. *J Thorac Cardiovasc Surg* 1990, 38:196–200.

23. Sezai Y: Tumors of the heart: incidence and clinical importance of cardiac tumors in Japan and operative technique for large left atrial tumors. *J Thorac Cardiovasc Surg* 1990, 38:201–204.

24. Blondeau P: Primary cardiac tumors: french studies of 533 cases. *J Thorac Cardiovasc Surg* 1990, 38:192–195.

25. Fisher J: Cardiac myxoma. *Cardiovasc Rev Rep* 1983, 9:1195.

26. Colucci WS, Braunwald E: Primary tumors of the heart. In *Heart Disease: A Textbook of Cardiovascular Medicine*, ed 4. Edited by Braunwald E. Philadelphia: WB Saunders Co; 1992:1451–1464.

27. Carney JA: Differences between nonfamilial and familial cardiac myxoma. *Am J Surg Pathol* 1985, 9:53–55.

28. Peters MN, Hall RJ, Cooley DA, *et al.*: The clinical syndrome of atrial myxoma. *JAMA* 1974, 230:694.

29. Hall RJ, Cooley DA: Neoplastic diseases of the heart. In *Hurst's The Heart*, ed 5. Edited by Logue RB, Rackley CE, Schlant RC, *et al.* New York: McGraw-Hill; 1982:1403–1421.

30. Krikler DM, Rode J, Davies MJ, *et al.*: Atrial myxoma: a tumor in search of its origins. *Br Heart J* 1992, 6:89–91.

31. Guereta LG, Burgueros M, Elorza MD, *et al.*: Cardiac rhabdomyoma presenting as fetal hydrops. *Pediatr Cardiol* 1986, 7:171–174.

32. Mehta A: Rhabdomyoma and ventricular preexcitation syndrome. *Am J Dis Child* 1993, 147:669–671.

33. Heath D: Pathology of cardiac tumors. *Am J Cardiol* 1968, 21:315–327.

34. Yabek SM: Cardiac fibroma in a neonate presenting with severe congestive heart failure. *J Pediatr* 1977, 91:310–312.

35. Glancy DL, Morales JB, Roberts WC: Angiosarcoma of the heart. *Am J Cardiol* 1968, 21:413–419.

36. Monma N, Satodate R, Tashiro A, *et al.*: Origin of so-called mesothelioma of the atrioventricular node. *Arch Pathol Lab Med* 1991, 115:1026–1029.

37. Robertson AL: The origin of primary tumors of the atrioventricular node. *Arch Pathol Lab Med* 1990, 114:1198.

38. Duray PH, Mark EJ, Barwick KW, *et al.*: Congenital polycystic tumor of the atrioventricular node. *Arch Pathol Lab Med* 1985, 109:30–34.

39. Balasundaram S, Halees A, Duran C: Mesothelioma of the atrioventricular node: first successful follow-up after excision. *Eur Heart J* 1992, 13:718–719.

40. King SJ, Smallhorn JF, Burrows PE: Epicardial lipoma: imaging findings. *AJR Am J Roentgenol* 1993, 160:261–262.

41. Rienmueller R, Tiling R: MR and CT for detection of cardiac tumors. *J Thorac Cardiovasc Surg* 1990, 38:168–172.

42. Loffler H, Grille W: Classification of malignant cardiac tumors with respect to oncological treatment. *J Thorac Cardiovasc Surg* 1990, 38(special issue):173–175.

43. Reece IJ, Cooley DA, Frazier OH, *et al.*: Cardiac tumors: clinical spectrum and prognosis of lesions other than classical benign myxoma in 20 patients. *J Thorac Cardiovasc Surg* 1984, 88:439–446.

44. Reynolds RD: Medical management of cardiac tumors. In *Cancer and the Heart*. Edited by Kapoor AS. New York: Springer-Verlag; 1986:110–117.

45. Vergnon JM, Vincent M, Perinetti M, *et al.*: Chemotherapy of metastatic primary cardiac sarcomas. *Am Heart J* 1985, 110:682–684.

46. Bertolini B, Meisner H, Paek SU, *et al.*: Special considerations on primary cardiac tumors in infancy and childhood. *J Thorac Cardiovasc Surg* 1990, 38:164–167.

47. Flipse TR, Tazelaar HD, Holmes DR: Diagnosis of malignant cardiac disease by endomyocardial biopsy. *Mayo Clin Proc* 1990, 65:1415–1422.

48. Adachi K, Tanaka H, Toshima H, *et al.*: Right atrial angiosarcoma diagnosed by cardiac biopsy. *Am Heart J* 1988, 115:482–485.

49. Waller DA, Ettles DF, Saunders MR, *et al.*: Recurrent cardiac myxoma: the surgical implications of two distinct groups of patients. *Thorac Cardiovasc Surg* 1989, 37:226–230.

50. Mesnildrey P, Bloch G, Cachera JP: Atrial myxoma: a new surgical approach using neodymium:yttrium-aluminum-garnet laser photocoagulation. *J Thorac Cardiovasc Surg* 1989, 98:313–314.

51. McCarthy PM, Piehler JM, Schaff HV, *et al.*: The significance of multiple, recurrent, and "complex" cardiac myxomas. *J Thorac Cardiovasc Surg* 1986, 91:389–396.

52. Wada A, Kanda T, Hayashi R, *et al.*: Cardiac myxoma metastasized to the brain: potential role of endogenous interleukin-6. *Cardiology* 1993, 83:208–211.

53. Jourdan M, Bataille R, Seguin J, *et al.*: Constitutive production of interleukin-6 and immunologic features in cardiac myxomas. *Arthritis Rheum* 1990, 33:298–402.

54. Kuroki S, Naitoh K, Katoh O, *et al.*: Increased interleukin-6 activity in cardiac myxoma with mediastinal lymphadenopathy. *J Intern Med* 1992, 31:1207–1209.

55. Takahara H, Mori A, Tabata R, *et al.*: Left atrial myxoma with production of interleukin-6. *J Jpn Assoc Thorac Surg* 1992, 40:326–329.

56. Seino Y, Ikeda U, Shimada K: Increased expression of interleukin-6 mRNA in cardiac myxomas. *Br Heart J* 1993, 69:565–567.

METASTATIC TUMORS OF THE HEART

16
CHAPTER

John C. English, Michael F. Allard, Shelina Babul, and Bruce M. McManus

The heart, like all organs in the body, is a potential site for metastatic tumors. Metastasis or tumor extension may occur on the epicardial surface, within the cardiac chambers, or by infiltration throughout portions of the myocardial walls. The frequency with which the heart is involved by a metastatic tumor is strikingly higher than the frequency of primary cardiac tumors [1]. Nearly all malignant tumors from every organ or tissue can metastasize to the heart, the exception being primary tumors of the central nervous system [1–14]. Although the origin of metastasis is diverse, it reflects geographic juxtaposition (lung, breast), the systemic nature of certain malignancies (lymphoma, leukemia), and the general metastatic behavior of solid tumors.

The physiologic and clinical consequences of cardiac metastatic tumors are similar to those of primary tumors in many respects. However, the possibility of encasement of the heart by neighboring tumors (primary lung and breast) is particularly distinct. In addition, because lung and breast tumors generally present in midlife and later, the corresponding metastasis correlates distinctly with demographics and age groups. The recent dramatic increase in the number of malignant lung tumors in women–largely as a function of the increase in cigarette smoking in this group–as well as the slight increase in breast cancer have led to a corresponding increase in the absolute numbers of cardiac metastatic tumors and the overall likelihood that lung and breast tumors will metastasize to the heart. In contrast, over the past two decades, the frequency of other malignant tumors (such as invasive cancer of the uterine cervix) has decreased, so the likelihood of metastasis may similarly decrease [15].

In this chapter, we focus on the most common metastatic tumors that involve the heart and emphasize their protean clinical signs and symptoms as well as their pathologic features. Improved outcomes for these malignant conditions will depend on advances in the early recognition and definitive treatment of primary extracardiac tumors.

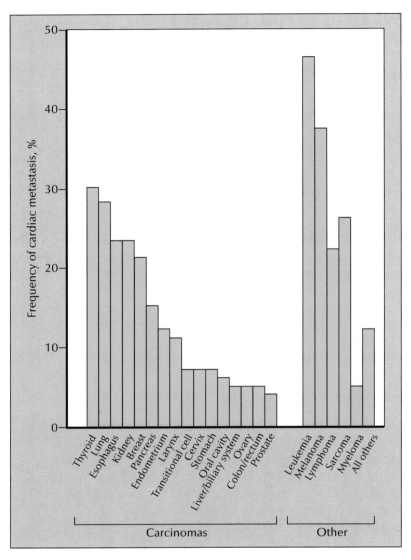

FIGURE 16-1. Frequency of metastatic tumors of the heart and pericardium found in one large autopsy series between 1950 and 1970 in one metropolitan area of the United States. Metastatic tumors of the heart are much more common than primary cardiac tumors. Certain tumors involve the heart by virtue of their proximity, while others do so based on the general frequency of a particular histopathologic type and its propensity to metastasize. Leukemia and melanoma have the greatest metastatic potential, involving the heart in over 40% and 30% of patients, respectively. Carcinomas of the thyroid gland and lung metastasize to the heart more than 25% of the time. (*Adapted from* McAllister and Fenoglio [1]; with permission.)

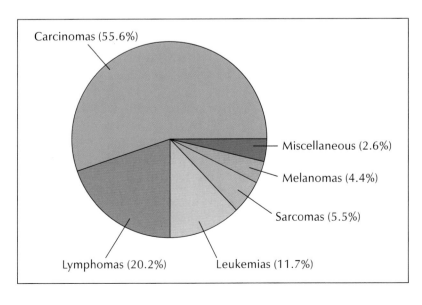

FIGURE 16-2. When the frequency of tumors that have metastasized to the heart is evaluated according to the type of tumor, carcinomas—themselves common—were clearly the most common metastases to the heart (56%). Lymphomas (about 20%) and leukemias (about 12%) were the second and third most common types of neoplasia found during evaluation for metastasis [2,4–6,9,10,12–14,16–25].

AUTOPSY EXPERIENCE

STUDY	TOTAL AUTOPSIES, n	AUTOPSIES OF CANCER CASES, n	TOTAL CARDIAC METASTASES, n	INCIDENCE FROM TOTAL AUTOPSY EXPERIENCE, %	INCIDENCE FROM MALIGNANT CASES, %
Fine [2]	3352	3352	377	11.2	11.2
Chan et al. [3]	790	3641	59	5.7*	1.6
Goudie [4]	4687	1270	126	2.7	9.9
McAllister and Fenoglio [1]	3877	3248	546	14.1	16.8
Malaret and Aliaga [5]	294	250	38	12.9	15.2
Roberts et al. [6]	402	420	156	38.8	37.1
MacGee [7]	2455	1311	57	2.3	4.3
Lam et al. [8]	12,485	—	154[†]	1.23	—
Abraham et al. [9]	3314	806	95	2.9	11.8
Young and Goldman [10]	1400	586[‡]	91	6.5	15.5
Prichard [11]	4375	4375	146	3.3	3.3
Scott and Garvin [12]	11,100	1082	118	1.1	10.9
Deloach and Haynes [13]	2547	980	137	5.4	14.0
Harrer and Lewis [14]	3710	1164	147	4.0	12.6
	54,788	22,485	2247	4.1 (Range 1.1–38.8)	9.9 (Range 1.6–37.1)

*Of the 59 cases, 14 diagnoses were made pre- or intraoperatively and 45 were made at autopsy. The incidence of secondary tumor involvement was 5.7% in the autopsy series.

[†]Some cases involve more than one location in the heart, thus having a greater number of involved sites (192) than the total number of cases (n = 154).

[‡]476 cases, excluding leukemias and brain tumors, since the former shows cardiac infiltrations frequently and the latter almost never metastasizes outside the central nervous system, the residual incidence being 19.1%.

FIGURE 16-3. Results from separate autopsy series from 15 hospitals and universities in six countries in which the frequency of cardiac metastasis was emphasized [1–14]. The experience encompassed 75 years (1916 to 1991) and more than 54,000 autopsies. Over this period, the frequency of tumors reported as cardiac metastases varied. Of the 22,485 extracardiac tumors reported, 2247 metastasized to the heart, for an overall rate of 10%.

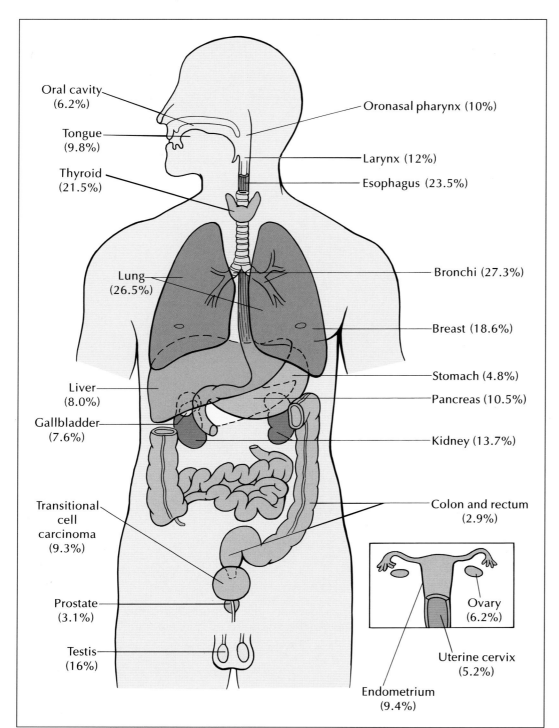

FIGURE 16-4. Prevalence of cardiac metastases by original site of carcinoma. Carcinoma is the tumor type that most commonly metastasizes to the heart (*see* Fig. 16-2). The primary tumor locations are designated, and the rate of cardiac metastasis is given in parentheses. As depicted, the bronchus (lung), esophagus, thyroid gland, and breast are all relatively close to the heart and are the sources of the greatest number of cardiac metastatic carcinomas.

Labels in figure:
Oral cavity (6.2%)
Tongue (9.8%)
Thyroid (21.5%)
Lung (26.5%)
Liver (8.0%)
Gallbladder (7.6%)
Transitional cell carcinoma (9.3%)
Prostate (3.1%)
Testis (16%)
Oronasal pharynx (10%)
Larynx (12%)
Esophagus (23.5%)
Bronchi (27.3%)
Breast (18.6%)
Stomach (4.8%)
Pancreas (10.5%)
Kidney (13.7%)
Colon and rectum (2.9%)
Ovary (6.2%)
Uterine cervix (5.2%)
Endometrium (9.4%)

CARDIAC TRANSPLANTATION

HEART ALLOGRAFT PATIENTS WITH PTLD

PATIENTS, n	CUMULATIVE OKT3 DOSE, *mg*	INTERVAL TO PTLD, *mo*	OUTCOME
5	<75	18.5	3 dead, 2 alive
5	>75	1.3	4 dead, 1 alive
		Range: 1–50 mo	

FIGURE 16-5. Posttransplant lymphoproliferative disorder (PTLD) is another sequela of cardiac transplantation. In recent reports 32 heart transplant patients developed PTLD [26–28]. In one study of 10 patients, those who received a cumulative dose of more than 75 mg of OKT3 had a very short interval between transplantation and the appearance of PTLD [26]. The correlation between large doses of OKT3 and short disease-free intervals was highly significant ($r=0.91$, $P=0.0006$).

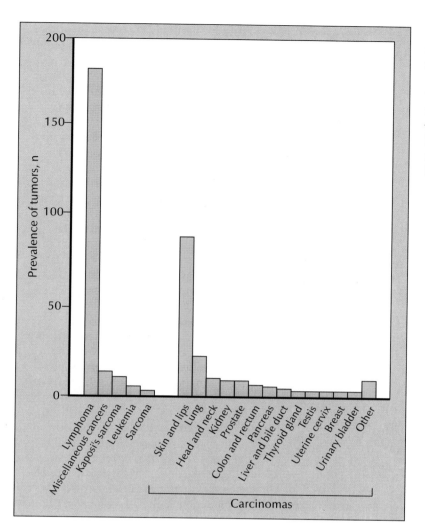

FIGURE 16-6. Prevalence of the most common extracardiac malignant tumors in cardiac allograft recipients, all of whom receive immunosuppressive and intensive induction therapy [29,30]. Although reports examined thus far have not established the frequency with which these tumors involve the heart, it is nearly certain that it will be at least equal to that of patients with extracardiac tumors who have not undergone transplantation. Lymphoma and squamous carcinoma of the skin and lips are most common in cardiac allograft recipients. The category "other" includes stomach, ovary, vulva, perineum, penis, and scrotum.

CLINICAL FEATURES AND DIAGNOSIS

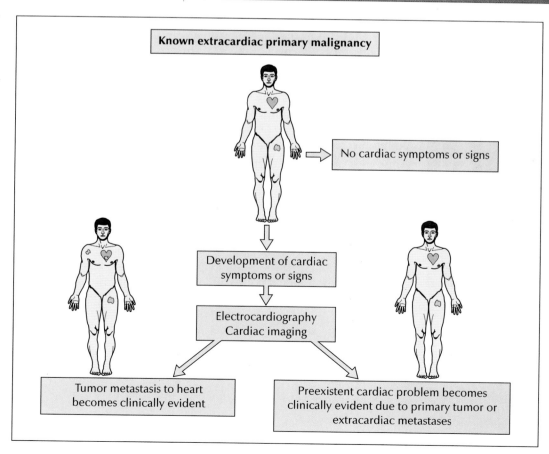

FIGURE 16-7. If a cancer patient without heart disease begins to experience cardiac symptoms or signs, metastasis of a tumor to the heart or sequelae of cancer therapy (*eg*, irradiation) are immediately suspected. Once cardiac symptoms or signs become evident, however, it is important to distinguish metastatic disease or anticancer treatment sequelae from preexisting cardiac disease, particularly in older patients who may have atherosclerotic or valvular disease. The differential diagnosis can be narrowed through use of various imaging modalities, particularly echocardiography, computed tomography, and magnetic resonance imaging. Once diagnosis has been made visually, endomyocardial (or pericardial) biopsy or needle aspiration may be useful in confirming metastatic involvement [31].

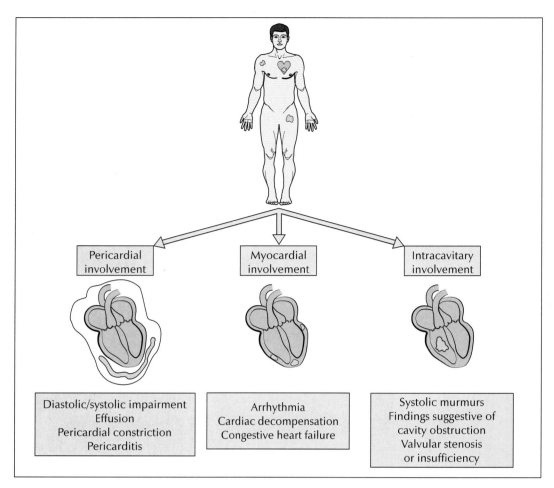

carditis, which is often discovered at autopsy.

Arrhythmias are the most common manifestation of metastatic tumors to the myocardium; those most commonly seen are atrial fibrillation or flutter, paroxysmal atrial tachycardia, nodal rhythms, heart block, and ventricular tachycardia or fibrillation [1,32]. The second most common manifestation is cardiac decompensation with congestive heart failure. Early signs of replacement of the myocardium or invasion by tumor include gallop rhythms, pulsus alternans, and changes in heart sound intensity. Generally, more prominent signs can be expected as the tumor replaces more of the myocardium. Congestive heart failure, enlargement of the heart with unusual configuration on chest radiographs, and electrocardiographic clues (including nonspecific ST-segment and T-wave changes) are common.

Although rare, a number of metastatic cardiac tumors consist mainly of an intracavitary mass with little invasion of the underlying myocardium [1,32]. Intracavitary tumors usually arise as implants of tumor cells on valve apparatus or endocardium. Systolic murmurs and findings that suggest obstruction are common. Direct valvular involvement is frequent and may mimic or actually cause stenosis or insufficiency. The presence of valvular insufficiency may help differentiate metastatic or primary malignant tumors from benign tumors of the heart. Occasionally, ischemic sequelae, including myocardial infarction, may be caused by intracoronary tumor emboli or compression of a coronary artery.

FIGURE 16-8. In 25% of patients with pericardial metastasis, cardiac function is significantly impaired [1]. Effusion and cardiac enlargement are the most common findings on radiographs. Other findings include occasional constrictive pericarditis, right-sided congestive heart failure, ST-segment depression on electrocardiogram, and T-wave abnormalities. Sinus tachycardia develops in 10% to 15% of patients, while other types of atrial arrhythmia are rare. A large percentage of patients with pericardial friction rub also have acute peri-

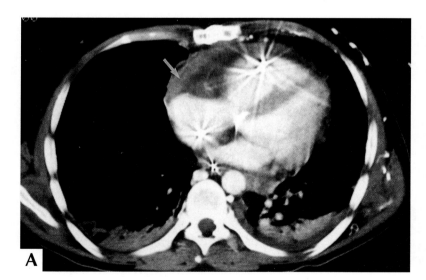

FIGURE 16-9. Computed tomographic scan with contrast medium enhancement at the level of the heart in a patient with adenocarcinoma of the lung. **A,** Thickened pericardium with an irregular contour (*arrows*) is shown. These findings are characteristic of infiltrative processes involving the pericardium.

B, The adenocarcinoma, which appears as a lobulated mass in the mediastinum (*large arrow*), encircles and compresses the right main pulmonary artery (*double arrows*) and the superior vena cava (*double arrowheads*). This case illustrates the use of computed tomography in evaluating the relationship of neoplasms to the heart and great vessels as well as in determining the extent of involvement by neoplastic disease. Although magnetic resonance imaging provides similar information in this regard, its image resolution is slightly lower. In certain patients, such as those with renal failure and allergies to contrast media, magnetic resonance imaging may be the preferred imaging modality to evaluate involvement because contrast enhancement is not required. (*continued*)

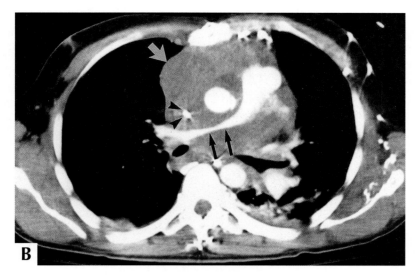

FIGURE 16-9. (*continued*) In addition, several imaging planes can be used. The propensity for metastatic adenocarcinomas to involve the atria accounts for the increased frequency of supraventricular arrhythmias. A wide variety of electrocardiographic abnormalities may be found, including ST-T wave changes, premature atrial contractions, premature ventricular contractions, left and right bundle branch block, atrial fibrillation or flutter, a short PR interval, sinus tachycardia, and left axis deviation [33]. Lung tumors may invade the heart and pericardium by several routes, including direct extension, vascular spread, and lymphatic spread, the last being the most common [33]. When the primary tumor focus is close to the heart, it often becomes difficult to distinguish direct extension from lymphatic spread. Although pulmonary vein involvement by bronchogenic carcinoma may be common [34,35] and is a major source of systemic tumor embolization, the hematogenous route of spread to the heart is the least well recognized of the metastatic pathways noted above.

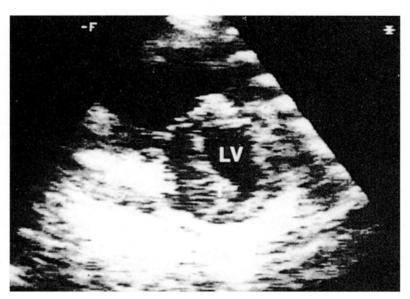

FIGURE 16-10. Two-dimensional echocardiogram showing an echo-dense, mobile mass attached to the left ventricular (LV) aspect of the ventricular septum. This mass was later proved to be malignant melanoma that had metastasized to the heart (*see* Figs. 16-15 to 16-17) [36]. As with benign cardiac tumors, echocardiography is particularly useful for identifying and defining those

with significant intracavitary involvement. Melanoma is recognized as the tumor with the highest relative frequency of secondary cardiac involvement (65%), reflecting the likelihood that melanoma will spread [37]. In addition, the absolute load of metastatic tumor within the heart is often far greater than for any other tumor. The pattern of widespread tumor deposition, with greater involvement of myocardium relative to pericardium, is believed to represent vast hematogenous spread. Only 1% to 2% of patients may show any clinical evidence of cardiac dysfunction [37], and they may not demonstrate significant electrocardiographic abnormalities [16]. Cardiac dysfunction usually supervenes only with massive involvement.

Cardiac metastatic melanoma has been detected radiographically using coronary angiography (demonstrating neovascularization and a tumor blush) [38], echocardiography [39], and magnetic resonance imaging [38,40]. Echocardiographic findings that suggest an intracavitary malignancy as opposed to a thrombus include heterogeneous echo density and a lack of underlying myocardial wall thinning. The melanin content of melanomas warrants special consideration in interpreting magnetic resonance images. If melanin is present in large enough quantities, it may act as a ferromagnetic source, resulting in a more intense (brighter) image on T_1-weighted scans [40]. This is in contrast to most tumors that have darker T_1 images because of their long relaxation times. (*Adapted from* Sheldon and Isaac [36]; with permission.)

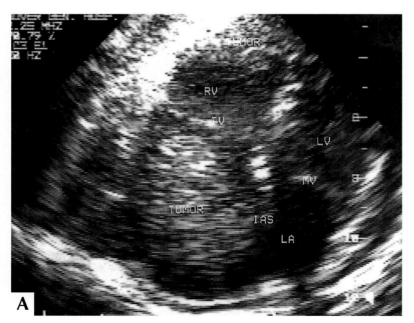

FIGURE 16-11. Echocardiograms of carcinoma that has metastasized from the cervix. A 62-year-old woman with a history of abnormal Pap smears was admitted for work-up leading to a cone biopsy. The patient developed shortness of breath and exertional dyspnea; a pulmonary embolus was suspected. She subsequently developed headaches and dysphasia. Upon examination, a pleural friction rub was noted, along with an accentuated second heart sound and tumor plop on auscultation. A computed tomographic head scan demonstrated a left parietal infarct, and the ventilation-perfusion scan revealed multiple segmental and subsegmental perfusion defects. The echocardiogram demonstrated a large right atrial mass, suggestive of myxoma. After surgical removal of the mass, however, the pathologic diagnosis was high-grade carcinoma consistent with a cervical origin. Subsequent vaginal and endocervical biopsies revealed high-grade, invasive, nonkeratinizing squamous cell carcinoma. The patient died several weeks after surgery. **A,** The off-axis four-chamber view demonstrates that the tumor virtually fills the right atrium (RA); an attachment point on the interatrial septum (IAS) can be seen. Additional tumor mass can also be visualized in the right ventricular (RV) apex. (*continued*)

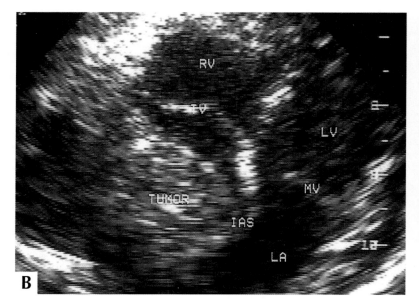

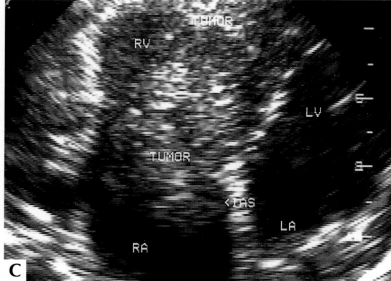

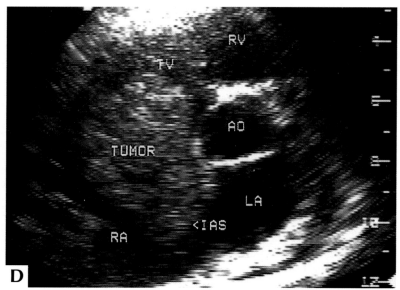

FIGURE 16-11. (*continued*) **B,** In systole, the off-axis four-chamber view demonstrates tumor mass in the RA. **C,** In diastole, the atrial tumor mass prolapses through the tricuspid valve (TV) to contact the RV apical tumor mass. **D,** On the parasternal short-axis view, the tumor mass can be seen in the RA with an attachment point to the IAS. AO—aorta; LA—left atrium; LV—left ventricle. (Courtesy of Dr. K. Gin, Vancouver General Hospital, Vancouver, BC.)

PATHOLOGY

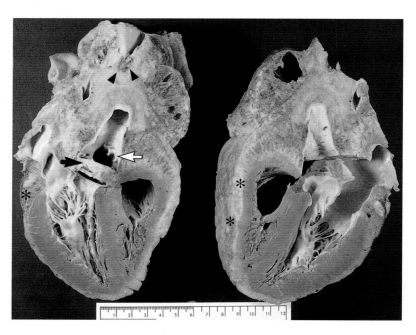

FIGURE 16-12. Gross specimens of metastatic adenocarcinoma of lung. The heart has been bisected in the four-chamber echocardiographic plane to reveal massive tumor infiltration around the base of the heart, encasing the great vessels and causing pericardial thickening (*asterisks in both specimens*). In the specimen on the left, the tumor has invaded and nearly obliterated the superior vena cava (*arrowheads*); the mechanical prosthetic valve is viewed parallel to the valve ring (*closed arrow*), and the orifice of a supravalvular pseudoaneurysm of the aortic root is visible (*open arrow*). Between 15% and 35% of patients with lung cancer have evidence of tumors that have metastasized to the heart demonstrated at autopsy [33,41,42]. Thus, bronchogenic carcinoma, a common malignancy with great potential for metastasis, is the solid tumor that most frequently involves the heart. Large cell anaplastic carcinoma (59%) and adenocarcinoma subtypes (41%) make up the highest percentage of metastatic cardiac tumors arising from lung [42]. Metastasis is more common in patients with extensive malignant disease at the primary site and in those receiving aggressive therapy. Involvement of the heart may take the form of 1) multiple nodular metastases, 2) intracavitary tumors or thrombi, and 3) diffuse myocardial replacement (on rare occasions).

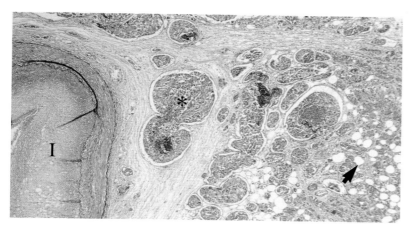

FIGURE 16-13. Photomicrograph showing metastatic lung adenocarcinoma. Extensive pericardial metastasis is evident in nests of tumor that infiltrate the pericardial fat (*arrow*) and lymphatics (*asterisk*). The histologic stain also reveals intra- and extracellular mucin (blue), which is characteristic of adenocarcinoma. Also present in this field is a portion of the left anterior descending coronary artery with significant intimal thickening (*I*; Movat pentachrome, × 100). Lung cancer is the most common cause of malignant pericardial effusion, accounting for more than 50% of cases [43,44]; some cases may present as cardiac tamponade [45]. Effusion may be serous, serosanguineous, sanguineous, or fibrinopurulent [41]. Tumor involvement may take the form of nodular studding or diffuse infiltration that transforms the pericardium into a thick pannus of tumor, as can be seen here.

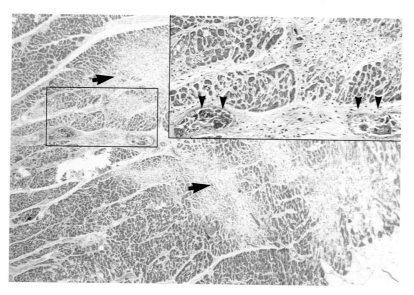

FIGURE 16-14. Photomicrograph of myocardial infarction and tumor emboli due to metastatic adenocarcinoma of lung. Tumor embolization (*arrowheads*) has caused widespread microinfarction of the myocardium. Patchy areas of myocyte loss with replacement by granulation tissue (*arrows*) can be seen close to several vessels containing tumor emboli (*inset*). (Movat pentachrome, × 40; inset, × 100). Coronary artery involvement by tumor may consist of narrowing secondary to external tumor compression, direct invasion by tumor, or tumor embolization. Lung carcinoma is the most common source of malignant emboli to coronary arteries (57% of cases) [46,47] and is associated with left atrial invasion in approximately 50% of cases. The likelihood of tumor embolization may increase with surgical lobectomy or pneumonectomy [48,49]. Despite the high degree of cardiac involvement, the presence of metastatic adenocarcinoma in the heart and pericardium often remains clinically undetected; however, causes of death in patients with bronchogenic carcinoma metastatic to the heart include intractable congestive heart failure, lethal dysrhythmias, and coronary involvement by tumor.

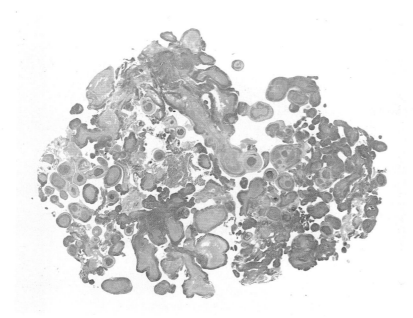

FIGURE 16-15. Whole-mount section of excised intracavitary mass of metastatic melanoma showing a papillary or frondlike configuration. Many of the papillae have central necrotic cores (*see* Fig. 16-19); necrosis promotes both thrombosis on the overlying surface and subsequent embolization. Intracavitary masses may become large, replacing most of one or both ventricles [50]. Although valvular involvement is uncommon [51], valvular stenosis [52] and insufficiency [53] produced by intracavitary melanoma have been reported.

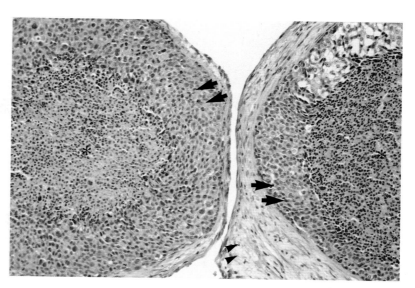

FIGURE 16-16. Two papillary tumor protrusions of metastatic melanoma contain central necrosis (*asterisks*) with a surrounding collar of viable tumor cells (*arrows*). The endothelialized tumor surface shows fibrous proliferation (*arrowheads*), which is more pronounced on the right. Intracardiac extension of the melanoma makes the tumor amenable to endomyocardial biopsy, and as with hematologic malignancies, melanoma is one of the more frequently biopsied tumors [31,50,53]. Fibrous encapsulation and tumor necrosis can interfere with the biopsy procedure, so care needs to be taken to ensure adequate sampling of the tumor.

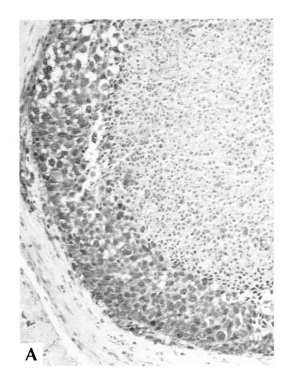 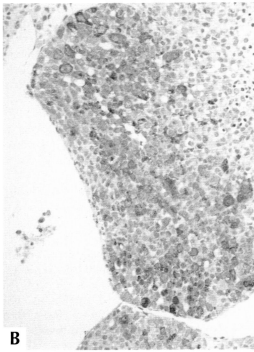

FIGURE 16-17. Positive immunohistochemical staining of tumor cells for S-100 protein (**A**) and with HMB-45 (**B**) is typical for melanoma. Tumor cells also stain positively with antibodies to the intermediate filament vimentin. This combination of immunohistochemical positivity (as well as the absence of staining with antibodies to the epithelial marker keratin) is virtually diagnostic of melanoma. Technetium-99m–labeled antibodies directed against melanoma-specific antigens, such as oncofetal antigen P97, have been used in combination with scintigraphic scans to detect metastatic lesions and determine their degree of spread [50].

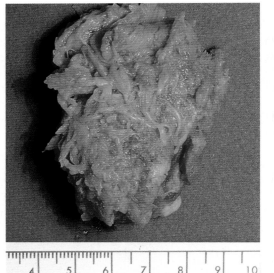

FIGURE 16-18. This specimen of metastatic carcinoma of the cervix that has been surgically excised from the heart has a friable, papillary appearance. Cervical carcinoma that has metastasized to the heart usually manifests as pericardial spread [54] either via lymphatic routes secondary to uncontrolled para-aortic nodal spread or from hematogenous dissemination [55]. Endocardial or intracavitary masses are less common, although a small number have been reported [54,56–58]. Bar = 1 cm.

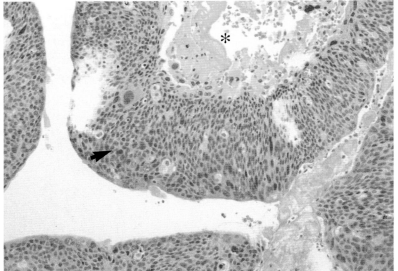

FIGURE 16-19. Viable malignant cells of metastatic carcinoma of the cervix are present on the superficial aspect of tumor mass projections (*arrow*). Note the projections' central necrotic core (*asterisk*). Necrosis and friability of this and similar intracavitary tumor masses promote thrombosis and embolism. Genital cancer in general and cervical cancer in particular are among those malignancies least likely to spread to the heart, despite an overall distant metastatic rate of 15% [59]. Based on autopsy studies, the rate of secondary cardiac involvement is between 1% and 4% [54,60–62]. Cardiac malignancy in the absence of widespread metastatic disease is rare, although pericardial involvement and tamponade have been the mode of presentation at first recurrence of squamous cell carcinoma [63]. Cardiac metastasis of squamous cell carcinoma of the cervix is rarely diagnosed before death; resection is palliative.

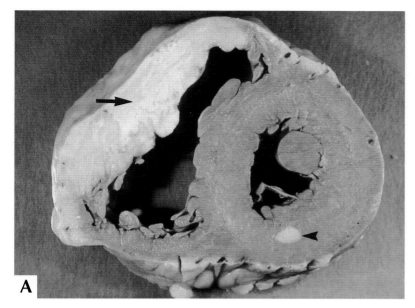

A

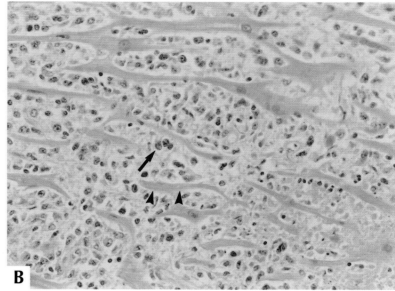

B

FIGURE 16-20. Lymphoma in a patient with AIDS. **A,** Metastatic neoplasms may extensively involve the myocardium, as shown in this transverse section of the ventricles of a 32-year-old man with HIV infection and large cell immunoblastic lymphoma. The right ventricular free wall is thickened and extensively replaced by a well-circumscribed homogeneous gray-white lymphomatous mass (*arrow*). A smaller mass can be seen in the mid-myocardium of the posterior left ventricle (*arrowhead*). **B,** Light micrograph showing infiltration of myocardium by large, malignant lymphoid cells, many of which have the cytologic features of immunoblasts typical

of large cell immunoblastic lymphoma (*arrow*). The neoplastic infiltrate separates and replaces atrophic, thin cardiac myocytes (*arrowheads*; hematoxylin and eosin, × 125). Malignant lymphomas in patients with AIDS are usually high-grade and either large cell immunoblastic or small, noncleaved (Burkitt's-like) in type [64–66]. Involvement of organs and tissues other than lymph nodes is common in AIDS, and lymphomatous involvement of the heart is well recognized [67,68]. The clinical findings in metastatic lymphoma, as in metastatic involvement of the heart by other neoplasms, are nonspecific in patients with AIDS.

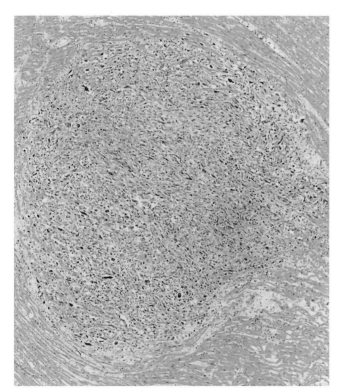

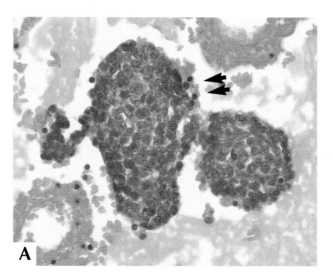

A

FIGURE 16-22. Cytologic examination of fluid from pericardial effusion may allow an etiologic diagnosis, specifically malignant effusion. **A,** In this cytologic cell block preparation, clusters of malignant epithelial cells (*arrows*) typical of small cell (oat cell) carcinoma can be seen against a bloody background (cell block, hematoxylin and eosin stain, × 100). **B,** Autopsy revealed a small cell carcinoma of the lung that encased the heart and great vessels (*double arrows*) and directly infiltrated the pericardium.

FIGURE 16-21. Light micrograph showing a poorly differentiated squamous cell carcinoma. In this case, the carcinoma was a primary tumor of the lung that had metastasized to the heart. The patient was a 62-year-old male cigarette smoker who died of widely disseminated disease (hematoxylin and eosin, × 50). Metastatic involvement of the heart by squamous cell carcinoma may be clinically insignificant and identified microscopically only as an incidental finding at autopsy.

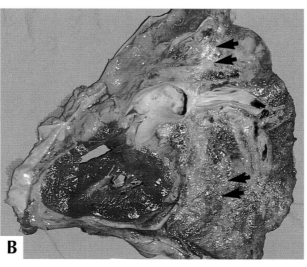

B

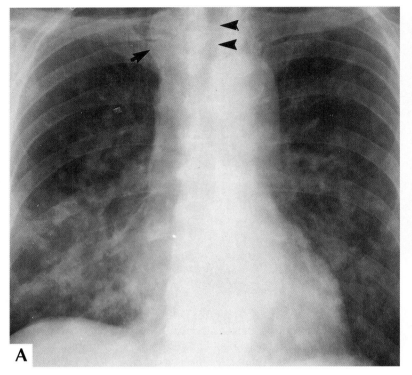

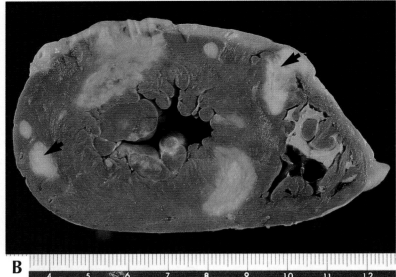

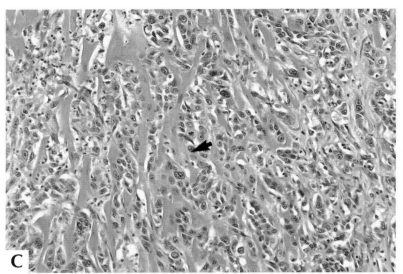

FIGURE 16-23. A, Chest radiograph of a 77-year-old man with carcinoma of the thyroid that was discovered 6 years previously. The patient was treated by thyroidectomy, radical neck dissection, and radiation therapy. He presented preterminally with difficulty swallowing and increased shortness of breath. A right paratracheal mass (*arrow*) and deviation of the trachea to the left (*arrowheads*) are shown. Both lung fields are studded with multiple, small nodular metastases. Heart size is normal. Autopsy revealed a mass in the right side of the neck that had infiltrated the trachea and adhered to the esophagus. The tumors had metastasized widely to multiple organs, including the heart, but there was no convincing evidence of a new primary site of malignancy. **B,** Transverse section of the left and right ventricular myocardium shows extensive involvement of the myocardium by several well-circumscribed tumor nodules (*arrows*). **C,** Photomicrograph of a representative tumor nodule in the myocardium showing a poorly differentiated carcinoma with marked cellular pleomorphism and evident mitotic activity (*arrow*; hematoxylin and eosin, × 100). Although immunohistochemical studies failed to demonstrate the presence of

thyroglobulin, a marker for thyroid differentiation, this carcinoma probably represents recurrence and metastasis of poorly differentiated thyroid carcinoma. This case illustrates that despite extensive cardiac involvement, clinical signs and symptoms may be nonspecific and possibly attributed to other causes or overshadowed by other clinical manifestations.

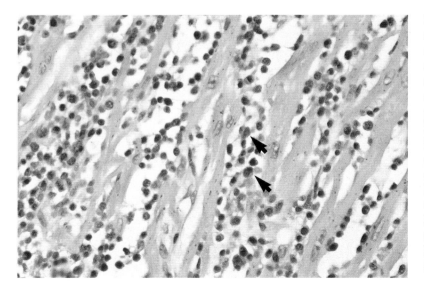

FIGURE 16-24. Myocardial tissue obtained from a failed heart allograft of a 60-year-old black woman. Lymphoproliferative cells have invaded the myocardium, and large, atypical lymphoid cells can be seen (*arrows*). Such infiltrates are composed primarily of immunophenotypic B cells. Posttransplant lymphoproliferative disorder (PTLD) occurs in the setting of cyclosporine immunosuppression in approximately 1% to 4% of heart transplant patients 3 to 4 months after transplantation [28–30]. However, when OKT3 is used for immunosuppression (particularly after a cumulative dose exceeding 75 mg), PTLD may occur in as many as 11% of cases [28]. The Epstein-Barr virus (EBV) has been implicated in PTLD [18,19] because EBV infection is often detected serologically or based on clinical parameters before PTLD becomes manifest. EBV may also be found in the cellular proliferation. One hypothesis suggests that decreased T-cell control allows proliferation of EBV-driven B cells in immunosuppressed patients [29] (hematoxylin and eosin, × 100).

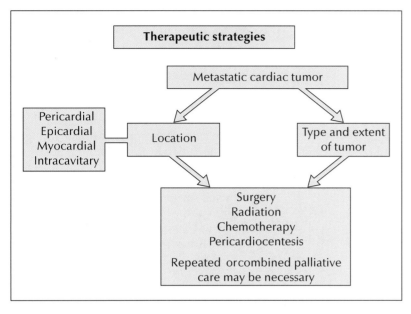

Therapeutic strategies

Metastatic cardiac tumor

Pericardial
Epicardial
Myocardial
Intracavitary — Location — Type and extent of tumor

Surgery
Radiation
Chemotherapy
Pericardiocentesis

Repeated or combined palliative care may be necessary

FIGURE 16-25. Therapeutic strategies for metastatic tumors of the heart. Metastatic cardiac neoplasms are becoming more prevalent, probably because more aggressive surgical and radiation therapy of primary lesions has increased survival rates [69]. Secondary malignant cardiac tumors occur 20 to 30 times more frequently than do primary neoplasms [70] and generally are associated with

a poor prognosis. Metastatic tumors of the heart are treated according to the location of the tumor (epicardial or pericardial, myocardial, intracavitary) and the type or extent of the tumor involved [70]. Surgical intervention is the therapy of choice and is most successful in patients with cardiac metastases that are localized to one portion of the heart and are obstructing intracardiac blood flow. Surgery would be expected to be most beneficial patients whose primary tumor is under control and who have had a significant disease-free interval between control of the primary tumor and detection of the cardiac metastases [71]. The metastatic neoplasm has also been controlled directly through radiation and chemotherapy; however, radiation is prescribed only after chemotherapy using single or multiple drugs have failed. Needle pericardiocentesis can relieve slowly developing clinical symptoms initially, especially when the tumor involves the pericardial space [70]. Because pericardial effusion tends to recur, repeat pericardiocentesis may be necessary, although the number of pericardiocenteses may be reduced by injecting tetracyclines, isotopes, or chemotherapeutic agents into the pericardial space [70]. Palliative measures are often applied in patients with metastatic tumors to the heart because cardiac involvement frequently indicates that the cancer has reached an advanced stage. Once this occurs, the emphasis should be on patient comfort. When targeted antitumor therapy (including genetic targeting) becomes available, the prognosis for patients with cardiac metastatic tumors should improve markedly.

CARDIAC TRANSPLANTATION IN PATIENTS WITH PREEXISTENT NEOPLASTIC DISEASES

EXTRACARDIAC NEOPLASMS	MAJOR SYMPTOMS AND SIGNS	OUTCOME
4 lymphomas (1 Burkitt's; 2 histiocytic)	2 CHF, 2 CMY	Asymptomatic
6 Hodgkin's disease	2 IHD, 1 CHF, 3 CMY	5 asymptomatic 1 dead/respiratory failure
2 Lymphoblastic leukemias (1 acute)	CHF	1 asymptomatic 1 dead/sepsis
2 Adenocarcinomas	IHD	1 asymptomatic 1 dead/cancer*
7 Carcinomas (3 breast; 1 basal cell; 1 transitional cell; 1 embryonal cell; 1 testicular)	1 IHD, 6 CMY	6 asymptomatic 1 symptomatic†
3 Sarcomas: (2 Ewing's; 1 osteogenic)	CMY	Asymptomatic

*Epidural mass found on back revealed a tumor consistent with metastatic adenocarcinoma from the colon. Spinal cord compression developed, and the patient died of respiratory failure.
†Basal cell carcinoma lesions reappeared on two occasions on the skin, but they were removed.

FIGURE 16-26. Summary of experience with cardiac transplantation in 24 patients with preexisting neoplastic disease [72,73]. Mean age at diagnosis was 29.5 years, and mean age at transplantation was 41.9 years (based on available data from 18 cases). The ratio of male-to-female patients was 8:6 (based on available data from 14 cases). Average follow-up was 21.8 months (range, 0 to 50). Only two of the 24 patients (8%) presented with subsequent malignancy—one patient had basal cell carcinoma that was treated successfully; in the other, a tumor consistent with metastatic adenocarcinoma resulted in death. Two other patients died of causes unrelated to malignancy,

and the remaining patients were asymptomatic. In the past, a history of cancer was considered a contraindication to heart transplantation because of concern about the possible adverse effects of therapeutic immunosuppression on cancer recurrence. However, recent studies have indicated that immunosuppressive therapy has not been associated with an increased risk for neoplastic recurrence [72–74]. These data indicate that previously treated neoplastic disease may not adversely affect graft rejection rates or survival of patients undergoing heart transplantation. CHF—congestive heart failure; CMY—cardiomyopathy; IHD—ischemic heart disease.

FUTURE DIRECTIONS

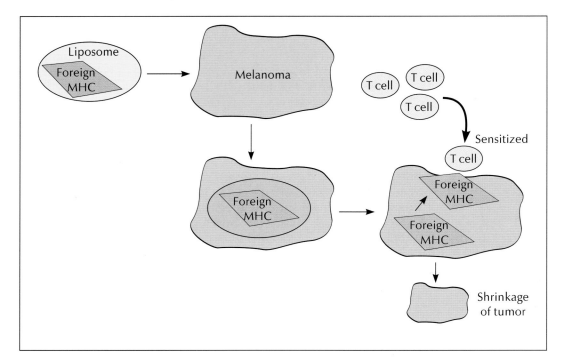

FIGURE 16-27. Effect of gene therapy in metastatic melanoma. Gene therapy is being used increasingly as an alternative in the treatment of numerous human diseases. Nabel *et al.* [75,76] have recently developed a method by which a foreign major histocompatibility complex (MHC) gene can be introduced into malignant tumors *in vivo* using liposomes. The foreign MHC molecule then stimulates the host immune system and elicits a cytotoxic T-cell response. This response decreases tumor growth and, in some cases, causes complete regression of the tumor. Such approaches are likely to become applicable to metastatic cardiac tumors.

The authors gratefully acknowledge the extensive editorial assistance of Janet E. Wilson and Karolyn Redenbach. Dr. Ian Dunn, Department of Radiology, St. Paul's Hospital, generously provided images and advice for several clinical cases.

REFERENCES

1. McAllister HA, Fenoglio JJ: Tumors of the cardiovascular system. In *Atlas of Tumor Pathology*, ed 2. Washington, DC: Armed Forces Institute of Pathology; 1978:111–119.

2. Fine G: Neoplasms of the pericardium and heart. In *Pathology of the Heart and Blood Vessels*, ed 3. Edited by Gould SE. Springfield, IL: Charles C. Thomas Publishers; 1968:851–883.

3. Chan HSL, Sonley MJ, Moes CAF, *et al.*: Primary and secondary tumors of childhood involving the heart, pericardium and great vessels: a review of 75 cases and review of the literature. *Cancer* 1985, 56:825–836.

4. Goudie RB: Secondary tumors of the heart and pericardium. *Br Heart J* 1955, 17:183–188.

5. Malaret GE, Aliaga P: Metastatic disease to the heart. *Cancer* 1968, 22:457–466.

6. Roberts WC, Glancy DL, DeVita VT: Heart in malignant lymphoma (Hodgkin's disease, lymphosarcoma, reticulum cell sarcoma and mycosis fungoides): a study of 196 autopsy cases. *Am J Cardiol* 1968, 22:85–107.

7. MacGee W: Metastatic and invasive tumors involving the heart in a geriatric population: a necropsy study. *Virchows Arch A Pathol Anat Histopathol* 1991, 419:183–189.

8. Lam KY, Dickens P, Chan ACL: Tumors of the heart: a 20-year experience with a review of 12,485 consecutive autopsies. *Arch Pathol Lab Med* 1993, 117:1027–1031.

9. Abraham JM: Neoplasms metastatic to the heart: review of 3314 consecutive autopsies. *Am J Cardiovasc Pathol* 1990, 3:195–198.

10. Young JM, Goldman IR: Tumor metastasis to the heart. *Circulation* 1954, 9:220–229.

11. Prichard RW: Tumors of the heart: review of the subject and report of one hundred and fifty cases. *Arch Pathol* 1951, 51:98–128.

12. Scott RW, Garvin CF: Tumors of the heart and pericardium. *Am Heart J* 1939, 17:431–436.

13. Deloach JF, Haynes JW: Secondary tumors of heart and pericardium: review of the subject and report of one hundred and thirty-seven cases. *Arch Intern Med* 1953, 91:224–249.

14. Harrer WMV, Lewis PL: Metastatic tumors involving the heart and pericardium. *Penn Med* 1971, 57–60.

15. Li FP, Schneider JA, Kanter AF: Cancer epidemiology. In *Cancer Medicine*, ed 3. Edited by Holland JF, *et al.* Philadelphia: Lea and Febiger; 1993:324.

16. Waller BF, Gottdiener JS, Virmani R, *et al.*: The "charcoal heart": melanoma to the cor. *Chest* 1980, 77:671–676.

17. Roberts WC, Bodey GP, Wertlake PT: The heart in acute leukemia. *Am J Cardiol* 1968, 21:388–412.

18. Chow WH, Chow TC, Chiu SW: Pericardial metastases and effusion as the initial manifestation of malignant thymoma: identification by cross-sectional echocardiography. *Int J Cardiol* 1992, 37:258–260.

19. Hunkeler N, Canter CE: Antemortem diagnosis of gross cardiac metastasis in childhood leukemia: echocardiographic documentation. *Pediatr Cardiol* 1990, 11:225–226.

20. Seibert KA, Rettenmier CW, Waller BF, *et al.*: Osteogenic sarcoma metastatic to the heart. *Am J Med* 1982, 73:136–141.

21. Fleisher AG, Tyers FO, Hu D, *et al.*: Dumbbell metastatic cystosarcoma phyllodes of the heart and lung. *Ann Thorac Surg* 1990, 49:309–311.

22. Daisley H, Charles WP: Fatal metastatic calcification in a patient with HTLV-1–associated lymphoma. *WI Med J* 1993, 42: 37–39.

23. Moon TD, Fox LS, Varma DGK: Testicular teratocarcinoma with intracaval metastases to the heart. *Urology* 1992, 40:368–370.

24. Scully RE, Galdabini JJ, McNeely BU: Case records of the Massachusetts General Hospital. *N Engl J Med* 1976, 295:1367–1374.

25. Gottdiener JS, Maron BJ: Posterior cardiac displacement by anterior mediastinal tumor. *Chest* 1980:77:784–786.

26. Swinnen LJ, Costanzo-Nordin MR, Fisher SG, *et al.*: Increased incidence of lymphoproliferative disorder after immunosuppression with the monoclonal antibody OKT3 in cardiac transplant recipients. *N Engl J Med* 1990, 323:1723–1728.

27. Nalesnik MA, Jaffe R, Starzl TE, *et al.*: The pathology of post-transplant lymphoproliferative disorders occurring in the setting of cyclosporin A–prednisone immunosuppression. *Am J Pathol* 1988, 133:173–192.

28. Armitage JM, Kormos RL, Stuart RS, *et al.*: Posttransplant lymphoproliferative disease in thoracic organ transplant patients: ten years of cyclosporine-based immunosuppression. *J Heart Lung Transplant* 1991, 10:877–887.

29. Couetil JP, McGoldrick JP, Wallwork J, *et al.*: Malignant tumors after heart transplantation. *J Heart Transplant* 1990, 9:622–626.

30. Penn I: Tumors after renal and cardiac transplantation. *Hematol Oncol Clin North Am* 1993, 7:431–445.

31. Flipse TR, Tazelaar HD, Holmes DR: Diagnosis of malignant cardiac disease by endomyocardial biopsy. *Mayo Clin Proc* 1990, 65:1415–1422.

32. Hall RJ, Cooley DA: Neoplastic diseases of the heart. In *The Heart, Arteries and Veins*, ed 5. Edited by Hurst JW, Logue RB, Rackley CE, *et al.* New York: McGraw-Hill; 1982:1403–1424.

33. Tamura A, Matsubara O, Yoshimura N, *et al.*: Cardiac metastasis of lung cancer: a study of metastatic pathways and clinical manifestations. *Cancer* 1992, 70:437–442.

34. Ballantyne AJ, Clagett OT, McDonald JR: Vascular invasion in bronchogenic carcinoma. *Thorax* 1957, 12:294–299.

35. Hinson KFW, Nohl HC: Involvement of the pulmonary vein by bronchogenic carcinoma. *Br J Dis Chest* 1960, 54:54–58.

36. Sheldon R, Isaac D: Metastatic melanoma to the heart presenting with ventricular tachycardia. *Chest* 1991, 99:1296–1297.

37. Glancy DL, Roberts WC: The heart in malignant melanoma: a study of 70 autopsy cases. *Am J Cardiol* 1968, 21:555–571.

38. Emmot WW, Vacek JL, Agee K, *et al.*: Metastatic malignant melanoma presenting clinically as obstruction of the right ventricular inflow and outflow tracts: characterization by magnetic resonance imaging. *Chest* 1987, 92:362–364.

39. Hanley PC, Shub C, Seward JB, *et al.*: Intracavitary cardiac melanoma diagnosed by endomyocardial left ventricular biopsy. *Chest* 1983, 84:195–198.

40. Vetto JT, Heelan RT, Burt M: Malignant melanoma metastatic to the right atrium: an asymptomatic solitary metastasis diagnosed incidentally by magnetic resonance imaging. *J Thorac Cardiovasc Surg* 1992, 104:843–844.

41. Bisel HF, Wroblewski F, LaDue JS: Incidence and clinical manifestations of cardiac metastases. *JAMA* 1953, 153:712–715.

42. Strauss BL, Matthews MJ, Cohen MN: Cardiac metastases in lung cancer. *Chest* 1977, 71:607–611.

43. Fraser RS, Viloria JB, Wang N: Cardiac tamponade as a presentation of extracardiac malignancy. *Cancer* 1980, 45:1697–1704.

44. Yazdi HM, Hajdu SI, Melamed MR: Cytopathology of pericardial effusions. *Acta Cytol* 1980, 24:401–412.

45. Haskell RJ, French WJ: Cardiac tamponade as the initial presentation of malignancy. *Chest* 1985, 88:70–73.

46. Franciosa JA, Lawrinson J: Coronary artery occlusion due to neoplasm: a rare cause of myocardial infarction. *Arch Intern Med* 1971, 128:797–801.

47. Ackerman DM, Hyma BA, Edwards WD: Malignant neoplastic emboli to the coronary arteries: report of two cases and review of the literature. *Hum Pathol* 1987, 18:955–959.

48. Aylwin JA: Avoidable vascular spread in resection for bronchial carcinoma. *Thorax* 1951, 6:250–267.

49. Karlsberg RP, Sagel SS, Ferguson TB: Myocardial infarction due to tumor embolization following pulmonary resection. *Chest* 1978, 74:582–584.

50. Gindea AJ, Steele P, Rumancik WM, *et al.*: Biventricular cavity obliteration by metastatic malignant melanoma: role of magnetic resonance imaging in the diagnosis. *Am Heart J* 1987, 114:1249–1253.

51. Hanfling S: Metastatic cancer to the heart: review of the literature and report of 127 cases. *Circulation* 1960, 22:474–483.

52. Thomas JH, Panoussopoulos DG, Jewell WR, *et al.*: Tricuspid stenosis secondary to metastatic melanoma. *Cancer* 1978, 39:1732–1737.

53. Gosalakkal JA, Sugrue DD: Malignant melanoma of the right atrium: antemortem diagnosis by transvenous biopsy. *Br Heart J* 1989, 62:159–160.

54. Ritcher N, Yon J: Squamous cell carcinoma of the cervix metastatic to the heart. *Gynecol Oncol* 1979, 7:394–400.

55. Charles EH, Condori J, Sall S: Metastasis to the pericardium from squamous cell carcinoma of the cervix. *Am J Obstet Gynecol* 1977, 129:349–351.

56. Dibadj A: Intracavitary cardiac tumor secondary to squamous cell carcinoma of cervix: report of a case and review of the literature. *Am J Clin Pathol* 1967, 48:58–61.

57. Schaefer S, Shohet RV, Nixon JV, *et al.*: Right ventricular obstruction from cervical carcinoma: a rare single metastatic site. *Am Heart J* 1987, 113:397–399.

58. Itoh K, Matsubara T, Yanagisawa K, *et al.*: Right ventricular metastasis of cervical squamous cell carcinoma. *Am Heart J* 1984, 108:1369–1371.

59. Nelson JH: The incidence and significance of paraaortic lymph node metastasis in late carcinoma of the cervix. *Am J Obstet Gynecol* 1974, 118:749–756.

60. Kountz DS: Isolated cardiac metastasis from cervical carcinoma: presentation as acute anteroseptal myocardial infarction. *South Med J* 1993, 86:228–230.

61. Badib AO, Kurohara SS, Webster JH, *et al.*: Metastasis to organs in carcinoma of the uterine cervix. *Cancer* 1968, 21:434–439.

62. Peeples WJ, Amar Inalsingh CH, Hazra TA, *et al.*: The occurrence of metastasis outside the abdomen and retroperitoneal space in invasive carcinoma of the cervix. *Gynecol Oncol* 1976, 4:307–310.

63. Rudoff J, Percy R, Benrubi G, *et al.*: Recurrent squamous cell carcinoma of the cervix presenting as cardiac tamponade: case report and subject review. *Gynecol Oncol* 1989, 34:226–231.

64. Acierno LJ: Cardiac complications in acquired immunodeficiency syndrome (AIDS): a review. *J Am Coll Cardiol* 1989, 13:1144–1154.

65. Ziegler J, Beckstead J, Volberding P, *et al.*: Non-Hodgkin's lymphoma in 90 homosexual men: relation to generalized lymphadenopathy in the acquired immunodeficiency syndrome. *N Engl J Med* 1984, 311:565–570.

66. Levine AM, Meyer PR, Begandy MK, *et al.*: Development of B-cell lymphoma in homosexual men: clinical and immunologic findings. *Ann Intern Med* 1984, 100:7–13.

67. Ziegler JL, Bragg K, Abrams D, *et al.*: High-grade non-Hodgkin's lymphoma in patients with AIDS. *Ann NY Acad Sci* 1984, 437:412–419.

68. Joachim HL, Cooper MC, Hellman GC: Lymphomas in men at high risk for acquired immunodeficiency syndrome (AIDS): a study of 21 cases. *Cancer* 1985, 56:2831–2842.

69. Cooley DA: Surgical treatment of cardiac neoplasms: 32-year experience. *Thorac Cardiovasc Surg* 1990, 38(Special Issue):176–182.

70. Loffler H, Grille W: Classification of malignant cardiac tumors with respect to oncological treatment. *Thorac Cardiovasc Surg* 1990, 38(Special Issue):173–175.

71. Piehler JM, Lie JT, Giuliani ER: Tumors of the heart. In *Cardiology: Fundamentals and Practice*. Edited by Brandenburg RO, Fuster V, Giuliani ER, *et al.* Chicago: Year Book Medical Publishers; 1987:1671–1693.

72. Dillon TA, Sullivan M, Schatzlein MH, *et al.*: Cardiac transplantation in patients with preexisting malignancies. *Transplantation* 1991, 52:82–85.

73. Edwards BS, Hunt SA, Fowler MB, *et al.*: Cardiac transplantation in patients with preexisting malignancies. *Am J Cardiol* 1990, 65:501–504.

74. Armitage JM, Kormos RL, Griffiths BP: Heart transplantation in patients with malignant disease. *J Heart Transplant* 1990, 9:627–630.

75. Nabel GJ, Fox BA, Plautz GE, *et al.*: Direct gene transfer and nonviral vectors for human cancer and AIDS. *J Cell Biochem* 1994, 18A:218.

76. Nabel GJ, Nabel EG, Plautz GE, *et al.*: Molecular genetic interventions for malignancy and AIDS. *J Cell Biochem* 1994, 18A:7.

INDEX